Counselling in HIV Infection and AIDS

Counselling in HIV Infection and AIDS

SECOND EDITION

EDITED BY

JOHN GREEN
Department of Clinical Health Psychology,
Clarence Wing, St Mary's Hospital, London W2 1NY and
National AIDS Counselling Training Unit

and

ALANA McCREANER
National AIDS Counselling Training Unit,
St Charles Hospital, London W10

Blackwell
Science

© 1989, 1996 by John Green and Alana McCreaner

Blackwell Science Ltd
Editorial Offices:
Osney Mead, Oxford OX2 0EL
25 John Street, London WC1N 2BL
23 Ainslie Place, Edinburgh EH3 6AJ
238 Main Street, Cambridge
   Massachusetts 02142, USA
54 University Street, Carlton
   Victoria 3053, Australia

Other Editorial Offices:
Arnette Blackwell SA
   224, Boulevard Saint Germain
   75007 Paris, France

Blackwell Wissenschafts-Verlag GmbH
   Kurfürstendamm 57
   10707 Berlin, Germany

   Zehetnergasse 6
   A-1140 Wien
   Austria

First published 1989
Reprinted 1989, 1990, 1992
Second edition published 1996

Set in 10 on 13pt Ehrhardt
by DP Photosetting, Aylesbury, Bucks
Printed and bound in Great Britain by
Hartnolls Ltd, Bodmin, Cornwall

The Blackwell Science logo is a trade mark of Blackwell
Science Ltd, registered at the United Kingdom Trade
Marks Registry

DISTRIBUTORS

Marston Book Services Ltd
PO Box 269
Abingdon
Oxon OX14 4YN
(*Orders:* Tel: 01235 465500
         Fax: 01235 465555)

USA
Blackwell Science, Inc.
238 Main Street
Cambridge, MA 02142
(*Orders:* Tel: 800 215-1000
           617 876-7000
         Fax: 617 492-5263)

Canada
Copp Clark, Ltd
2775 Matheson Blvd East
Mississauga, Ontario
Canada, L4W 4P7
(*Orders:* Tel: 800 263-4374
           905 238-6074)

Australia
Blackwell Science Pty Ltd
54 University Street
Carlton, Victoria 3053
(*Orders:* Tel: 03 9347 0300
         Fax: 03 9347 5001)

A catalogue record for this title is available
from the British Library

ISBN 0–632–03605–2

Library of Congress
Cataloging-in-Publication Data
Counselling in HIV infection and AIDS/edited by John
   Green and Alana McCreaner. — 2nd ed.
McCreaner.—2nd ed.
      p.   cm.
   Includes bibliographical references and index.
   ISBN 0–632–03605–2 (pbk.)
   1. HIV-positive persons—Counseling of.
   2. AIDS (Disease)—Patients—Counseling of.
   I. Green, John, clinical psychologist.
   II. McCreaner, Alana.
   RC607.A26C683   1996
   362.1′969792—dc20   96-7395
                                                CIP

Contents

Preface

Since the first edition of this book was published six years ago there have been many changes in HIV counselling. Some of these have been changes in emphasis. For instance, HIV disease is conceptualised much more as a continuum rather than a series of stages. Other changes have been more profound, for instance our increasing knowledge about mother–child transmission of HIV and the first glimmerings of an understanding about how we might reduce the risk of such transmissions.

If some things have changed, much remains the same. The disease continues its global spread at an alarming rate. There have been some successes. In the UK the rate of infection of drug users has been lower than elsewhere, which is probably largely attributable to the early introduction of harm minimisation strategies. There have been other successes, but they must be offset against the larger failure to control the disease in so many different places and in so many different populations.

We still have no effective cure for the disease. There have been advances in the treatment of opportunistic infections, but we still lack an antiviral which controls the virus in the medium term. There is still no effective vaccine and, at the time of writing, no sign that a really effective vaccine is about to go on trial. Such is the time scale of these things that if an effective vaccine were developed tomorrow, it would be years before it could be distributed on a global scale.

At the present moment avoidance of the behaviours which transmit HIV remains the only hope for the control of the disease. HIV counselling should, we believe, be a key part of the global and national control of HIV infection. We badly need more research in the area; there are so many gaps in what we know. Nonetheless, in this book we have tried to outline what we believe is good practice in HIV counselling.

HIV counselling is not simply about changing behaviours to prevent spread. Equally important is helping all those affected by HIV – including their carers, families and friends – to maximise their quality of life. We have tried to pick this up in the book.

Most of the chapters in this edition are new; others have been brought up to date with extensive revisions. Some chapters we have retained with minor changes because the information contained in the first edition has not changed; however, these are very much the minority. A few chapters we have left out altogether in the second edition, not because we felt that they were not valuable, but because there is a limit to the number of pages any book can have before it becomes too expensive, or too unwieldy, for most readers.

Inevitably authors have addressed in different ways the issues they were asked to write about. However, we believe that all the chapters fulfil the one essential criterion we set when we embarked on this edition: that the book should above all be useful. We have asked authors to keep references to a minimum, using them only when required and avoiding referencing the obvious. We have also asked them to try to address the issues which will generally interest, and hopefully inform, the person carrying out counselling with those affected by, or at risk of, HIV disease.

Counselling, in the context in which it is used in this book, is not something which only trained counsellors do; it is something which anyone working in any capacity with people affected directly or indirectly by HIV, not only can but must do.

Readers may not agree with everything in the book but we do hope they will find it stimulating and interesting, whether they have been working in the field for years or are new to it.

Dedication

This book is dedicated to the memory of our friends and colleagues Kenneth Fortune and David Sinclair.

John Green
Alana McCreaner

Chapter 1

HIV and AIDS – an Introduction to the Virus and the Disease

Barry Peters

History and background to the disease

AIDS was first recognised as a new condition in 1981. Three patients, all of them homo-sexual men, had a very rare form of pneumonia, *Pneumocystis carinii pneumonia* and a very rare form of cancer, *Kaposi's sarcoma*. All three of these men were previously healthy, and all three were found on laboratory testing to be severely immunosuppressed. Hence this condition was termed the Acquired Immunodeficiency Syndrome, or AIDS.

Many more cases of AIDS were described over the next few months, and it became clear that this disease was assuming epidemic proportions. The hunt was on for the cause of the condition. It was more than two years before the infectious agent was finally found to be a virus. This virus is now known as the human immunodeficiency virus, or HIV.

The HIV virus invades those cells which bear a special receptor site on their surface. This site is called the CD4 antigen. Chief among these cells are the white blood cells, the T-4 or T-helper cells. T-helper cells act to switch on the immune system when the body is under attack by infectious agents. They also play a key role in the body's defences against cancer by mobilising immune system processes which kill cancer cells.

In AIDS many of the T-helper cells are invaded by the virus and killed, or rendered ineffective. The result is that the immune system – the body's defence against disease – does not switch on properly in response to infection or to cancer cells. Not all aspects of the immune system are heavily impaired, since not all aspects rely on the action of T-helper cells, but the damage is extensive. The result is that the person with AIDS becomes vul-nerable to infections and tumours which a person with a normal immune system can easily fight off. These infections and tumours are called 'opportunistic' because they take the opportunity to invade the body when its immune defences are weakened.

The virus

HIV belongs to the family of viruses known as the retroviruses. There are actually two main types of HIV: HIV-1 and HIV-2. HIV-1 is the most common type worldwide; HIV-2 is rarer and found mainly in West Africa. Both viruses cause AIDS and for most practical purposes they can be regarded as the same virus. Earlier names for HIV that are still sometimes used include HTLV-III and LAV.

Other types of retroviruses to infect man include two leukaemia viruses, HTLV-I and HTLV-II. Several other forms of retroviruses are found in other mammals, such as the feline leukaemia virus found in the cat. Of most interest is the Simian Immunodeficiency Virus, or SIV, which is almost identical to HIV-2 and causes an AIDS type disease in monkeys. SIV infection in monkeys was probably the forerunner of AIDS in man, and provides a valuable tool for studying AIDS in humans.

The virus particle itself consists of a core of genetic material, which is the blueprint for the virus to reproduce itself. The core is in the form of a double strand of RNA. Attached to the RNA is a special enzyme unique to this group of viruses, called reverse transcriptase. Surrounding the core are two layers of proteins, and surrounding these is a layer of lipid. This lipid layer must be intact for the virus to be able to survive outside the host cell. A large number of things can damage this lipid layer, including heating, bleach and a wide range of disinfectants. Studding the membrane are molecules of glycoprotein; these are one of the chief substances that the body recognises as foreign.

Figure 1.1 shows the way in which the virus invades the cell. As noted above, it invades cells which carry the CD4 antigen on their surface. A number of cells of the immune system carry CD4, but the greatest concentration of CD4 appears on T-helper cells.

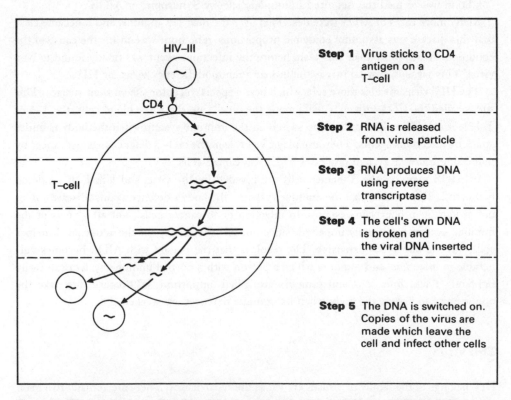

Fig. 1.1   The infection of a T-cell by HIV (Source: Green, J. & Miller, D. (1986) *AIDS The Story of a Disease*. Grafton Publications).

The virus first fuses with the CD4 receptor site. It is then pulled inside the cell. The outside of the particle is stripped off and the viral RNA with its attached reverse transcriptase is released into the cell. Once free, the RNA makes a copy of itself in DNA, the material from which human chromosomes – the genetic material of the cell – are made. DNA copies can only be made from RNA with the help of the reverse transcriptase enzyme.

Once the virus has made a copy of itself in DNA it breaks the DNA in the cell's own chromosomes and then builds itself into the break. Once a person is infected with the virus, the virus material actually becomes part of the cells of that person. The virus then uses the cells it has invaded to make more virus material. This virus material then leaves the cell, 'stealing' part of the cell wall to make its membrane, thus completing a new virus particle. The virus can now go on to infect other cells or other people. Eventually the infected cell dies, and there is one less T–helper cell to fight infections and tumours.

The routes of transmission of the virus are covered in detail in Chapter 4. It is worth stressing here that, in the real world, the virus has only been shown to be transmitted by sex, by blood-to-blood contact, by the mother to her unborn child *in utero* or during childbirth, and also occasionally through breast milk. There is no evidence, despite intensive study, that this fragile virus can be passed on by casual contact.

After infection

There are four main stages of infection with HIV, known as groups 1 to 4. There is the process of becoming infected for the first time (group 1); a long period when the patient has no signs of HIV disease and is usually perfectly well (group 2); a period when the lymph glands are swollen (group 3); and the last stage (group 4) when the patient develops one or more of the diseases resulting from HIV infection. This four stage classification was introduction by the Centers for Disease Control (CDC) in the USA, and is widely used. This classification has already had several additions and revisions. We shall look at each of these stages in more detail. We shall concentrate here on the clinical features as the laboratory tests are discussed in the next chapter.

Group 1: becoming infected

The majority of people who become infected with HIV remain well, and have no reason to suspect that they have been infected. Approximately 20% do develop clinical features around the time of acute infection; these are often identical to glandular fever, with enlarged glands in the neck, a sore throat, a red skin rash and fever. The features of infection might be quite mild, but occasionally might be very severe with features of meningitis or generalised brain infection (encephalitis).

Antibodies will not be produced against HIV in the early stages of infection, although the vast majority of cases will give a positive HIV antibody test three months after exposure to HIV. There are tests which can look for the presence of the virus itself but these are not always readily available.

Group 2: the asymptomatic period (period without symptoms)

The symptoms of acute HIV infection, if present, usually disappear within a few weeks. The individual then remains well and there is no evidence that this person is infected with HIV just by examining him. The only means of knowing with certainty that the person is infected with HIV is to do laboratory tests; the HIV antibody test is a very reliable and cheap test to confirm infection.

Although to outward appearances there is no physical abnormality, the immune system will usually continue to deteriorate. The rate of this deterioration varies greatly between individuals. A few people have had no apparent damage to their immune system even 15 years after their initial infection. Indeed it is still not known if everyone will develop AIDS following HIV infection. The large majority of people do, however, develop AIDS within 15 years of infection with HIV. The average time to AIDS is about 10 years.

During the first part of the 1980s people who were asymptomatic were not given treatment, but were reviewed to make sure that they had remained well. Although there remains controversy over the best time to begin certain treatments, particularly the anti-HIV drugs, the asymptomatic patient with low CD4+ counts will certainly be offered prophylactic antibiotics to prevent the common AIDS pneumonia, *Pneumocystis carinii pneumonia* (known as PCP). Bringing the asymptomatic seropositive patients into the therapeutic arena at this stage means that they have to make decisions about treatment whilst they are feeling well. This is an example of advances in therapy leading to a requirement for earlier counselling.

Group 3: PGL (persistent generalised lymphadenopathy)

A proportion of patients will develop enlarged lymph glands throughout the body, and these glands can persist for months or even years – hence the name persistent generalised lymphadenopathy, or PGL. The patients most commonly notice these glands in the neck, armpits or groin. The patient usually remains well throughout this stage, and the development of these swollen glands is not thought to herald a worse prognosis. Patients will eventually progress from PGL to the next group, although it might be many years before this happens.

Group 4: disease

When patients develop one of the many diseases secondary to HIV infection, they have progressed to the next group. Some patients develop a collection of symptoms that was known under the original classification of AIDS-related complex (ARC). Patients with this syndrome develop features such as weight loss, fevers, night sweats, and loss of energy. They might also have one of the oral conditions: oral candidiasis, or hairy oral leucoplakia (HOL).

Oral candidiasis (or 'oral thrush') is often one of the first signs of HIV infection. It is a white fungal infection that affects any part of the mouth and can be easily scraped off. Oral candidiasis might suggest HIV if risk factors are present, but it can occur in a variety of other conditions or states. These include diabetes, alcohol excess, general malnourishment or immunosuppression from any cause. It can also occur with ill fitting dentures or following antibiotic use. Hence it is important not to equate oral candidiasis with HIV infection until other causes have been considered.

Oral candida can be treated with nystatin or amphotericin B lozenges. Ketoconazole or fluconazole tablets are used if these simple measures do not work.

Oral hairy leucoplakia is almost always associated with HIV infection (very rarely it can be associated with other causes of immunosuppression). It is also white, often affecting the sides of the tongue, and can only be scraped off with difficulty. It is not usually necessary to treat this condition, and the therapies for candida do not work.

AIDS

An individual is diagnosed as having AIDS on the basis of three criteria:

● Opportunist infections
● Opportunist tumours
● Other AIDS defining conditions.

Opportunist infections

A person with AIDS becomes prone to certain diseases caused by organisms which are common in the environment, but which do not usually make us ill. The opportunist infections that individuals get depend on what organisms they are exposed to. Someone living in a temperate country like England will be exposed to a different range of conditions from someone living in the tropics. Exposure to infections also varies with lifestyle; genital herpes which fails to heal is common in gay men with AIDS, but is rare, say, in haemophiliacs. The fact that *Kaposi's sarcoma* is common in gay men but rare in intravenous drug users (see below), is probably explained by their different levels of exposure to sexually transmitted organisms.

The commonest conditions to occur in the UK or the USA are mentioned below.

Protozoal infections

Pneumocystis carinii pneumonia (PCP) is a chest infection and one of the commonest conditions in AIDS. If the patient presents with the early symptoms, such as dry cough and general tiredness, the condition is usually mild and the patient can even be treated as an outpatient. If recognised late, the infection can be life-threatening and the patient might need ventilation. The treatment of choice is cotrimoxazole, although if an allergy develops, other drugs such as intravenous pentamidine can be used. Prophylaxis is given in the form of tablets, such as cotrimoxazole, or pentamidine in the form of a fine mist by mouth (aerosolised or nebulised pentamidine).

Cryptosporidiosis can cause a profuse and persistent diarrhoea. There is no good specific treatment for this condition.

Toxoplasmosis is a common infection in the general population, acquired from eating raw meat or from contact with cat faeces. In people with AIDS it can cause extensive lesions in the brain. Treatment is available, but mortality and morbidity remain high and recurrence is frequent.

Fungal infections

Oesophageal candidiasis   When candida affects the oesophagus, it implies that the patient has more severe immunosuppression than someone with oral candidiasis, hence they are classified as having AIDS.

Cryptococcal meningitis   is a fungal inflammation of the covering of the brain. The long term outlook from this condition is poor, even though specific treatment may prove very successful initially.

Bacterial infections

Tuberculosis   is a mycobacterial infection that attacks not just the lungs but other major organs as well.

Atypical mycobacteria   (caused by organisms known as MAC or MAI, *mycobacterium avium complex/intracellulare*). These are opportunistic infections par excellence. They were exceedingly rare prior to the days of HIV infection, but are one of the commonest types of infection in someone with AIDS. Like tuberculosis, this disease can affect many parts of the body and the patients usually have fever and malaise. Several treatments are available but none are very effective and response is often slow. Some physicians offer patients pro-phylaxis against MAC infection if their CD4+ count is very low (below 50 or 75 mm). Drugs used as treatment or prophylaxis include rifabutin or clofazamine.

Recurrent Salmonella septicaemia   This common bowel pathogen often causes a severe infection of the blood in patients with HIV infection. Recurrent septicaemia due to this organism signifies that the individual's immune system cannot keep the organism under control, and hence classifies an HIV positive person as having AIDS.

Recurrent bacterial pneumonia   (two or more attacks of proven bacterial pneumonia in 12 months). This was introduced as an AIDS defining event in the 1993 revision because bacterial pneumonia is rare in someone who is well and has an intact immune system; hence repeated attacks in an HIV positive individual signify the progression to AIDS.

Viral infections

Herpes simplex infections   lasting more than one month signify that the patient has AIDS; a normal immune system would have cleared herpes simplex in a much shorter time.

Cytomegalovirus   is common in the general population, but in people with AIDS it commonly affects the eye and the bowel. Less commonly it can affect the brain, lungs or other sites. It is important that patients receive treatment if the eye is affected, otherwise they are likely to lose their sight. The two specific treatments for cytomegalovirus are ganciclovir or foscarnet.

Progressive multifocal leucoencephalopathy (PML) This condition looks and acts like a brain tumour, although it is caused by a virus infection, the JC virus. There is no good treatment available, although chemotherapy or radiotherapy might ameliorate the condition in certain cases.

There are other infections which lead to an AIDS diagnosis but these are only common in certain parts of the world. The infections include histoplasmosis, which is a protozoal infection, and two fungal infections: coccidioidomycosis and isosporiasis.

Opportunist tumours

There are three tumours that are strongly associated with AIDS.

Kaposi's sarcoma This tumour is exceedingly rare in people without HIV infection, but it is common in AIDS. It usually affects the skin first and presents as a purplish raised lesion. Eventually, if the patient survives long enough, the tumour might affect the internal organs, such as the lymph glands, lungs and bowel. The skin lesions can be treated with local radiotherapy, as well as being camouflaged with cosmetics. Severe skin lesions, or internal disease, often respond well to chemotherapy.

Lymphoma As patients with AIDS live longer, so more cases of this tumour are occurring. The commonest site to be affected is the brain but other sites can be involved, such as the bowel and the lungs. This tumour often responds well to chemotherapy or radiotherapy, even in patients with AIDS. Lymphoma occurring in AIDS is usually fast growing, however, so the prognosis is generally poor.

Cervical carcinoma occurs more commonly in women who are infected with HIV, and signifies them as having AIDS. It is important that women who are HIV positive have cervical smears performed regularly (e.g. every six months) to enable the early detection and treatment of pre-malignant or malignant change.

Other AIDS defining conditions

AIDS dementia, or HIV encephalopathy Some individuals with AIDS develop dementia due to a direct involvement of the nervous system with HIV. This is discussed in more detail in Chapter 6.

Wasting syndrome Some patients literally waste away with HIV, without any opportunistic condition being found. This wasting condition is in itself an AIDS diagnosis. In Africa a similar condition is known as Slims disease.

CD4+ count of 200 mm or less The USA and some other countries have adopted this as a definition of AIDS. The UK and most European countries have not so far decided to include this laboratory finding as AIDS-defining, but continue to rely on clinical events.

Other conditions occurring in HIV infection

There are several conditions that are common in the general population but are even more common, or more severe, in HIV infection. Examples of this are skin conditions such as seborrhoeic dermatitis, folliculitis, warts, and shingles; other examples include bacterial infections of the chest, and sinusitis. The relative severity of many of these conditions in HIV infection is once again explained by the disordered immune system.

The natural history of HIV infection and AIDS

As mentioned previously, people develop AIDS at different intervals following infection with HIV. It is not known why some people develop AIDS more quickly than others. Part of the explanation might lie with the HIV virus; there is evidence that those patients with a more aggressive strain of HIV might develop disease more quickly. Another cause probably lies in genetic differences between different individuals, and in the way they care for themselves in terms of nutrition and hygiene. There are various laboratory tests that suggest which patients are likely to progress more quickly, and these are discussed in Chapter 2.

Once an individual has developed AIDS, there is great variation in their survival. The average survival has increased over the years, and provided patients have access to good medical care, the average survival now approaches three years. There are three main reasons for increased survival in AIDS:

- Patients present to the hospital earlier than before. This prevents treatable conditions such as PCP becoming more severe or life-threatening and is probably much more important in prolonging survival than the following two reasons:
- The use of prophylaxis against conditions such as PCP.
- The use of specific anti-HIV drugs. Zidovudine (AZT/Retrovir) was introduced in 1987, but new drugs include DDI and DDC.

Prognosis depends on the particular AIDS diagnosis. For example, patients often develop oesophageal candida when they have only slight damage to the immune system, and the prognosis is good. Conversely, patients only develop cytomegalovirus infection or atypical mycobacteria if they have severe immune damage; the outlook is therefore comparatively bad. However, many patients seem to progress much worse or much better than our expectations.

Measures of the immune system, such as the CD4+ count, are also an imperfect guide. Although someone with a high CD4+ count generally does better than someone with a low CD4+ count, there are many examples of people with CD4+ counts too low to measure who have remained well for long periods.

In summary, AIDS has a course that varies greatly from individual to individual. Hence there is often cause for reasoned optimism when discussing the outcome with a patient.

Epidemiology of AIDS

Different countries have a different pattern of spread of HIV infection. In America and Europe the two largest categories infected are homosexual men and intravenous drug abusers. Haemophiliacs and those receiving contaminated blood have been infected in the past; the use of heat treated factor VIII concentrate and the screening of blood should ensure that infections in this category will be rare in the future. A small number of health professionals have been infected by exposure to blood at work, for instance through needle stick injuries, but this is an extremely rare event.

In Africa and some other areas of the world, heterosexuals are the main risk category. Heterosexual transmission of HIV is much rarer in the western world, but it does occur. It would be folly to predict that heterosexual spread of HIV will not become a significant problem in the western world; at this stage we simply do not know. It has emerged that anal intercourse is probably a greater risk factor for the transmission of HIV than vaginal intercourse. Nonetheless, HIV can be transmitted by normal vaginal intercourse, even if the vagina is healthy and undamaged.

At present the number of AIDS cases is increasing considerably, particularly in Africa. There are also several developing countries where HIV and AIDS are just emerging as a problem, such as Thailand, Burma and India. For example, in Thailand there were very few HIV positive cases reported until the early 1990s. Now it is estimated that there are between 200 000 and 400 000 people with HIV infection; although most of these are well at present, many will develop AIDS over the next few years.

Recent progress in anti-HIV treatment

There are no immediate prospects for either a cure or a vaccine against HIV. Much progress has been made, however, in both these areas. There are now alternatives to zidovudine that have successfully passed through the clinical trials stage and are being used both singly and in combination with zidovudine, such as DDI and DDC.

It is still not clear, however, what is the best stage to start treatment with antiretrovirals such as zidovudine. Should we wait until patients have symptomatic disease such as AIDS, or should we intervene earlier when the patient is asymptomatic? If we wish to give treatment when the patient is asymptomatic, do we offer this when they have mild, or moderate or severe immunosuppression?

In the early 1990s, studies from the USA suggested that giving zidovudine to asymptomatic positive patients who had a CD4+ count <500 mm slowed progression to AIDS and prolonged survival. The larger European 'Concorde' study demonstrated that any beneficial effect was temporary and that after one to two years patients who had not taken zidovudine did just as well as those who had taken the drug. Currently, therefore, patients are usually offered zidovudine when they have symptoms or when the CD4+ count has fallen to low levels (around 200 per cubic mm).

More recent studies have focused on combination therapy, that is, using several drugs at one time for the treatment of HIV infection. The results from these studies suggest that combinations of antiretroviral drugs are more effective than single drugs. Further work is going on in combination therapy at the time of writing and several novel drug combinations have shown considerable early promise. There are many more drugs and other therapeutic approaches in the developmental stage.

There are still obstacles to overcome before a vaccine to prevent HIV is developed. One of the greatest difficulties is that there is a huge degree of variation in the outer protein coat of the virus. Hence a successful vaccine will need to protect against all the variant strains of the virus.

There are many more people infected with HIV in the developing world than the western world; similarly, in the future the majority of new infections will occur in developing countries. Therefore, when a vaccine or cure is developed, it is our utmost moral duty to make sure that it is made freely available to the developing world.

Until the vaccines and drugs appear, counselling and health education are the only tools available to us to prevent transmission and, as far as possible, to keep well those already infected. Counselling is an important part of maintaining the quality of life of those who already have the disease, and will remain so until a cure is found.

Chapter 2

Laboratory Tests for HIV

D.J. Jeffries, BSc, MBBS, FRCPath.

Introduction

A range of laboratory tests is now available for the diagnosis of HIV infection, and their sensitivity and specificity is continually being refined. These tests may be performed for a number of purposes, including:

(1) Diagnosis in an individual, who may benefit from early medical intervention
(2) Public health and infection control in the context of epidemiological surveillance, health care provision and public health policy-making
(3) Potential benefit to another person who may have been exposed to the virus by one of several routes, e.g. sexually, by transfusion, by inoculation injury, etc.
(4) Regulations introduced for certain specific reasons, e.g. immigration control, insurance applications.

Serious implications of confidentiality, public and occupational health and safety, civil rights and liberties and ethics are involved in approaches to HIV testing. Testing should never be performed without adequate provision for pre- and post-test counselling (Centers for Disease Control 1987). Details of the counselling process are presented in the following chapters.

HIV antibody tests

Testing for HIV antibody is used as the routine method for diagnosing infection. Commercially available tests, which were first introduced in 1985, have been based on the detection of antibodies in serum; plasma can be used as an alternative. A volume of 5–10 ml of clotted blood should be sent to the laboratory. If there is likely to be a delay in transit, the sample can be kept in a refrigerator (4°C), but it must not be frozen unless the serum has previously been separated from the cellular elements. Recently, tests for HIV antibody in saliva have been introduced. This non-invasive approach to HIV testing has been valuable for epidemiology studies but it must still be regarded as experimental and requires further evaluation before it could be considered for routine diagnostic use.

The use of HIV antibody testing to determine a person's HIV status is based on two assumptions:

(1)   People who have been infected with HIV produce detectable antibody
(2)   Those with detectable HIV antibody are infected with HIV.

With certain conditions, these assumptions have stood the test of time. Providing the person has had time to develop antibody following exposure, the occurrence of infection without antibody is extremely rare – a phenomenon that appears to be restricted to a small percentage of HIV-infected children (< 3%). The time to the appearance of antibody is within three months of contact in at least 95% of individuals, and if it has not appeared by six months after exposure, infection is normally excluded. At present, a confirmed positive antibody test indicates the presence of virus. From our knowledge of the nature of HIV infection, this must imply that the individual concerned will be persistently infected and potentially infectious for the remainder of his/her life.

The situation may change with scientific advances. The introduction of vaccines for HIV may lead to the occurrence of persistent HIV antibody positivity in individuals who are not infected. This situation may require the use of other tests, such as virus culture and poly-merase chain reaction (PCR) (see later in this chapter) to distinguish between immunisation and infection. Also, the implications of being HIV-antibody positive may alter if therapeutic strategies to control, and possibly eliminate, the infection can be developed.

In many countries, including the UK, procedures have been introduced to ensure accurate testing. Assay systems are carefully evaluated to determine precisely the levels of sensitivity and specificity of the many different products, and this is carried out indepen-dently of the manufacturers' assessment. Laboratories engaged in testing take part in external quality control schemes to ensure that standards are maintained. To reduce the danger of sampling errors, particularly the mislabelling of blood bottles, it is essential to confirm positivity by re-testing on a further sample taken on another occasion. Any positives detected in screening assays must be confirmed by the use of other, methodologically independent, HIV antibody tests (see later section on confirmatory tests). This process of confirmation of repeatedly positive antibody tests virtually eliminates the risk of false positive results.

Although HIV-2 is rarely encountered, except in West Africa and in Europeans who have lived in West Africa, a small number of cases have been reported from many other countries and there has been secondary spread in European and Asian cities. For this reason, modern screening tests detect both HIV-1 and HIV-2 antibody and further tests are then used to distinguish the infections.

HIV antibody tests can be developed from large amounts of whole virus grown in cell culture from which antigens are purified and incorporated in assay systems. Similar antigens can be made by DNA cloning technology or by polypeptide synthesis based on knowledge of the genetic sequence of the virus.

Other accounts (Mortimer & Clewley 1987; Wilber 1987) and manufacturers' literature give technical details of specific assays but the principle of each test is outlined in the following sections.

ELISA tests

The enzyme-linked immunosorbent assay (ELISA) is by far the most widely used test for screening and diagnostic purposes. There are several possible formats for this type of assay but the principle is adequately illustrated by the following description.

HIV antigen (whole viral lysate, cloned viral DNA, or synthetic peptides) is coated on to the well of microtitre plates or on to polystyrene beads that are then placed into the wells. This is known as the solid-phase of the assay. The patient's serum is then placed into the well and incubated to allow time for any HIV antibody to combine with antigen on the solid phase. Any unbound antibody is then washed away. Next, an indicator conjugate consisting of an anti-human antibody coupled to an enzyme, e.g. horseradish peroxidase, is placed in the well. Excess anti-human antibody in the indicator conjugate is removed by washing. The enzyme incorporated in this complex is available to catalyse a colour-producing reaction when the substrate for the enzyme is added to the well. The colour change is measured with a spectrophotometer and if it exceeds a calculated threshold, the test is considered specifically reactive. Control positive and negative sera are included in the test run and this simple and versatile system is normally scaled up to incorporate dozens or even hundreds of samples in one batch. The relatively short duration of the test means that results can be available within a few hours. This has been found to be valuable for units providing a rapid testing service for the 'worried well'.

The sensitivity and specificity of current commercial ELISA tests for HIV are both over 98% and may approach 100%. When screening low risk populations, such as blood donors, the assays have a low predictive value when compared to their use in high risk individuals. In other words, there is more likelihood that a 'positive' result will prove to be a false positive. Although less common with the latest tests, false positive reactions have been attributed to the presence of antibodies to class H histocompatibility antigens (particularly HLA-DR4) and they have occurred occasionally in individuals with a history of multiple pregnancies or blood transfusions. The fact that sera yielding false positive results do not generally react in another test system highlights the importance of confirmatory testing.

Confirmatory tests

The immunoblot or western blot was, for several years, the most widely used confirmatory assay for sera found to be HIV antibody positive in ELISA screening tests. Some workers used immunofluorescence assays. There has been an increasing trend towards using alternative ELISA systems for confirmation. With careful selection of assays it is possible to ensure that the ELISA used for confirmation is based on a totally different source of antigen to that used in the screening test. This approach has proved to be satisfactory in eliminating false positive reactions.

Western blot

The principle of the western blot is the demonstration of antibodies in a patient's serum to individual specific proteins of the virus (HIV-1 or HIV-2). Denatured, concentrated virus is electrophoresed in polyacrylamide gel and this separates and distributes the individual proteins as a series of bands according to their molecular weights. The proteins are then transferred (blotted) on to nitrocellulose paper by another electrophoretic procedure and the paper is cut into a series of thin test strips, each with a set of HIV protein bands. A test strip is incubated with serum from a patient and then washed prior to further incubation with a labelled anti-human globulin (an antibody to human immunoglobulin).

The label is usually an enzyme e.g. horseradish peroxidase, that will react with its substrate to produce a coloured band on the strip. Thus if antibody to a particular protein is present in a patient's serum it will bind to that protein. The anti-human globulin will itself combine to anti-HIV antibodies bound to the protein and the enzyme reaction will highlight these reactions. Most sera from HIV antibody positive individuals have antibodies to many or all the proteins and multiple bands are obtained in positions which correspond to those seen in a parallel test performed with a positive control serum. Figure 2.1 illustrates the pattern of bands produced in a western blot for HIV-1.

Early and late in HIV infection, a patient may not react to some of the bands in a western blot. In addition, some HIV-negative individuals have antibodies in their blood which crossreact in the western blot with HIV proteins, particularly the core protein p24. Thus stringent criteria have been introduced to assist laboratory staff in interpreting sera yielding

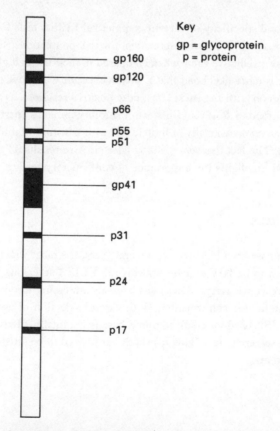

Key

gp = glycoprotein
p = protein

gp160
gp120
p66
p55
p51
gp41
p31
p24
p17

Fig. 2.1 Diagram to demonstrate the distribution pattern of HIV-1 protein bands in a western blot test.

an incomplete banding pattern, with two or three defined antigen/antibody reactions being necessary for confirmed positivity (Hausler 1988; Centers for Disease Control 1989). Repeat sampling from a patient with an indeterminate result on the western blot may clarify the picture. The generation of indeterminate reactions is a major drawback to the use of western blotting as a confirmatory test for HIV antibody, as significant numbers of individuals may be left with a tentative diagnosis of HIV infection without confirmation.

Immunofluorescence assay

This is a relatively simple procedure which has been used as a confirmatory assay in the past (McHugh *et al.* 1986). A sample of the patient's serum is placed on to fixed, HIV infected lymphocytes on a glass slide. After incubation, the cells are washed and then treated with a fluorescein labelled anti-human globulin. A further incubation step follows, followed by further washing. If the patient's serum contains anti-HIV antibody this will bind to infected cells, and the adherent antibody will be bound by the anti-human globulin. Inspection in a UV microscope will reveal the apple green fluorescence of fluorescein localised to the infected lymphocytes. No fluorescence is seen with uninfected cells or in parallel preparations using known HIV-negative sera. The disadvantage of this method is its subjective nature. It also requires the availability of HIV culture facilities for preparing the slides.

HIV antigen testing

Commercial tests are available for the detection of the major core protein of HIV, p24 antigen (24 000 daltons molecular weight) in serum, plasma and CSF of infected individuals. The assays are also used to detect the growth of virus in cell cultures. As shown in Fig. 2.2, p24 antigen may be present early in the course of HIV infection, prior to the detection of antibodies. It frequently reappears much later, following the decline of anti-p24 antibody and, at this stage, the reappearance of p24 antigen is a prognostic marker for the development of AIDS and other HIV-related disease (Lange *et al.* 1986). Approximately 70% of AIDS patients are positive for p24 antigen (Kenny *et al.* 1987). Antiviral agents, e.g. zidovudine have been shown to suppress p24 antigen levels, and quantification of p24 levels has been valuable in assessing short-term anti-viral efficacy.

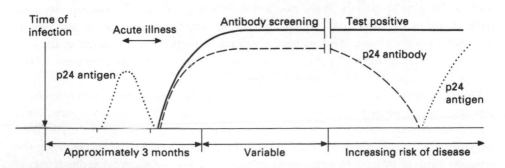

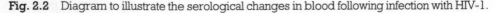

Fig. 2.2   Diagram to illustrate the serological changes in blood following infection with HIV-1.

Another important use of the p24 antigen test is for the diagnosis of HIV infection in babies and children under 15 months of age. During this period, the persistence of trans-placental maternal antibody means that antibody testing of the offspring is largely unreliable. Although the sensitivity is low (approx 50%), a positive p24 antigen test confirms infection of the baby.

Measurement of p24 antigen in CSF is sometimes used to assess CNS involvement with HIV. The assays are based on modifications of the ELISA technology described earlier. By adsorbing specific anti-p24 antibody to the solid phase, it is possible to capture antigen present in a patient's serum. This is then identified by the addition of further anti-p24 antibody conjugated with the enzyme horseradish peroxidase, and addition of the substrate yields a colour reaction which is measured with a spectrophotometer.

The full potential of p24 antigen testing is still being assessed. Its use has been considered in blood transfusion centres as a way of detecting donors who may be in the so-called 'antigenic window' before they become antibody positive (Allain *et al.* 1986). Several large surveys have shown that in areas of relatively low HIV seroconversion rates, the chance of a donor presenting at this critical time is extremely low. In areas where HIV infection is spreading very rapidly, the problem may be more critical. However, the duration of the 'antigenic window' has decreased as a result of increasingly sensitive HIV antibody tests which can detect low positives at an earlier stage than the older tests.

Some infected individuals who have been shown to be p24 antigen negative with the standard assays become positive if their sera are treated with acid. This is thought to release p24 antigen bound in circulating immune complexes, and modification of the test increases the sensitivity by 5–20%. The significance of the detection of these additional p24 antigen positive individuals is uncertain and is currently being assessed.

HIV isolation

The lentivirus causing AIDS was first isolated from a patient with persistent generalised lymphodenopathy and was reported in 1983 (Barre-Sinoussi *et al.* 1983). This early work was carried out by co-cultivation with normal human T lymphocytes and the virus was detected by the demonstration of reverse transcriptase production.

Further work led to the confirmation of this discovery and also provided a description of adaptation of the virus to continuous T cell lines (Popovic *et al.* 1984). This, in turn, allowed bulk culture of HIV which facilitated the production of antigens for diagnostic tests and material for genetic analysis. With modified techniques, HIV can be isolated from the lymphocytes of the majority of seropositive individuals and, depending on the stage of infection, from the plasma of many; plasma viraemia is particularly prominent in the pre-seroconversion stage and is also increasingly common when patients have very low CD4+ counts and become ill with HIV-related disease.

Despite refinements in technology, HIV culture remains a work-intensive and expensive procedure which, because it requires high-containment laboratories (category 3 status in the UK), is usually only available in specialised units and reference centres. At present, the need for virus culture is relatively limited. It has been a valuable technique for assessing the infection status of infants. As mentioned earlier, the presence of maternal antibody means that other tests are necessary to determine whether a baby has acquired HIV from the mother; p24 antigen testing is reliable but insensitive, and virus isolation has been the 'gold standard'. In the follow-up of babies born to HIV-infected women, some have been seen to lose antibody positivity but they have retained viable virus in their lymphocytes.

Virus isolated from HIV-infected individuals can be stored in liquid nitrogen (or at −70°C) and these isolates provide a valuable source of material for molecular genetic analysis to monitor virus mutation. Recent work suggests that the growth characteristics of HIV in MT-2 cell culture may be correlated with disease progression and possibly response to antiviral therapy. The phenotypic change from non-syncytium forming isolates (NSI) to syncytium forming (S1) mutants, which produce larger amounts of virus in culture, has been strongly associated with rapid progression to AIDS and, possibly, with failure to respond to zidovudine. If this proves to be true, virus culture is likely to become more important as a method of monitoring disease progression.

By quantitative culture techniques it is possible to measure the amount of virus in a patient's cells and/or plasma (Coombs *et al.* 1989; Ho *et al.* 1989). This approach, which is cumbersome and expensive, is currently being explored as a direct method of detecting the effects of antiviral drugs on circulating HIV in patients.

The techniques of virus isolation have been described elsewhere (Jackson *et al.* 1988). Blood is collected into preservative-free heparin (10 i.u/ml) and transferred to the laboratory as quickly as possible, certainly within the same day. The volume of blood required depends to an extent on the patient's lymphocyte count. Normally one would collect 20 ml from an adult and 5–6 ml from an infant.

The plasma may be inoculated directly into normal T lymphocytes (which have previously been activated with phytohaemagglutinin), and blood mononuclear cells are separated from other blood components on a Ficoll-Hypaque gradient prior to inoculation. The plasma/donor T cell cultures and/or mononuclear cell/donor T cell cultures are incubated in the presence of interleukin-2 (IL-2). Supernatants are analysed every two to three days for the presence of reverse transcriptase activity or the production of p24 antigen. To maintain the cultures over a prolonged period, additional donor lymphocytes are added to the cultures. A positive isolate, as detected by reverse transcriptase or p24 antigen, can be passaged into fresh donor lymphocytes or continuous cell lines for further studies.

Nucleic acid detection

Some viruses can be detected by the use of nucleic acid hybridisation techniques. This involves the binding of labelled nucleic acid probes, homologous to known sequences of the viral genome, with either an extract of viral DNA deposited on filters or gels or directly on virus-infected cells (*in situ* hybridisation). The binding of the probe can be demonstrated by autoradiography if a radiolabel is used, or by an enzyme-induced colour reaction. The technique of *in situ* hybridisation has had some applications as a research procedure in HIV infection, particularly in the examination of fixed tissues. It has proved to be insensitive for demonstrating virus in circulating blood samples due to the small percentage of cells bearing HIV nucleic acid. This varies between patients and at different times after sero-conversion, but typically between 0.01% and 0.1% of the lymphocytes contain HIV proviral DNA. The introduction of the polymerase chain reaction, which allows the amplification of very small amounts of nucleic acid, provides the basis for highly sensitive and versatile nucleic acid detection systems which are now being developed for many infectious agents including HIV.

Polymerase chain reaction

The first applications of the polymerase chain reaction (PCR) were to detect small known sequences of DNA amid much larger amounts of DNA, e.g. the identification of single genes or virus genomes in cell extracts that also contain enormous numbers of copies of the entire human genome. This is done by selectively and repeatedly making copies of the target DNA sequence until there is a sufficiently large amount to demonstrate by conventional detection systems, such as nucleic acid hybridisation with labelled probes (Ou *et al.* 1988; Schochetman *et al.* 1988). The technique can also be used to synthesise large amounts of a specific DNA sequence for detailed analysis and for the construction of expression systems to obtain synthetic proteins.

As a prerequisite to performing PCR, the DNA sequence of the target area and its flanking regions must be known. This allows the synthesis of oligonucleotide primers, which are short single-stranded DNA sequences (20–25 base pairs in length) complementary to the target DNA sequences. The size of DNA fragment to be amplified is usually several hundred base pairs in length. First, the double stranded DNA is separated into single strands by heating and, on cooling, the primers hybridise to sequence at the 3' end of each strand. When nucleotide triphosphates and a thermostable DNA polymerase are added, the enzyme synthesises complementary DNA sequences for each of the strands of the target DNA sequence. Thus the original two strands of DNA have become four. By repeating this process many times, for which automated thermocyclers are now available, the original DNA fragment can be amplified millions of times.

The breakthrough that allowed this technique to be considered for diagnostic use was the discovery and characterisation of a heat-stable Taq DNA polymerase, in the bacterium *Thermus aquaticus*, which could survive the high temperatures necessary to separate the DNA strands and could, therefore, be retained in the reaction mixture during multiple temperature changes. Further development led to the availability of the technology for RNA detection. This is achieved by converting RNA to DNA by the retroviral enzyme, reverse transcriptase, prior to amplification of a DNA copy.

PCR offers tremendous potential as a basis for extremely sensitive diagnostic tests and its use for many different agents is being explored. Theoretically it should be useful for detecting HIV-1 or HIV-2 RNA or proviral DNA and, indeed, it is widely used experimentally for these purposes. There are, however, major drawbacks associated with the inherent sensitivity of the process. It is very prone to contamination and if the system is contaminated with minute amounts of extraneous DNA, they will be amplified along with the patient's material. False positives may occur and, because the technique is potentially far more sensitive than any other, there may be no way of confirming these apparent positive results.

Secondly, the primer pairs chosen may not be specific to HIV and there may be cross reactions with cellular DNA sequences or other infectious agents – another potential source of false positivity. Regional variation in the genetic sequence of HIV isolates means that primer pairs appropriate for one isolate may not be homologous to sequences in isolates from other regions. This lack of specificity resulting from genomic variation may be a cause of false negative results.

Thus, at the time of writing, PCR remains a research tool and is not a routine diagnostic test. It is likely, however, that it will soon be introduced for certain aspects of HIV diagnosis, and the investigation of babies born to HIV-infected women is an attractive area for use of PCR.

Overview

In the short time since the isolation and characterisation of HIV, diagnostic tests have been refined to a remarkable degree. Antibody tests provide by far the most useful means of diagnosing infected individuals and the availability of many different technologies facilitates the choice of adequate confirmatory tests. The introduction of sensitive antigen tests and the association of p24 antigen positivity with disease progression, provide a marker, albeit of limited value, for disease progression. The suppression of p24 levels has been valuable in antiviral drug assessment.

Virus culture remains difficult and expensive and, although the sensitivity has been improved, it is not of major use in routine diagnosis. PCR has enormous potential but must still be regarded as experimental. The difficult area of neonatal and paediatric diagnosis is currently covered by virus culture and p24 antigen detection; PCR is likely to be the routine in future.

References

Allain, J-P., Laurien, Y., Paul, D.A., & Senn, D. (1986) Serological markers in early stages of human immunodeficiency virus infection in haemophiliacs. *Lancet*, ii, 1233.

Barre-Sinoussi, F., Chermann, J.C., Rey, F. *et al.* (1983) Isolation of a T lymphotropic retrovirus from a patient at risk of acquired immune deficiency syndrome. *Science*, **220**, 868.

Centers for Disease Control (1987) Guidelines for counselling and antibody testing to prevent HIV infection and AIDS. *Morbidity & Mortality Weekly Report*, **36**, 509.

Centers for Disease Control (1989) Interpretation and use of the Western blot assay for serodiagnosis of human immunodeficiency virus type 1 infections. *Morbidity & Mortality Weekly Report*, **38**, 5–7.

Coombs, R.W., Collier, A.C., & Allain, J-P. (1989) Plasma viraemia in human immunodeficiency virus infection. *New England Journal of Medicine*, **321**, 1626.

Hausler, W.J. (1988) Report of the Third Consensus Conference on HIV testing sponsored by the Association of State and Territorial Public Health Laboratory Directors. *Infection Control and Hospital Epidemiology*, **9**, 345.

Ho, D.D., Moudgh, T., & Alam, M. (1989) Quantitation of human immunodeficiency virus type 1 in the blood of infected persons. *New England Journal of Medicine*, **321**, 1621.

Jackson, J.B., Coombs, R.W., Sannerud, K. *et al.* (1988) Rapid and sensitive viral culture method for human immunodeficiency virus type I. *Journal of Clinical Microbiology*, **26**, 1416.

Kenny, C., Parkin, J., Underhill, G. *et al.* (1987) HIV antigen testing. *Lancet*, i, 565.

Lange, J.M., Paul, D.A., Huisman, H.G. *et al.* (1986) Persistent HIV antigenaemia and decline of HIV core antibodies associated with transition to AIDS. *British Medical Journal*, **293**, 1459.

McHugh, T.M., Stiles, D.P., Casavant, C.H. *et al.* (1986) Evaluation of the indirect immuno-fluorescence assay as a confirmatory test for detecting antibodies to the human immunodeficiency virus. *Diagnostic Immunology*, **4**, 233.

Mortimer, P.P., Clewley, J.P. (1987) Serological tests for human immunodeficiency virus. In: *Current Topics in AIDS* (eds M.S. Gottlieb, D.J. Jeffries, D. Mildvan, A.J. Pinching, T.C. Quinn & R.A. Weiss), p.133. John Wiley, Chichester.

Ou, C-Y., Kwok, S., Mitchell, S.W. *et al.* (1988) DNA amplification for direct detection of HIV-1 in DNA of peripheral blood mononuclear cells. *Science*, **239**, 295.

Popovic, M., Sarngadharan, M.G., Read, E., & Gallo, R.C. (1984) Detection, isolation and continuous production of cytophathic retroviruses (HTLV-III) from patients with AIDS and pre-AIDS. *Science*, **224**, 497.

Schochetman, G., Ou, C-Y., & Jones, W.K. (1988) Polymerase chain reaction. *Journal of Infectious Diseases*, **158**, 1154.

Wilber, J.C. (1987) Serologic testing of human immunodeficiency virus infection. *Clinical Laboratory Medicine*, **7**, 777.

Chapter 3

Pre-test Counselling

Alana McCreaner

The HIV antibody test has been freely available throughout the UK since October 1985. All western countries and many developing countries either have introduced, or will shortly introduce, facilities for HIV testing. In most countries in the world the incidence of HIV in the population has steadily risen and with it the need for expert counselling of people who are considering taking the test.

The aims of pre-test counselling are:

- To ensure that any decision to take the test is fully informed and based on an under-standing of the personal, medical, legal and social implications of a positive result. At one level, this is simply a practical application of the traditional medical ethic of informed consent to a new procedure. While it is not a legal requirement to obtain consent in writing, it is often helpful.
- To provide the necessary preparation for those who will have to face the trauma of a positive result. Such preparation is vital in that patients who have been prepared for a positive result are able to face that result much more equably.
- To provide the individual with necessary risk reduction information on the basis of which he or she can reduce the risk of either acquiring HIV infection or passing it on to others. This needs to be done with anyone who has been, or may be, at risk. It needs to be done whether he or she eventually elects to be tested or not, and if tested, whether the individual is found to be positive or negative.

It is crucial in pre-test counselling to gain the trust which is clearly essential in the discussion of the more intimate areas of the person's life. It is always advisable to provide assurances that what is discussed between the counsellor and the individual will be kept confidential.

In some agencies, confidentiality is guaranteed, as it is in the UK National Health Service by the NHS (Venereal Diseases) Regulations 1974; this regulates disclosure of any relevant information by employees of the health authority (and since NHS reorganisation by other health care staff). Other agencies may have limits on the extent of confidentiality they can offer, for example, social services staff who work within the Children Act 1989 may find that, under certain circumstances, they have some limitations on the degree of confidentiality they can offer where a child is involved.

Some HIV testing is done in GP surgeries and health centres. One special problem which faces GPs is that they may have to fill in medical forms about a patient for insurance companies or for employers. If they are aware that a patient is seropositive they will legally be bound to reveal this if they are to fully complete the form. Clients seeking HIV tests from a GP need to be aware of any difficulty in this area.

It is important that any restrictions or limitations on confidentiality should be made explicit at the outset of counselling so that the patient knows exactly where he or she stands (see Chapter 17).

Pre-test counselling is sometimes done in a formulaic fashion. At its worst it can degenerate into a 'reading of rights' to a patient – a trotting out of a standardised recitation of information and advice. At its best, however, pre-test counselling is an interaction between counsellor and patient as they try to solve various problems and reach sensible conclusions about particular courses of action. This does not necessarily mean that it always takes a long time; indeed the hallmark of good pre-test counselling is likely to be that the amount of time differs according to the needs of the patient. An individual who is well-informed about HIV, has thought extensively about the issues and has already taken appropriate steps to reduce their risk (and there are many such patients) is unlikely to take as long in pre-test counselling as an individual who shows the reverse pattern. An individual with little or no risk behaviour is usually not going to take as long to pre-test counsel as someone with extensive risk, simply because they are likely to have less to say about the issue.

Each person will have distinctive needs and the discussion should develop towards identifying these needs. Once a session is under way an effective counsellor will remain alert to the danger of over-directing the individual and particularly of anticipating his or her decision about whether to take the test. There are several stages in providing pre-test counselling; the order in which these will be covered will probably differ from individual to individual. However, it is always important to be consistent and ensure that, by the end of the session, all necessary areas have been covered.

Finding out why the client wants a test

It is helpful to establish why the client wants or perceives the need to have an HIV test. While reasons given will be individual, they may give the counsellor some insight into other problem areas that may need to be addressed, for example:

● The client has a well established risk, e.g. having unprotected sex, sharing needles etc.
   This is a fairly straightforward reason for requesting a test. However, it needs to be approached with some caution. Is the client saying that he realises that his risk behaviour carries a danger of being infected and that he would like to be tested so that he can start changing his behaviour? Or, is he hoping the test will be negative so as to justify his continuing his present behaviour? The approach to counselling about risk reduction will clearly differ in these two cases.

● The client wants the test prior to starting a family or new relationship
   The client will need to be made aware of the limitations of the test – for instance in terms of 'window period' (time before measurable antibodies appear) – and a frank assessment of past and current risks will need to be made.

- The client has just seen a programme on HIV on the television or an article in the newspaper and has decided to seek testing on the basis of this

Media coverage of HIV issues often results in large numbers of people coming forward to be tested. Some will have few risks or no risk and will come only because they saw the programme. Some will be hypochondriacs and their worries about their health will have focused on HIV. Others will use the programme as an excuse for coming forward for testing and will have had very real risks.

- The client has been informed by a past sexual partner or 'works' (drug injecting equipment) sharing partner that they are HIV positive

Dealing with contacts of known cases (or supposed cases) is always difficult. Contacts often assume – quite wrongly – that if they have had sex with, or shared works with, an HIV infected individual, it is certain that they are themselves infected. There is also the issue of how they are going to feel about the person who may have infected them if they turn out positive. It is not always clear, of course, that that partner is the only person they have slept with/shared works with who is infected. The client themselves may have infected the partner, rather than the other way round.

- The client who is complaining of symptoms which he is convinced are caused by AIDS

Of course, he may be correct. However very often the individual turns out to be 'worried well', and the symptoms turn out to be those of anxiety. Sometimes the symptoms turn out not to be HIV-related but to be caused by some other physical condition. Obviously, anyone presenting with symptoms needs to be properly evaluated. It is worth remembering that even if a client turns out to be seropositive, his symptoms may not necessarily be caused by HIV.

- The client is seeking an HIV test in order to meet some legal or financial requirement, perhaps in order to live in countries requiring a negative test result or in order to obtain insurance

Situations like this are very difficult. Where people need to live abroad because their job demands it, there can sometimes be little or no choice for them. Unfortunately a proportion of tests in such people turn out to be positive, leaving an individual who is not only seropositive but also, sometimes, jobless.

These are common reasons for people seeking an HIV test. Each reason is likely to lead to a different approach to pre-test counselling. A standardised approach which deals with pre-test counselling of a hypochondriac in the same way as pre-test counselling of a woman who has just found out that her lover is HIV positive, somehow misses the point!

These are only a few of the reasons why people seek testing. There are other less common ones. Some clients are more or less 'sent' by partners.

Peter came asking for an HIV test. His wife came with him and sat, stony faced, in the waiting room. At first he said he was afraid that he had been at risk and was seeking the test for his own reassurance. However, it transpired that he had had a brief affair with a woman who worked with him and his wife was 'teaching him a lesson' by making him have an HIV test.

Obviously, it is always wise to be cautious with clients who are seeking to have an HIV test at the behest of someone else. There may be good reasons for such a situation. Perhaps the partner is negative and wants to know whether the couple can have unprotected penetrative sex. Sometimes the partner is positive and wants to know whether they have given their partner HIV. However there can, as in the example above, be other reasons which need handling with tact. It sometimes happens that people wanting the HIV test (and screening for other sexually transmitted diseases) have no known risk factor except that they suspect their partners are being unfaithful. Clearly such a situation needs approaching with great caution.

Anyone involved with HIV pre-test counselling will fairly quickly be able to come up with a list of unusual reasons given by patients for seeking a test. Whether the reason seems a weird one, or just downright bad to the counsellor, does not really matter. The patient can still have the test if they want it. However, the way the counsellor seeks to carry out pre-test counselling is likely to differ with the reason given for seeking testing.

Assessing a client's level of risk

It is important to assess the actual level of risk of the individual as opposed to their perception of the risk. The most important risk factors will vary from country to country and often from area to area within a country. An awareness of the most common types of passage of infection in an area is vital to the counsellor carrying out pre-test counselling.

However, in pre-test counselling it is always necessary to guard against being 'blinded by statistics' and pre-judging the risk factors of any person on the basis of superficial questioning. The counsellor should also be aware of the fact that the importance of different risk factors may change over time. Sometimes the first warning of such a shift comes with finding that someone thought to have little risk is, in fact, infected. For instance, even in areas where heterosexual spread is uncommon, occasional cases will occur. While some individuals are 'low risk', far fewer will be 'no risk'. It is therefore essential to take a history. This should cover:

- The sexual behaviour of the individual. Where known to the individual, the sexual and other risk behaviours of any partners
- Any history of injecting drug use

There are also some less common ways of getting infected which should be routinely enquired about:

- Past blood transfusions prior to the introduction of screening of donations, although in most western countries new identifications of such cases will be rare.
- Use of blood products for the treatment of haemophilia prior to the introduction of screening and/or heat treatment. Again, in the west at least, most such cases will already be known.
- Invasive procedures carried out under non-sterile conditions such as cosmetic procedures, ritual scarification and circumcision. This will also include repeated injections carried out with the same equipment with inadequate sterilisation procedures, as they are by unqualified (and sometimes qualified) healers in some countries.

In taking a history of risk behaviour it is important to be straightforward and clear.

Mary, a 45 year old married woman, attended for an HIV test following a sexual encounter with a man she met while on a business trip. Mary was very distressed and felt extremely guilty as she felt she had betrayed her husband's trust after 16 years of marriage. She had seen this man once only and had little information about his background.

COUNSELLOR: 'You said you had seen this man once only; how often did you have sex?'
PATIENT: 'I spent one night with him.'
COUNSELLOR: 'Did you have sex once only during the night?'
PATIENT: 'Well, we had normal sex about three times during the night.'
COUNSELLOR: 'Did he put his penis in your vagina?'
PATIENT: 'Yes.'
COUNSELLOR: 'Did he put his penis in your back passage?'
PATIENT: 'No, but he did put it in my mouth.'
COUNSELLOR: 'Did he wear a condom?'
PATIENT: 'No. I am on the pill.'

It is important to get a clear picture of what actually happened in a person's sex life. In this case a particular incident concerned the patient. Vague discussions about whether Mary 'had sex' without being explicit about what the counsellor means by the term can leave a gulf of misunderstanding between patient and counsellor. Also, by asking very direct questions, the counsellor helps the patient. It is much easier, if one is embarrassed, to say 'yes' or 'no' to the question 'did he put his penis in your back passage' than to volunteer the information in answer to a vague question such as 'what did you do?'

On the basis of such an assessment it is helpful to give the individual an estimation of the likely risk their behaviour has put them at. Obviously this is not going to be in the form of an exact numerical set of odds, but in terms of whether their behaviour has been putting them at higher or lower risk. This is important because it leads naturally into discussion of risk behaviour and risk reduction.

Estimating risk is also important because it allows the counsellor to take an intelligent approach to test results; mix-ups do occur in laboratories and it is important to be cautious about positive results in an individual who does not seem to have been at risk. It is also important in dealing with individuals who are seronegative 'worried well', and who may seek to engage the counsellor in elaborate questions about the possibility of late seroconversion and other hypothetical exotica. The counsellor's response is likely to be much more robust in the presence of a good history showing little or no risk.

However, it is important to acknowledge that clients may withhold information about themselves that would alter the estimation of likely risk. It can be helpful to remind clients that any assessment of risk given will be based on the information they have given the counsellor. Where the risk appears minimal the person should be told so. On the other hand no actual risk, however slight, should be dismissed out of hand. The odds of being struck by lightning in the UK are several million to one, but every year several people in the UK *are* struck by lightning. Given enough people, even the most unlikely event tends to happen at least once.

Explaining about HIV and the HIV test

Confusion over what the test can actually tell us is very common. It is essential to be able to explain, in jargon-free language, exactly what the test does and does not establish. Visual material illustrating the process involved is most helpful and the use of written materials that the patient can take away with them is of great value.

A clear account of the limitations of the test should be included. In particular it is important to discuss the length of time which it can take before measurable antibodies appear (the window period). These issues are considered in more detail in Chapter 2. Clearly a man who has had risky sex the day before cannot rely on a negative test result on sera collected that day to show him that he is not infected. This sort of consideration can be unsettling for those who look to the test to resolve their anxieties once and for all, but it must be stressed that the test brings with it no guarantees.

Another matter which often needs clarification is the difference between being HIV positive and having AIDS. Many people coming for the test still believe that it is a test for AIDS rather than for HIV infection. The test cannot indicate how advanced an individual's HIV disease is, nor can it give any clue as to when they might have been infected.

Some individuals come forward for an HIV test because they believe that they have been at risk when, in fact, they have not. For instance we saw an elderly woman who came in to say that her lodger had developed AIDS and she was concerned that she had been sharing cutlery and crockery with him. Simple factual information saw her going home untested but perfectly happy.

Explaining a little about HIV and its transmission can be very helpful, as long as it does not turn into a lecture. It can give counsellor and client a common basis for discussion, can help the client to answer questions appropriately by helping them to understand why particular questions are being asked, and it can sometimes provide considerable reassurance.

The advantages and disadvantages of an individual client having the test

The decision about whether to be tested or not is, essentially, a matter of balancing advantages and disadvantages. The balance will differ from individual to individual.

People coming for the test have sometimes thought through what a negative result would mean for them but have not thought through the repercussions of a positive result. The advantages and disadvantages of being tested, for the particular individual, have to be fully explored. In the end it will be that person's choice whether to be tested, and the process of choosing will involve an assessment for that person of the advantages and disadvantages.

The advantages and disadvantages of being tested are not fixed. They may vary over time. Should an effective treatment for HIV infection become available, clearly the advantages of being tested would, for the vast majority of people, be overwhelming.

For the pregnant woman, one issue she will need to consider when deciding whether to be tested is that trials have indicated that AZT administration during pregnancy, childbirth and to the neonate may affect the risk of the child being infected (see Chapter 9). This fact will not necessarily decide whether she should have the test; it is one factor she needs to balance against the advantages of having it.

Other advantages of being tested for an individual might include, if they are positive, such things as:

- Providing information for a differential diagnosis in someone with symptoms. This is often a powerful reason for being tested, particularly when awareness of a client's status will affect the treatment they receive.
- The client being able to arrange regular monitoring of their health to identify any problems early.
- The client having the possibility of prophylaxis against common opportunist infections when their CD4+ count falls to an appropriate level, and possibly starting on antivirals.
- Possible influences on decisions about how the client will live their life (for instance a decision to retire early on a lower pension).
- For some individuals, a positive influence on their risk behaviours leading to a reduction of their risks of infecting others and of getting intercurrent infections, particularly sexually transmitted infections or infections spread by syringe–sharing. Notice, however, that a positive test result does not in itself necessarily reduce risky behaviour (Chapter 4).
- The ability for a woman to decide potentially to avoid pregnancy or to terminate an existing pregnancy.

These are merely examples; there are many other possible reasons why finding out that one is seropositive may confer benefits. Finding out that one is negative can also have advantages, which might include:

- Being able to live in countries demanding a negative HIV test
- Feeling less anxious about HIV
- Knowing that one can engage in unprotected sex with a partner who is themselves negative (assuming that both parties are going to take steps to stay that way).

On the other hand, there are usually disadvantages to finding that one is positive. These might include:

- A worsening of quality of life caused by awareness of infection with HIV and consequent adverse psychological consequences. Some clients respond with great distress to a positive result.
- Problems in getting financial services, particularly insurance and mortgages.
- The inclusion of specific questions about HIV is becoming more common in health questionnaires and medical examinations for job applicants. If these questions are answered inaccurately contracts of employment may be voided. While many employers will employ individuals who know they have HIV infection, many others will not.
- Being put in the dilemma of having either to tell friends and family of one's status or to keep a secret which may reduce closeness to them.

There can even be disadvantages to finding that one is negative. Some clients – indeed quite a lot of clients – treat having a negative result as a licence to continue to engage in their existing sexual or other risk behaviours. Indeed, they may become more risky, having 'got away with it so far'. It is hard to think of a more adverse outcome of testing than that.

It is important to bear in mind that there is seldom any public health interest in testing an individual, however many governments and other organisations may behave as though there is. HIV testing is helpful in so far as it benefits the individual, and it is for the individual to balance the advantages and disadvantages and take a decision about what is best for them. It is not for the counsellor to seek to persuade them either way, but to seek to get the client to bring out the advantages and disadvantages for them personally.

Helping the client to plan for behaviour change

Pre-test counselling is a good point at which to start the process of thinking through risk reduction (if there are risk behaviours). There are several good reasons for choosing pre-test counselling rather than leaving it to the post-test counselling:

- Discussion of risk reduction follows on naturally from an exploration of the reasons for wanting a test
- A client may decide not to have the test having had pre-test counselling
- A proportion of individuals who opt to be tested fail to return for their results
- People who are seronegative are usually too relieved to give much attention to issues such as risk-reduction
- Regrettably many services allocate little time to post-test counselling negatives.

Behaviour change is one of the key elements in HIV pre-test and post-test counselling. In many cases, although not in all, the individual will need to make the same risk-reduction changes whether they test positive, negative or opt not to be tested.

Risk reduction is covered in more detail in Chapters 4 and 8.

Preparing for a possible positive result

It is important to get a client to start to think through some of the things they might have to do if they find out that they are positive. It is difficult for someone who has just been told that they are seropositive to start to take a whole string of difficult decisions. Sometimes it is difficult even to take simple decisions like how to spend the rest of the day. Advance preparation can be reassuring and helpful. The points can be picked up after the test, but it helps at least to make a start on them before the result comes back.

Of course one would not spend the same time on preparation with a 'worried well' individual with no risk factors, as one would with someone who has been at risk. However, for those who have had risks, even if these do not seem particularly great, it is worth doing some forward planning. It could be on the basis that a positive result is unlikely but no harm is done by preparing for a slight chance of the individual being positive. There are several areas of action which are helpful.

Planning for the visit to get the results

It is surprising how many people plan to come and get their HIV test results and then go straight on to work or a social occasion. Obviously if the result is positive they may be faced with difficulties. Creating some space is important.

Some people feel safer if they bring someone with them to the clinic. This obviously means they will have to find a trusted individual who can come and whom they feel able to tell that they are having the test. Others, of course, would prefer that no-one knows they are being tested.

Planning what they will do after getting the result is important. It is helpful to explore what they might do if they get a positive result and feel bad about this. Do they have people to turn to? Or will they end up on their own at home faced with a long anxious weekend? Making a definite plan about how to spend the time is very helpful.

Telling other people

It can be very helpful to think through with the client who they might want to tell about their HIV status. Some clients will not want anyone to know if they are positive. Others, however, will feel the need to talk to other people about the issue, to get support and perhaps help. Some clients will want to tell particular friends, and it is helpful to establish at this stage who they might be. Others may want to tell family. Still others want to meet individuals who have themselves had similar experiences and they can be put in touch with voluntary agencies or self-help groups.

Most clients find that those they tell about their HIV status are supportive. However this is by no means universal; adverse reactions do occur and sometimes these can rebound. I have seen a number of patients who have lost jobs or had other adverse consequences from letting 'friends' know that they are HIV seropositive, and then finding that the information spreads rapidly and widely. It is a difficult path to negotiate; telling no-one leaves the client short of social support, but once someone has been told they cannot be un-told.

It is also helpful to start the process of thinking through the issue of telling partners. It is important to establish whether an individual's current partner is aware that they have come for the test. If they are aware, what has the client told them about possible risk factors, what explanation has the client offered to the partner about why they are having a test? Where an individual's partner is not aware that he is being tested, why has the client not told them? If the client has, in fact, been at risk, would it be better if they did tell their current partner they were being tested? If they do turn out to be infected, how will they go about telling their partner and what is the likely reaction?

It is also helpful to discuss the need to inform past partners. At pre-test counselling there is little point in getting too deep into this issue. There is time to explore it in more detail if the results are positive, but at least some idea of how many individuals might be involved and what difficulties the issue might present, can be established.

Taking a decision

There is no reason why a client has to decide there and then whether to have the HIV test. They can almost always return at another time and be tested then. This needs to be made explicit.

In practice, most individuals coming forward for the HIV test do elect to be tested after pre-test counselling. However, there will always be some clients for whom being tested is of little or no value. In some settings, where most clients have been at little or no risk, such individuals may be in the majority. Even amongst populations where risk of HIV infection is high, some individuals may decide that there is little personal advantage in being tested while they remain well, if they have made lifestyle changes which mean they do not put themselves or others at risk. They may even feel that not knowing their status helps them to maintain, say, safer sex.

The success of a pre-test counselling service is sometimes measured by what proportion of individuals have the test, but this is not a sensible criterion. One would expect that in most successful services a number of clients will decide not to be tested and in some the proportion of individuals not electing to be tested may be quite high; it just depends on the circumstances.

Written material summarising the main points covered in pre-test counselling should be available for all. It is particularly useful for those who need more time to consider before reaching a decision. It is helpful to tell the individual that they do not necessarily have to make a decision there and then; they can always return later to have the test.

Explaining the procedure

It often helps to explain the physical procedure for HIV testing, since most clients have only the haziest idea what the test consists of. Some clients expect to get an instant result and it is important to explain how long it will take to get test results back. At the time of the last edition of this book waits of a few days were common, but now many clinics offer same day or next day results and really long waits are uncommon. However, there can be variations in procedure and the arrangements need to be explained to the client. Where there is an extended wait it can be helpful to enquire how the client will cope with this. Some clients are so anxious during the wait that they need extra support, or there may be a case for trying to speed things up at the laboratory.

It is always important to make a definite time for the client to come back for their test results. Giving clients the results over the telephone or by letter is not a good idea. Whether the result is positive or negative, proper post-test counselling is needed.

Dealing with other issues

Staff doing pre-test counselling are often working under pressure, which limits the time available for each client. Where time is short, it is necessary to concentrate on the task at hand – dealing with the issues around testing itself. However, many individuals coming for possible HIV testing have other issues which it is just not appropriate or possible to follow through in a pre-test counselling session. Clients often bring other issues into the pre-test session, either knowingly or unknowingly. The counsellor needs either to rebook the client, to see them at another time to address these issues, or to refer them on.

Overview

The term pre-test 'counselling' is often misleading. It is not only counselling, although there is a strong counselling element, but also a sharing of information which may alter the client's perception of being tested.

Obviously many of the same issues come up again and again in pre-test counselling sessions. It is tempting to reduce the procedure to a formula which can be repeated with each client. To do so, however, provides the client with a second-rate service and loses a key opportunity to help and educate them and meet their needs.

Chapter 4

Counselling People Infected with HIV

John Green

Reactions to HIV infection

Figure 4.1 shows a hypothetical graph of distress in an individual with HIV infection. Like all hypothetical graphs it applies to no-one in particular; however it does show a typical pattern of distress. The source of the data is our own research and the published literature and I include it because it has implications for the way that services might be organised for those with HIV (Green & Hedge 1991).

The typical pattern seen in someone who becomes aware of the fact that they have HIV is in several phases. The time of peak distress is when people have just decided to have a test and when they are waiting for the result. If the result is negative most people rapidly resolve their distress. For those who are positive there is a period of gradual adjustment, when they try and sort out the implications for them and for their lives. This typically takes from three to six months but more rapid or slower adjustment sometimes occurs (Jadresic *et al.* 1989;

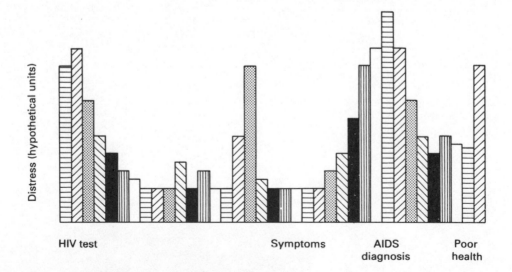

Fig. 4.1 Hypothetical graph of distress in HIV disease.

Pery *et al.* 1990). Over this time the level of distress of the individual drops, though not always back to what it was before the test. An individual who continues to be highly distressed over a period of months needs extra time and attention. Usually they have issues which they have not been able to sort out.

People continue to get their lives in order and to adjust to the diagnosis over the next few months or years. By and large most seropositives have successful and enjoyable lives. They are still aware that they are infected and they may have days when they are anxious or depressed, but they function well. However, during this period people often have upsurges in distress caused by events in their lives associated with HIV (as well as the ups and downs that everyone has in their life). They may, for instance, find that they split up with their partner and have to try to form a new relationship in the context of HIV infection, or they may be unable to change jobs because of their status, or they may find that the death of a friend from AIDS throws their own status into stark relief. These sorts of event tend to cause a sharp upsurge in distress which then resolves, providing they are able to sort out the problem either alone or through friends or formal counselling.

At some point symptoms may start to appear. The person with HIV may find that they are suffering increasing fatigue, or they may notice changes in the speed with which minor ailments resolve, or they may develop skin problems. It is not usually the symptoms as such which are the issue. The person with HIV sees these things as a sign that the virus is gaining ground. We provide artificial symptoms for our patients sometimes by providing them with information on their CD4+ count. A patient may feel well but see their CD4+ count inexorably declining.

This period when they move from asymptomatic to symptomatic is a moment of considerable distress for many people. They may over years have continued well and have hoped that they might be a 'non-progressor'. They may have been able, by and large, to put the issue out of their minds for most of the time. Now they are confronted with the fact that their disease is progressing. As their symptoms become more severe, their distress is likely to increase. One of the elements in this is the feeling of uncertainty about whether and when they will move to having AIDS. In spite of the essentially arbitrary nature of the AIDS diagnosis, it is hard for the individual not to see it as a significant milestone in the disease.

Paradoxically, the diagnosis of AIDS itself – despite usually coming as a shock – sometimes also comes almost as a relief. At least there is something which can be adjusted to and dealt with, a certainty rather than simply waiting for the 'axe to fall'. After the AIDS diagnosis most people adjust again and their level of distress falls once more. They usually find that, except when they are actually ill, they are able to lead a more or less normal and fulfilling life.

Distress rises again as the person finds that their health is declining. Bouts of illness become more severe and closer together and the residual disability after each illness is greater. They are faced with the greater immediacy of death and with adjustment to greater physical problems and the reactions of others.

It is important to stress several points about this analysis. These 'stages' are points on a continuum. The disease itself is highly variable and does not always show the smooth pattern of progression described above. Not everyone has the same experience of the disease or shows the same pattern of distress. It is, however, probably the single most common pattern and, as such, has implications for organising a counselling service.

Organising counselling

It follows from the pattern of progression described above that counselling the individual with HIV is an ongoing activity, not a matter of a once-and-for-all post-test counselling session or sessions. There are times when it is necessary to be proactive and actively offer counselling to the patient. These times are pre-test and post-test, when the patient starts to have symptoms or their CD4+ count starts to fall, when they have their AIDS diagnosis, and when their health declines badly in late-stage disease. It should not be necessary to wait for the patient to request a service at these times; it should be actively offered.

Patients are likely to remain well and have little distress for long periods when they are HIV seropositive. There is no point in having repeated counselling sessions with a patient who does not need them; it is a waste of the counsellor's time and the patient's. On the other hand it is important that they should know where to make contact if they do need help, and it is important to ensure that they get a prompt service if they do make contact. For that reason we do not ever completely discharge a patient; we simply terminate that episode of contact (by mutual agreement) and make it clear to patients that they can come back if they feel it would be helpful. Not all problems will be related, directly or indirectly, to HIV. People with HIV have the same life problems as everyone else; the HIV problems are additional to these.

It is important to try to monitor patients even when they are not having formal counselling. Because most patients will come back for routine medical screening from time to time, there is an opportunity for the doctor or nurse to enquire how they are, and if there are any problems to refer them back for further counselling.

Patients may require different sources of counselling for different problems and they may find some sources more congenial than others There is a need to provide definite inputs at definite times, but as far as possible it is helpful to fit in with what they want. The other side of the coin is that the counselling of patients is a function of the service rather than of an individual. That is not to say that there should not be specialist counsellors or that the function should not be undertaken by psychologists, nurses, doctors, health advisors, or volunteers allocated to that role. However, it is important to understand that much of the counselling role takes place outside those specialities. The doctor who reassures a patient about their CD4+ count, the nurse who spends time with a patient when they are in hospital, the buddy from a voluntary organisation and many others are all involved in the same process of contributing to the patient's psychological well-being. That being so, the service has to have a way of co-ordinating its care for the individual. Whether this is done through formal meetings at which patients are reviewed, or through a well-established network of joint working between individuals, is a matter of local practice. In the absence of arrangements for an integrated approach we are likely to fail our patients.

Patients have a life outside hospital. Formal counselling is only one source of support and help for them. Friends, family and social organisations all play a part in how the patient feels and how they adjust to the disease. This can be as important, or more important, than what happens to them when they are being 'counselled' or otherwise dealt with by a hospital service. Counselling can augment but never replace these other sources of support.

The description of the counselling service given above is in terms of the patient. However, services also have to take into account the needs of partners, family and the other formal and informal carers of those infected with the disease. These people are often as distressed or more distressed than the patient themselves. They too may need support and help.

Alan had AIDS and was extremely ill. He lived with his sister, Sarah, who had moved down from Scotland to look after him. She found the burden of caring for him very difficult. Not only did she have to look after the practical aspects of his care – doing most of the domestic work, supervising his medication, cooking special meals for him and ferrying him to hospital appointments – but she had also taken on the main task of organising his life for him, taking virtually all the decisions about what they would do and how he would spend his time. The more she did for him, the more she felt she had to do. She never felt satisfied with what she was doing. She became anxious and, as his health continued to decline in spite of all her efforts, depressed.

Obviously Sarah needed both counselling and practical support in dealing with Alan.

For most counsellors, the first contact with people with HIV infection often comes at around the time of the HIV test. Managing this time well is important.

Post-test counselling

The foundation of good post-test counselling is laid in pre-test counselling (Chapter 3). If pre-test counselling is not carried out or is skimped or reduced to 'reading the patient their rights' (i.e. mechanically going through some set patter) then good post-test counselling becomes very difficult. If pre-test counselling is done well, the counsellor will already have a relationship with the patient, will have laid the ground for any necessary changes in behaviour or planning for the future, and will know quite a lot about the patient.

Most patients are distressed at the time when they come back for their test results; they are anxious and apprehensive. Some patients anticipate the results, expect to be positive and so are calm. Even so, it usually still comes as something of a shock to find that they really are positive. Patients may have difficulty taking in what they have been told or deciding what to do next at the first session, and it may be necessary to arrange a second session very soon after when outstanding issues can be picked up.

We have usually found it useful, even in the calmest of patients, to arrange a follow-up appointment within a few days of the first appointment, to check how things are going, since distress sometimes builds up when the patient has time to think things through. They usually have issues that they want clarified in any case. After that it is a matter of agreement between counsellor and patient what, when and how frequently further appointments are needed. It is good practice to arrange to see patients at three months post-test and this can usually be fitted in with routine clinical monitoring. However, many – perhaps almost all – seropositive patients will need more than two sessions early on.

The first post-test session

The first session after the test results come back is a crucial one. The patient is likely to be highly anxious and may be distressed by a positive test result. In the first session time is bound to be limited. There is seldom enough time to get everything possible in and it can be very difficult to decide how to structure the session. Table 4.1 sets out a suggested structure. This is simply a suggested structure not a prescription; it is not going to be applicable to all patients or all situations.

Table 4.1   Suggested structure for first post-test counselling session

---

(1) Give result clearly and concisely.
(2) Encourage patient to express their own issues. Try to encourage them to range reasonably widely over issues and not get stuck on a single one, but try to stay with their agenda.
(3) Ensure that key areas of finding out about the patient have been covered. These are likely to include: primary relationship, social life, health, finances, work, sex and other partners, accommodation, family, leisure. These are key background areas. The counsellor should end the session with an idea of whether there are any problems in each of these areas that will need to be addressed in future sessions.
(4) Identify any issues that need to be dealt with in that session and try to establish a plan of action.
(5) Identify with the patient what key issues they need to address, and work out a plan of action.
(6) Sort out with the patient a plan of future meetings.
(7) Ensure that any linkages to other services are made, including necessary referrals.
(8) Ensure that the patient knows how to contact the counsellor if there is a problem.
(9) Ensure that if the patient has any factual questions about HIV, they are answered there and then.

Taking Table 4.1 as a model, we will now look at each element in turn.

Giving the results

The first task is usually to give the patient their results.

COUNSELLOR: 'Hello, Peter (shaking hands), come in and sit down. Have you come back for your HIV test results?'

PATIENT: 'Yes, that's right.'

COUNSELLOR: 'We have the results back and you are positive; you are infected with HIV.'

This approach may, at first sight, appear rather bald, even brutal. The counsellor checks whether the patient has come back for the results, gives the result clearly and simply and stresses that the positive result means an infection.

Giving bad news, whether of seropositivity or AIDS or another health event is difficult for both the patient and the health professional. Counsellors sometimes seek to 'soften the blow' by wandering around verbally, seeking to find a way to put the result kindly. There is no way to make a positive result acceptable and no form of words which can soften the blow. Trying to fudge the issue can make it look as though the result is so awful that the counsellor is unable to bring themselves to give it straightforwardly. It can also easily appear patronising. In other words, trying too hard to put things kindly can easily end up making the patient feel worse. I have also seen more than one patient who has been given an HIV result by a health professional who hedged about the issue so much that the patient ended up not knowing what he was being told.

The next thing to do is to wait for the patient to say something. This can take some time. It is not easy, however prepared a patient is, for them to get their mind around the fact that they are infected with HIV. It is very important to listen to what the patient says next. When people are under stress they tend to produce the most important issues for them either directly, or indirectly through connected issues. Consider this example from a patient who was told he was HIV positive:

PATIENT: 'What is going to happen to my dog?'

At first sight the example seems strange. Why would anyone's first thought be about their dog at such a time? In fact, there are all sorts of possible links. The patient may be particularly fond of their dog; they may be conveying the fact that they have no close friends who might look after it; it might be an expression of their feeling that they are going to die very soon and not outlive the dog; or the patient may be afraid of infecting the dog or catching some opportunistic infection from the dog. Whatever issue the patient raises, it is best to start there.

COUNSELLOR: 'You're worried about your dog?'
PATIENT: 'I live alone. He's only a puppy and if I have to go into hospital there is no-one to look after him. There's no-one to look after me if I get sick for that matter.'

Reactions of patients are entirely unpredictable. It is never possible to predict what they are going to say. Various types of response can be picked up:

● *Statements, e.g. 'I never thought that I could be positive' or 'It's what I expected' or 'I was so careful and I still got infected.'*
They need to be responded to by encouraging the patient to go on in some way, e.g. by echoing the statement: 'You didn't think that you could be positive?', or by rephrasing: 'it comes as a surprise to you?', or just by saying 'uh-huh' or 'go on'.

● *Questions about facts, e.g. 'Does that mean I've got AIDS?' or 'Can I pass it on to the people I share the house with?'.*
It is best to answer these as briefly as possible without unnecessary qualification or detail, and then get the patient to go on talking. At this stage, in most cases, it is important to get the patient to talk to the counsellor, rather than vice versa. Factual issues can always be expanded on later.

● *Expressions of concern expressed as questions, e.g. 'How will I tell my wife?'.*
This may be a straightforward question but ninety times out of a hundred it is likely to be an expression of anguish or anxiety, and needs to be responded to by saying, for example, 'You are worried about your wife's reaction' or 'she doesn't know you've been tested?', depending on how it seems the question is intended.

● *Reactions, e.g. instead of saying anything, the patient bursts into tears or stares out of the window or at the counsellor.*
This is rare but extremely unnerving. The counsellor should usually sit tight and just wait until the patient has thought what they want to say. A brief statement such as 'it's often a shock, take your time' can help if silence goes on for a long while. In the case of tears I usually

provide tissues in as unobtrusive a way as possible and then wait. It is easy to assume that patients responding with these silent reactions have simply blanked out. It helps to realise that they are trying to come to terms with a sudden shock and their minds are usually racing. It is best to avoid asking questions, which would stop that process as they would have to switch their attention to what the counsellor is saying. All the silent patients I have ever had have eventually said something, so waiting and listening is what is required.

One of the greatest temptations at this point is to launch into a set patter, as in this extract from a counsellor transcript from some training I carried out:

COUNSELLOR: 'You have the AIDS virus.'
PATIENT: 'What about my wife and family?'
COUNSELLOR: 'There are five ways in which HIV can be transmitted.'

It is easy to see how this situation arose. The counsellor was stumped by the patient's reply and panicked. Like most people who are anxious, they fell back on what they knew best – in this case 101 useful facts about HIV. The fact that this was a wholly inappropriate response did not stop them doing it. We are all tempted to do this when stuck: to take control of the session and launch into some pre-arranged patter. We do it because it makes *us* feel better but we can easily deceive ourselves into the belief that it is for the patient's benefit.

The only certain point about the reactions of people to a positive HIV test is that you can never predict what those reactions will be. Some people will have good reason to suppose that they are HIV positive, will have thought through the issue and will react quite calmly. Others will seem to have given the issue just as much thought, and to have expected the result just as much, but will react with great distress.

Carrying on

Once a session is under way, there is not usually any difficulty in keeping going. At first the patient is likely to express their concerns, fears, questions and issues which are important to them. These are likely to come out in a haphazard way with no particular structure. This does not matter; there is no need to impose a particular structure but there is a need to try to help the patient say what they want to say in a way that the counsellor can understand. Typically, patients raise all sorts of points in a rush and it is not possible to follow everything through at the same time.

PATIENT: 'This is going to make a real mess of my life. Not only have I let Ralph down, my parents are old and my father has been ill with his heart and I don't know how he'd take it. I'm moving flat on Monday and it's much more expensive. My boss is a homophobic guy who'll sack me if he finds out. If I can't work how can I pay the rent?.... Do you think I'm going to get sick soon?'
COUNSELLOR: 'OK, you've raised a lot of issues there; let's work our way through them one by one. Shall we start with Ralph? You say you've let him down?'

Trying to respond to all the patient's points at once is hopeless. The counsellor acknowledges that they have heard all the issues, and then picks on one to start with. It does not usually matter which one is chosen; all will be reached eventually. If the patient wants to start somewhere else they usually say so, which is fine. However it is important for the counsellor either to have a good memory or to take notes – even just jottings of key words as an *aide memoir* – otherwise issues get lost.

Different counsellors have different ways of encouraging their patients to talk to them; some ask questions, others seek to reflect back what the patient is saying. These different styles are the subject of strong feelings amongst some counsellors, but the two approaches often lead to the same result.

PATIENT: 'I don't feel able to tell the people at work about being HIV positive; I don't feel I'd get the response I wanted.'
COUNSELLOR: 'You feel the people at work may not be sympathetic?'
or
COUNSELLOR: 'How do you think the people at work would respond if you told them?'

Either of the above approaches is likely to end up at the same place in the end; it is very much a matter of style and what feels comfortable.

Asking the patient how they feel is not necessarily wrong at this stage, but is often unhelpful. It is sometimes a subtle form of avoidance by the counsellor, and appears to be the sort of thing that counsellors 'should' say:

PATIENT: 'I never thought I could have HIV.'
COUNSELLOR: 'How do you feel about that?'
PATIENT: 'Bloody awful, how do you expect me to feel?'

Asking people how they feel about things in order to 'get them to express their feelings' is often not very helpful early on. There is no hard and fast rule about it and it may be helpful in the right context, but as in the above case it usually does not take the discussion forward On the other hand, asking them how they feel about something because the counsellor genuinely wants information for a purpose, as in 'How do you feel about telling your mother?', can be very helpful. But even that sort of question is best left until later in the session. The main drawback of continually asking people about their feelings is that they have to stop thinking about what concerns them, and start examining their feelings. This interrupts their agenda, replacing it with the counsellor's agenda.

Occasionally I have seen counsellors do very well for ten minutes, then run through some particular issue and get no response, and they panic and terminate the interview by making another appointment for some days hence. The problem here is usually that the counsellor feels they have a number of issues to address, they run through their own agenda and get no response, and they then feel that they have run out of anything to ask or say. If the counsellor concentrates on what the patient is saying, rather than thinking about what they are going to ask next, they will usually find that the patient provides ample material for any number of sessions. The issue then becomes one of trying to address the issues within limited time. The central point of the opening of the first session should be about the patient saying what the issues are for them. It should not be the basis for a lecture on safer sex, on telling their partner or similar matters.

Making sure key areas are covered

At some point the patient is likely to exhaust their immediate reaction to the news. Alternatively time may be getting on and the end of the session looming. At this stage it is helpful to go through things in a more systematic way. It should not be assumed that a patient will spontaneously mention all the most important or pressing issues in their life in respect of HIV. Also the counsellor will want to get a more general understanding of the patient and their world, not simply in terms of HIV but as a person.

It helps therefore to review what has been covered and try to cover areas which have not yet been covered. Table 4.1 suggests a convenient way of identifying whether key areas have been covered. The key areas are derived from interviews with patients about what they saw as the key parts of their lives for some research we have been carrying out.

COUNSELLOR: 'You've talked a bit about your worries, about your job, and you said that you thought that it might reduce your chances of promotion because you might not be able to work abroad in some countries which have restrictions. That's obviously very important to you and we are going to have to talk about it some more, perhaps spend a session just looking at that. I just want to pick up on some other areas of your life to see whether being HIV positive might have any impact there, and also to try to get a bit of a wider picture of your life generally.'

The counsellor summarises what has been said, shows that they have understood the importance of the work issue to the patient and intend to go into it in more detail, and explains why they are moving on.

COUNSELLOR: 'Let me just ask you about your relationship. I know you told me pre-test that you were living with Mary...'
PATIENT: 'That's right.'
COUNSELLOR: 'And you told me that she knew you had come for the test...'
PATIENT: 'Yes.'
COUNSELLOR: 'How do you think she is going to react to your being positive?'
PATIENT: 'She's going to be very upset. She knew it was likely that I would be positive, given my history, but I think it will still be a shock. We've talked about it a lot.'
COUNSELLOR: 'How will you tell her?'
PATIENT: 'She's taken the afternoon off work and I shall go home and meet her as soon as I've finished here. We've been through a lot and I don't think I'm going to find it difficult to tell her – awful but not difficult.'
COUNSELLOR: 'How do you think that your being positive will affect the relationship?'
PATIENT: 'I think it's strong enough to survive it. We have talked about what would happen if I was positive.'
COUNSELLOR: 'Have you any concerns in that area?'
PATIENT: 'Maybe when I've told her I'll know a bit better. She might like to come and see someone herself; would that be possible?'
COUNSELLOR: 'Of course; if she wants to ring me I'll be happy to fix up to see her quickly, or I'll be happy to talk to her on the phone if it's something she wants to talk about there and then, and she can come in later.'
PATIENT: 'I'll tell her.'

COUNSELLOR: 'What about your friends? Have you told any of them you were thinking about being tested?'

PATIENT: 'That's a real problem. I haven't told anyone and I've been putting them off while I've been waiting for the result.'

COUNSELLOR: 'You mean you haven't seen any of your friends?'

PATIENT: 'I mean I have been avoiding them.'

COUNSELLOR: 'Are your friends important to you?'

PATIENT: 'Very important. A lot of them I've known for years. I'm close to maybe five or six people and have maybe a dozen more friends who I see regularly...'

The objective of the counsellor is to try to cover as much ground as possible in order to build up a broad picture of the patient's situation and identify any problem areas. These can be discussed at subsequent sessions; they don't necessarily have to be dealt with there and then. The important issues in different areas, and some counselling approaches to these, are covered in more detail later in the chapter.

Identifying issues which must be dealt with in the first session

Thankfully most patients do not have anything that they absolutely must resolve in the first session. There is time to meet them again to look at important issues. However they do sometimes raise issues which they need to sort out at the first session because these will be immediate problems for them before the next meeting with the counsellor. It is important to ask specifically whether there are any such matters.

COUNSELLOR: 'Is there anything you will have to do, in relation to being HIV positive, before we next meet in a few days?'

PATIENT: 'I have to tell my partner tonight that I'm positive, and I just don't have a clue how I'm going to do it.'

COUNSELLOR: 'It has to be tonight?'

PATIENT: 'We're going away for the weekend. He's bound to know there's something wrong. He knows me too well.'

COUNSELLOR: 'And will he ask you what's wrong?'

PATIENT: 'Oh yes. And I don't want to lie to him.'

COUNSELLOR: 'Would it help if we looked at that now?'

PATIENT: 'Please.'

Unfortunately patients do not always spontaneously produce these pressing issues, so they must be asked about them. Patients are under stress and they are not always thinking in an organised fashion, which is hardly surprising under the circumstances.

When going through the different areas of the patient's life, it is best to ask, for each area, whether there is anything which they have to take action on quickly. Then it is important to enquire again at the end, to see if anything pressing has been missed. Obviously with pressing issues it is important to try to come up with a plan of action of some sort. Dealing with particular problems is dealt with in more detail below, and the issue generally is dealt with in Chapter 13.

Identifying other issues

The next stage is usually to try to work out the key issues that need to be addressed, and produce a plan of future sessions. This is probably best done by reviewing what the patient has said, in summary, and then trying to sort out with them which areas, if any, they want help with.

COUNSELLOR: 'Let me take you through what you've said and let me make sure that I've understood the important issues for you. Please tell me if I've misunderstood anything or left things out.'

PATIENT: 'Yes, OK.'

COUNSELLOR: 'You were an injecting drug user in the mid 1980s but you haven't used them for the last four or five years.'

PATIENT: 'Apart from a few smokes – cannabis – I've been clean for a long time.'

COUNSELLOR: 'Right, and you live on your own at the moment. You have a lot of friends and you'd like to tell at least some of them but you don't want to tell all of them.'

PATIENT: 'Right. I want to tell those I see a lot of as soon as I can. I think they'll be OK about it. I've got good friends I don't see much because they don't live close. I want to tell them to their faces, not on the phone, and I don't want someone else telling them.'

COUNSELLOR: 'You're not sure how to tell people.'

PATIENT: 'I'm not sure *what* to tell them, what words. How do you say a thing like that. Some of them don't know about the drugs.'

COUNSELLOR: 'Would it help if we went through some of that?'

PATIENT: 'I don't know. I hope so.'

COUNSELLOR: 'You're living on your own at the moment. You are in good health and you have a job that pays enough to support you. You enjoy your leisure time and life generally. You'd like your parents to know about your health but not while you remain well. You said none of those are issues at the moment.'

PATIENT: 'Right. All that's OK. At least it's not a problem yet.'

COUNSELLOR: 'You also told me that you haven't got a sexual partner at the moment and you haven't had for some time.'

PATIENT: 'I haven't had a partner since about the time I gave up drugs, except for Annie. We came off together and then, right after we split, she told me she was positive. I didn't want to put anyone else at risk. I've been a long time getting round to being tested.'

COUNSELLOR: 'And you'd like to let her know that you're positive too?'

PATIENT: 'I want to, but I don't know if I can handle it.'

COUNSELLOR: 'Perhaps we could think that through?'

PATIENT: 'Yes.'

COUNSELLOR: 'So the main things for you at the moment are telling Annie and telling your friends.'

PATIENT: 'That's it. That's enough to be going on with, don't you think?'

Once the key areas are sorted out, the next stage is to sort out some sort of timetable to see the patient again.

Organising future sessions

Sorting out future sessions is a matter of deciding how many sessions are likely to be needed, how often and when. It is important to try to decide what the sessions are going to be about, although this need not be stuck to rigidly. Often it is not possible to know for sure how long things will take, so it is probably best to try to set out a number of sessions and then review it later.

COUNSELLOR: 'Suppose we meet a couple of times more and concentrate on the issue of telling other people. If other things come up or you have other concerns, then we can look at those as well. At the end of the second session we can think about how things are going and what we should do next. Does that seem like a good plan of action?'

PATIENT: 'That's fine with me. When?'

Making necessary referrals

Quite often the counsellor will want to get other services involved with the patient for one reason or another. It is important to agree these with the patient. Many referrals for all sorts of problems – not just HIV – made by hospitals, GPs and other workers simply end with the patient not turning up. This is often because they did not really want the referral anyway or were not sure why it was made. It is important to establish that the patient knows what the referral is for and actually wants it made.

COUNSELLOR: 'You were saying that you were socially rather isolated and that you wanted to meet other people who have had to deal with similar problems.'

PATIENT: 'That's right.'

COUNSELLOR: 'I can put you in touch with a support group if you think that would help. You could have a word first with the worker who leads the group. She could tell you what happens and you could see whether you'd like that or whether it wouldn't suit you, in which case we could think again. Would you like me to put you in touch with her, or would you like to think about it for a while?'

PATIENT: 'I'd like to think about it. I don't know if I'm ready to talk to a stranger about it. Can we do it later?'

COUNSELLOR: 'Of course, no problem. The offer is always open and we can come back to it any time you want.'

PATIENT: 'I'd like to leave it just now.'

COUNSELLOR: 'The other thing is the pain you're getting in your stomach. I think it might help if we got that checked out. I can get you into the clinic tomorrow to see Dr Smith and she can have a look at you, just to make sure that there is nothing wrong. You seem to be well otherwise at the moment and the pain doesn't necessarily have anything to do with HIV, but we should check it out. In any case, there's no point in being in pain if we can sort out the problem.'

PATIENT: 'Yes, please do that.'

Ensuring that the patient's questions about HIV are answered

It may appear strange to leave this issue to last, when it may get squeezed for time. Many people carrying out HIV counselling tackle this issue first in the post-test counselling session.

It is undoubtedly best if factual issues about HIV are put into pre-test counselling. Then, when the patient comes to the post-test counselling session, they should already have a reasonable grasp of issues such as the difference between HIV and AIDS, the significance of the test result, routes of transmission, safer sex and so on. The first post-test counselling session, with an anxious patient faced with many difficult issues, is not the ideal time to start education on basic information about HIV.

If you carried out the HIV pre-test counselling yourself, which is usually best, or you can depend on the quality of someone else's work which is second best, then things are usually all right. Some patients may be pretty well informed about HIV anyway, when they come for the test. However, where you feel the pre-test counselling has been skimped or done poorly, you may well be faced with providing information from scratch. Worst of all is the situation where the patient has been so confused that they have picked up completely misleading information. In this case there is nothing for it but to start on the information-giving with a heavy heart.

Where the pre-test counselling has been of a reasonable standard, it is usually possible simply to encourage the patient to raise any questions at the end of the session. Many patients will have some questions. It is usually helpful to give them written material about HIV at the same time. Some basic information about HIV is given in Tables 4.2 and 4.3.

All this is not to downgrade the importance of providing clear accurate information to the person with HIV. But post-test counselling should not be a mini-lecture on HIV/AIDS.

Subsequent sessions

After the first post-test counselling session it is likely that the counsellor will start to talk through with the patient practical and emotional issues to do with HIV. Both need to be addressed and enquiries about how people are feeling as well as how they are dealing with practical issues get to be more germane. Patients will in any case be able to sort out better how they feel when they are not in a state of immediate shock.

Not everything can, or needs to be, dealt with in the first post-test session. By the time the first batch of post-test counselling sessions ends, the counsellor would probably hope to have covered all the issues mentioned in the next section, if only to make sure that there are no problems which the patient and counsellor need to work on.

Terminating an episode of contact

At some point most patients have adjusted to some extent and sorted out the main issues resulting from their test result. At that stage there is usually little point in continuing to see patients on a frequent basis. Instead arrangements need to be made to ensure that if the patient does develop problems they can get effective help. The counsellor should:

Table 4.2 Routes of transmission of HIV.

The following are known routes of transmission:

Blood and blood products If infected blood from one person gets into the body of another person the recipient my contract HIV infection. Many cases of infection have occurred worldwide in the past through whole blood transfusion (now screened in most countries) and through Factor VIII concentrate used in the treatment of haemophilia (now heat-treated to inactivate the virus).

Injecting drug users can pass on HIV through blood contaminating a syringe that is shared with others. They may inject themselves, pull blood back into the syringe and then re-inject it, leading to particularly heavy contamination of the syringe. There is no evidence that infection can occur through blood contamination of intact skin but in very rare cases infected blood coming into contact with extensively damaged skin appears to have caused infection.

Tissue and organ transplants Similar considerations apply as for blood.

Semen Relatively large amounts of virus can be present in the semen of infected men. This can enter the sexual partner via the vagina, cervix and rectal mucosa, all areas that have cells related to T-cells present. Damage to these areas is thought to aid transmission but not to be necessary for infection to occur.

Vaginal and cervical secretions Can contain relatively large amounts of virus. In female to male infection the virus probably passes across the glans rather than the shaft which is skin-covered. Lesions to the penis are not necessary for transmission to occur.

Breast milk Can contain considerable amounts of virus. Breast milk is now considered to provide a substantial additional risk of infection to the child and so breast-feeding by an infected mother should be avoided *where safe alternatives are available*.

Other materno-foetal Transmission *in utero* and at birth occurs. The relative importance of the two is still not clear.

The following are *not* thought to be routes of transmission:

Saliva, tears, urine, faeces, sweat The levels of virus found in these body fluids are extremely low and, in the case of saliva, there is some evidence that enzymes in saliva may inactivate the virus.

Overall Transmission of the virus is dependent, in practice, on two things. The first is the amount of virus present in a body fluid or tissue – the higher the concentration, the greater the risk. The second is the fact that the virus has to get *into* the body to cause infection. There is no evidence that it is able to cross intact skin, therefore the virus must come into contact either with non-skin surfaces like the vaginal and rectal linings, or be carried through the skin, as with blood transfusions.

Millions of people are infected worldwide. It is impossible to rule out very rare cases of unusual transmissions but there have been so many cases that we can be confident about how the virus can and cannot be transmitted.

- Make sure that whoever is following up with routine medical care knows of the counsellor's involvement and enquires about the patient's mental wellbeing as well as their physical health, and refers back if necessary.
- Make sure that the patient knows they are welcome to come back at any time, that they know how to get in touch, and that they know they will be seen quickly if they do have a problem.

Perhaps one of the most pleasing aspects of this counselling is the extent to which patients you have not seen for some time, occasionally years, suddenly get in touch when they have a problem.

Of course, some patients need continuing counselling over an extended period for issues other than HIV. The diagnosis often makes people review their lives and look at issues they

Table 4.3   Infection control advice.

It is clear that individuals living with someone with HIV are not at any risk of contracting the infection through normal household contact. A person with HIV infection should:

Not donate organs, blood or body fluids or carry an organ donor card.

Not have any surgical or other invasive medical or cosmetic procedure carried out except under proper sterile conditions. This includes ear-piercing or skin-piercing, tattooing, skin-cutting, ritual scarification, ritual circumcision or any other procedure unless he knows that the practitioner is taking appropriate infection-control measures. In the case of acupuncture, for instance, the patient should seek assurances that either disposable needles are used or appropriate sterilisation procedures are in place. Otherwise there may be a risk of transmission of HIV to other patients/clients of the practitioner or of the acquisition of other infections by the individual with HIV.

Not share wet-shave razors or toothbrushes with others.

Not share syringes or needles with anyone else.

Not worry about transmission through casual contact, shaking hands, kissing, normal casual contact.

Not worry about others catching HIV from the WC, bath, toilet, towels, cups or crockery or other domestic items.

Lead a normal life.

If he cuts himself he should stop the bleeding and cover the cut with a clean dressing. He should mop up the blood using tissues, toilet paper, newspaper, leaves or any other absorbent material to hand and flush it down the lavatory or bury it or burn it or otherwise dispose of it safely. Surfaces can be washed down with a 10% bleach solution for extra safety. If anyone else mops up the blood they should wear household rubber gloves. Contaminated clothing can be washed in the normal way.

---

have avoided up until that point. There is no reason why help should not be provided, either by the counsellor who first sees them, or, if it is outside their time availability, remit or expertise, by someone else to whom the counsellor refers the patient.

At the end of post-test counselling, it is reasonable to expect that patients will:

- Be well-informed about HIV
- Be clear what steps they want to take in their lives in view of their infection
- Have started to act on any plans they have made and be making good progress
- Have notified any past partners they need to notify or be in the process of doing so
- Feel that they are coming to terms with the fact that they are infected with HIV
- Be reasonably free from distress.
- Be coping with their everyday lives.
- Know where and how to come back if they have problems.

It is reasonable to expect that they will feel it is right to terminate immediate contact at this point – in other words it is a joint decision. It would not be reasonable to assume that they will be happy about having HIV infection.

Counselling the seronegative patient

For most health workers involved in counselling and testing services, or involved in counselling those at risk, seronegatives outnumber seropositives by a large margin. In the UK today I would guess that fewer than 2% of HIV tests are positive, even excluding those done on blood donations. Figures are much higher in some London clinics and in clinics in a few other areas, but this is not typical of the country as a whole. Of those testing negative, many will have little or no risk of HIV infection, but there will be a fair proportion who have been at risk and continue to put themselves at risk.

It is reasonable to suppose that time spent attending to seronegatives who are at risk is extremely valuable. Avoiding someone becoming infected in the first place is the best possible outcome. But seronegatives often get only the most cursory of attention at many clinics and hospitals.

The situation is even broader than that. Many health professionals, people involved in personal social services and workers with voluntary organisations meet a wide range of clients, patients and users. They have the opportunity to enquire routinely about whether individuals are putting themselves at risk and then to offer some simple advice – and further counselling if this seems appropriate. Many workers I have spoken to about this are reluctant to start asking patients coming for something else about their risks of HIV and other sexually transmitted diseases, because such questions might be 'intrusive'. It is hard to think of anything which would be more intrusive to a patient than catching HIV.

It is important to try to identify those at risk of HIV and to try to work with them to reduce their risks of infection, whether those risks are sexual or injecting. Much of the work can be done at pre-test counselling, but this needs to be followed up at post-test counselling.

One of the worrying issues about HIV seronegatives is that there is no evidence that they reduce their risks of catching HIV after a negative test. There is plenty of evidence that seronegatives (and seropositives) carry on with high levels of sexual risk after HIV testing (Dawson *et al.* 1991; Higgins *et al.* 1991; Landis, Earp & Koch 1992; Zenilman *et al.* 1992). Indeed there is some evidence that they may actually increase their risk of sexually transmitted diseases after a negative HIV test (Otten *et al.* 1993).

It is not difficult to see why this might be so. An individual becomes concerned about HIV, they change their behaviour to reduce their risk of infection and to reduce their risk of infecting others if they are already infected. They go for an HIV test which turns out to be negative. So they never really had any reason to worry, did they? They have 'got away with it' so far, so why shouldn't they continue to do so. This sort of view of the situation, which is very natural, can easily be inadvertently reinforced by a perfunctory counselling session by an apparently disinterested counsellor. It is not necessarily what the counsellor says. If one only gets five or ten minutes after the test there really can't be that much to worry about, can there? After all, the clinic does not seem very bothered.

Specific issues for HIV individuals

This section deals with specific issues which come up in HIV counselling, sometimes at post-test counselling but also at other times.

The primary relationship

Many people are in what they would regard as a primary relationship. For some people it is the most important thing in their life. It is usually, but need not be, a sexual relationship. Sometimes people are in more than one primary relationship. Many hospital staff will be familiar with the situation where a patient is admitted and the spouse and lover turn up at the same time to see them on the ward.

For many individuals with HIV infection the primary relationship is their main concern. The partner may or may not know that the individual has come for a test, or even was at risk of HIV infection in the first place. Obviously things are easier when the two of them have discussed matters in advance, but the world is not always constructed for the counsellor's convenience. Particularly difficult is the situation where the patient has been having an affair, or worse has broken an understanding that the two of them have had about sex outside the relationship. If the patient has also put their partner at risk without the partner knowing, things are doubly difficult.

Simon and Bill had lived together for seven years. The frequency of sex between them had declined and they now had sex only occasionally. Both had occasional casual partners outside the relationship. They had agreed that when they had sex together they would not practise safer sex, but also that neither of them would have penetrative sex outside the relationship. This agreement was probably unrealistic but Bill had managed to stick to it; Simon had not. He had not felt able to renegotiate the arrangement with Bill and, unfortunately, contracted HIV infection. He had now not only broken their agreement but had put Bill at risk.

I have seen a number of cases like this over the years and they are extremely difficult to deal with, not least because the guilt felt by the patient makes it very difficult for them to adopt any sensible line of action.

There are other potential strains on a relationship. Where one member of a relationship becomes ill the whole balance of the relationship can change.

Alex and Elizabeth had been together for ten years. She relied on him to pay all the bills, arrange dealings with tradesmen and to take most of the decisions about their lives. When he developed HIV disease he was unable to work. For the first time she had to go out to work and to deal with almost all the day-to-day decisions. They had exchanged roles, and both of them found this very difficult to adjust to.

In dealing with any relationship the first thing for the counsellor to do is to find out about it in detail.

COUNSELLOR: 'How long have you known Tom?'
PATIENT: 'I've known him since we were at college together but we really only got together about two years ago when I came to London, after I divorced my husband.'
COUNSELLOR: 'Do you live together?'
PATIENT: 'No, I have my own place. I have my son, Elliott, with me from my previous marriage and I need to live close to his school. Tom lives close to work on the other side of town. Usually he stays over the weekend with me or I go over to his place.'
COUNSELLOR: 'Do you take your son with you when you go to his place?'
PATIENT: 'No, he usually goes to stay with his father at the weekends, or sometimes he stays with my mother.'

COUNSELLOR: 'Does he get on with Tom?'

PATIENT: 'He's pretty good with him, but we've been cautious about the situation. It's difficult for Elliott, with his father and me breaking up like that; he's only five and we've been cautious about him feeling that mummy has found a replacement for daddy.'

COUNSELLOR: 'How is the relationship between Tom and you?'

PATIENT: 'It's very good basically. But then we don't live together.'

COUNSELLOR: 'Is that just because of the practical issues?'

PATIENT: 'Not just that. After I split up with my husband I had an affair with a man which didn't work out. I thought he was the love of my life but all he gave me was a lot of heartache and HIV. I guess I'm cautious about taking a risk.'

It is important to find out what the partner is like and what the couple are like together.

COUNSELLOR: 'Tell me about Tom, what is he like?'

PATIENT: 'He's very different from me. He's very calm, he has a very well-ordered life. His flat is neat and tidy whereas my house is a wreck.'

COUNSELLOR: 'Do you have rows?'

PATIENT: 'Not really. One of the advantages of living apart is that you don't get the chance to let things build up into a row.'

COUNSELLOR: 'Have you ever had a row?'

PATIENT: 'We once went to a party at his work and I thought he was paying too much attention to some girl there and we had a row in the car.'

COUNSELLOR: 'What did he say?'

PATIENT: 'He said I was too sensitive, that she was just someone he worked with. I am a bit jealous. I can't stand the thought of him going off with someone else.'

COUNSELLOR: 'So this is a very important relationship to you?'

PATIENT: 'At first he was just someone I felt safe with. But I now love him.'

COUNSELLOR: 'And how are things when you are together?'

PATIENT: 'Very good. He's very kind and understanding. I think I'm good for him. I stop him working all the time; he's not very sociable and I get him out.'

It is important when looking at a relationship not just to look at the bad points but also to look for its strengths. In most relationships there tend to be good as well as bad aspects. It is as important to understand the strengths of a relationship as it is the weaknesses, because strengths are what can be built upon.

In looking at relationships it is important not to import too many prejudices about what makes a good and a bad relationship. There is a common cultural ideal in the UK of a relationship being one where the partners have an equal relationship in which they are sexually faithful, share their thoughts and feelings, have few rows, are never violent to each other and spend a lot of time doing things jointly. Relationships are supposed not to be about money or security, but about love and affection.

Counsellors, like anyone else, bring their own aspirations, experiences and feelings about relationships to bear on their view of what makes a good or a bad relationship. They also bring their own appreciation of published research. Some counsellors feel that a relationship is one where couples do more or less everything together; others feel that each partner needs to have 'a life of their own'. Some counsellors feel that heterosexual couples 'staying together for the children' is the right approach; others feel that it is better for a couple in severe conflict to split up, as this is less strain for the children. It is important to realise that these stereotypes of good and bad relationships do not necessarily bear on how an individual experiences their own relationship. People have different needs and aspirations and it is important to work with these. Different cultures and sub-cultures within the UK and across the world have different ideas about what is appropriate and have different values.

For instance, the belief that a relationship where there is significant physical violence must be a bad one is based on heterosexual couples where the weight, size and aggressiveness of the two parties is uneven. In a few gay couples I have seen, the partners have occasionally resorted to fighting it out when they could not solve matters in other ways. This does not mean that fighting is the right way to resolve issues, and the counsellor should look for other ways in which they might resolve problems, but it does not necessarily mean either that a relationship is doomed. It is not uncommon for gay couples to have a very good relationship and yet have little sexual activity with each other. Sometimes sex has stopped altogether. They may have outside partners. Yet the relationship can be a very close and positive one. Some heterosexual couples live apart, even in different countries, and see each other rather infrequently, but still have strong, positive relationships.

The most important issue is not how the counsellor sees a relationship but how the members of the couple see the relationship. There are various ways of looking at a relationship; one way that can be helpful is in terms of the costs and rewards of the relationship (Jacobson & Margolin 1979; Stuart 1980). How satisfied someone is with a relationship is dependent on the balance between what they put into the relationship and what they feel they get out of it. Of course this does not work in the short term. On any one day all the costs may run one way and all the rewards another. However, over days and weeks the balance works out.

A relationship which brings few costs and lots of rewards to a couple is likely to be one which is satisfying. Rewards are likely to be emotional, sexual, the opening of possibilities (like having someone to go to the cinema with) and material rewards like being able to afford a house or being better off with two incomes. Security is also a reward – the feeling that if one partner falls on hard times the other will support them. Just having company around, someone to talk to who is supportive, is a potential reward. Costs are likely to be emotional, sexual, the restriction of opportunities (not being able to do what one wants because of the other person) and material costs (such as having to support a partner financially).

However, satisfaction with a relationship is not necessarily what keeps it together. Studies on marriage, for instance, do not always find a strong relationship between the happiness of partners with a marriage and whether they stay together. That seems to be more a matter of the feelings of the partners about whether they might do better elsewhere.

A man may stay in an unhappy marriage if he feels that the alternative is living alone in a bedsit, or not being able to see his children regularly. He is likely to stay in the relationship if he feels he is unlikely to be able to form a happier one elsewhere. It is the same for women. The greater ease with which younger people can change relationships is probably at least part of the reason why they tend to have less stable relationships. It is also probably a factor in the rising post-war divorce rate as increasing affluence makes it easier for couples to afford the heavy financial burden of divorce and individuals find it easier to survive materially without a partner.

Many people stay in unhappy relationships because the short-term unhappiness of splitting up, with the attendant loneliness and financial problems, outweighs for them the possibility of having a happier life in the long-term. Where a relationship between a couple is very unhappy the counsellor can sometimes give the patient the freedom to break out of it by supporting them over the unhappy period of the actual break-up. This gives them the freedom to make a move to separate.

Understanding what keeps a relationship together and makes it prosper, or not, is an important step for the counsellor to take before seeking to help. For the counsellor looking at a relationship the key issues are what the patient gets out of the relationship, what they don't get out of it, and what they feel they should get out of it.

COUNSELLOR: 'What do you get out of the relationship with Tom; what does it give you?'
PATIENT: 'It gives me someone to talk to, someone I can rely on if things go wrong. It gives me someone to go out with who is interesting and amusing to be with. It stops me being lonely. Tom has been very generous. It is difficult to go out to work because of my young son. I'm freelance and I rely on being able to work evenings and weekends to make a decent living, and I haven't been able to do that. He's helped me out financially sometimes.'
COUNSELLOR: 'And what don't you like about the relationship?'
PATIENT: 'Don't get me wrong, I love him dearly, but sometimes he's a bit too staid for me. I have to drag him out to things. And he doesn't really fit in with my friends. A lot of them are artists, designers, that type. He just has nothing to say to them and really I think they bore him, and so I don't see them as often as I would like.'

It is interesting that finding out a partner is HIV positive rarely causes a negative partner to walk out on them. But it is not uncommon for the HIV positive partner to leave the negative one. The reason is, I believe, simple. Many people persist with a relationship which is troubled or dead because in the short term it is not worth the upset of ending it. When their horizons for the future are suddenly cut back by the prospect of premature illness or death, life suddenly seems too short to persist with something that is not giving them what they want.

Implementing safer sex

For the individual who finds that they are infected with HIV, the issue of safer sex is important. It does not simply protect the partner, it also protects the individual with HIV from other sexually transmitted infections and, perhaps, from infection with other strains of HIV (although this is a matter of uncertainty).

An outline of current safer sex guidelines is given in Table 4.4. It is important to discuss safer sex with every patient. In many cases it will only be necessary to check that the patient understands the necessary information. Many gay men I see have already implemented safer sex. They were infected in the past before the importance of safer sex was well understood.

Table 4.4   Current safer sex advice.

Vaginal intercourse HIV is transmitted from male to female and female to male in vaginal sex. The only entirely safe approach is to avoid such sex entirely. However, a condom provides protection providing it is used properly and does not break. Condoms should be used with water based lubricants; oil based lubricants will weaken condoms and therefore lead to breakages. The effectiveness of the female condom in this context remains to be established. The use of spermicidal agents such as nonoxynol-9 for additional antiviral protection is not supported by the available evidence. Women should be advised to use a second method of contraception, such as the pill or diaphragm, in addition to the condom in order to provide better protection against pregnancy.

Anal intercourse The receptive partner is at high risk in anal sex. However, the risks to the insertive partner appear to be much lower, although some still exist. The use of condoms provides protection to both partners providing there is no breakage. Breakages are probably more common in anal than in vaginal intercourse, but if condoms are used with care and with liberal amounts of water based lubricant, such breakages can be kept to a minimum. As with vaginal sex, the only completely safe way is to avoid anal sex altogether.

Oral sex This remains an area of debate. The difficulty of finding individuals who have only ever had oral sex makes it difficult to assess the potential risk. In fellatio it is likely to be the receptive partner who is at risk and this risk is markedly reduced if intra-oral ejaculation is avoided. Any risks could be further reduced through the use of a condom. Many prostitutes use a condom for this purpose, but many other people find condoms unaesthetic. A handful of reports on possible transmission in cunnilingus are difficult to evaluate, hence the value of dental dams etc. is uncertain.

Sharing sex toys For instance, dildos, vibrators. High risk and to be avoided.

Oral-anal contact (rimming) To be avoided because of risk of transmission of pathogens from the gut. These may be a particular risk to immunocompromised individuals, such as those with HIV infection.

Inserting hand into rectum (fisting) Can cause damage to anorectal area and, if followed up with anal sex, can potentially increase risks to both partners.

Water sports (urinating on to partner's body) Not a risk in itself.

Mutual masturbation Safe. Can be engaged in with as many people as desired, as often as desired.

Body rubbing (frottage) Safe if kept to rubbing genitalia against skin.

Other activities The ingenuity of the human mind knows no bounds when it comes to sex. However the risk of any behaviour can usually be assessed by analogy to one of the above items. Any activity involving contact between cervical or vaginal secretions, blood or semen and areas not covered in intact skin are probably best avoided.

Other infections The above advice is for protection against HIV. It is worth remembering that other sexually transmitted infections can be transmitted in other ways and that these may act as co-factors for HIV disease progression, as well as having adverse effects in their own right. While mutual masturbation and body rubbing are likely to be safe for more or less everything, other sexual behaviours may carry different risks.

In that case there is little need to spend hours going over information the patient already knows.

Many gay men, however, do not consistently apply safer sex, taking the occasional, or more than occasional, risk. Very few heterosexuals apply safer sex consistently.

Because of the importance of this area, helping people to change their sexual behaviour is covered in Chapter 15.

Telling sexual partners

Telling current sexual partners

Virtually every patient wants to tell their current sexual partner, and there are good reasons why they should. There is usually little debate on the subject. The partner may not be infected and may be able to take steps to ensure that they do not become infected. In the case of heterosexual couples, if the partner is female she may need to take steps to avoid pregnancy. If the partner is having relationships outside the couple they may have to take steps to protect or inform those other partners. The partner needs to take steps to protect his own health if he is infected.

Occasionally one comes across a patient who does not wish to tell his (or her) partner. It is not uncommon to find the partner of a person with AIDS saying that he does not want to tell his partner that he too is infected because it would only add to his partner's worries. This is an understandable reaction; whether it is the right reaction will depend entirely on the couple. However, it does no-one any harm.

Very occasionally one comes across the individual who does not wish to tell his or her sexual partner even though the partner has been at risk. Often this is out of a sense of guilt and overwhelming shame. The strength and irrationality of the reaction is nicely illustrated by a case in which a woman was diagnosed as having HIV disease and her husband (who had no idea he was infected) was subsequently found to be seropositive. He wouldn't tell his wife about his status even though he was the only man she had ever had sex with and she knew full well that she must have contracted it from him.

There is one other reason why patients are sometimes unwilling to tell partners; the fear of physical violence. This is an issue rarely referred to in published papers (Green & Kentish 1995). Women in particular sometimes fear that they will be physically attacked or even killed if they tell their partner of their status. Their fears are not always unfounded.

It can be a difficult situation if an individual has been putting a sexual partner at risk and does not wish to tell them. The first step is to try to find out why the patient is unwilling to tell their partner.

> Clive had been having unprotected sex with his long-term partner, Ben. Both of them knew they were negative, at least when they started out on their relationship. However Clive had also been having unprotected sex with various casual partners he met in gay bars, usually when he had been drinking or taking drugs, and he had been embarrassed about admitting this to his partner because he felt (rightly) that Ben would disapprove of his taking the risk. He had not been able to suggest to Ben that they should use a condom. When he found out that he was positive he became extremely anxious and tearful and swore point-blank that he would not tell Ben.

This case illustrates the two most common elements in those who do not wish to tell: embarrassment at having deceived the other person and a fear of the reaction of the other person. Quite often telling the other person about one's status means unfolding a whole tale of unfaithfulness, of past sexual adventures, of areas of sexual behaviour of which the partner has been blissfully ignorant. One of my patients found himself explaining that the past girlfriends he had told his wife about were, in fact, mostly men.

After discussion, most patients do decide to tell their partners. To refuse to do so is something which is understandable in the heat of the moment, but after a 'cooling off' period wiser counsels usually prevail. The most important role for the counsellor at this stage is to go through the reasons why the patient does not want to tell their partner and try to work round to getting the patient to voice the reasons why it might be a good idea. Giving the patient a lecture on moral responsibility or public health issues usually results in the patient not coming back.

If the main reason for not telling is their fear of the reaction of that partner, it can be helpful for the counsellor to offer to be with the patient when they tell their partner, or even, with the patient's agreement, to tell the partner for them. While this may not be ideal, sometimes it is the only way. It can also be important where the patient has a fear of violence. In this case it may also be important to try to plan to get the patient away somewhere safe, just in case their fears turn out to be justified.

But if a counsellor does have a patient who just will not tell his partner, what should the counsellor do then? Does the counsellor have a duty to tell the wife or lover of an individual that that person is infected with HIV? Suppose the partner is pregnant, or the patient is unwilling to adopt safer sex? There are legal issues here (see Chapter 17 for the UK situation). However there is also an ethical dilemma for the counsellor concerning their duty to the patient and their duty to the partner and a wider society.

Like all ethical dilemmas this one is difficult to resolve. Different people hold different views about where the balance of duty and responsibility lie. However it is easy to miss a central issue. The reason why the UK sexually transmitted disease system puts such a high premium on the right of the individual to confidentiality is not a moral one, but a practical one. By offering confidentiality one maximises the probability that a patient will seek, and comply with, treatment. If patients feel that we will tell their current, or past, sexual partners about their HIV status without their consent, they are less likely to come forward for HIV testing in the first place and are less likely to be truthful with us about who they have been having sex with. If they come forward, we can seek to persuade them to tell their partners. If they do not come forward in the first place, there is nothing we can do.

Whatever the position of the counsellor on the issue, it is important to make clear to the patient at the outset, before they get into the issues, what the limits of confidentiality are for the counsellor. That gives the patient the choice and there can be no misunderstandings further down the line.

Telling past sexual partners

Telling past partners is less straightforward than telling current partners. It can be difficult to know how far back to go and which partners have, in fact, been put at risk. Patients are seldom able to pinpoint exactly when they were infected. Obviously over-zealous partner notification is not only of no value but can be harmful. No-one wants to be suddenly revisited by a past partner from ten or fifteen years before if they have not been at any real risk.

It is also worth considering the purpose of partner notification. The objective of partner notification is to inform individuals that they have been at risk of infection with a sexually transmitted disease, in this case HIV. It follows that there is little point in putting huge efforts into partner notification programmes to reach individuals who already knew that they were at risk. This is important because resources are usually finite. I can think of several parts of the world where extensive resources are devoted to partner notification programmes, but once an individual is found to be positive there are hardly any resources available to help them. Such an approach defies common sense.

It is necessary to get the active co-operation of the patient to carry out self-notification (i.e. the patient themselves telling the partner) or contact-tracing (the health worker telling the partner on behalf of the patient). If patients do not want to inform their partners or tell the counsellor who they were, they have to lie or give false details.

There are other problems also. Early on in the HIV epidemic my colleague Alana McCreaner carried out some work on sexual links between gay men in a London cohort who were HIV positive. This work showed that there were many cross-links, so if there was rigorous partner notification the same individual might be notified many times as a result of sexual activity with different partners. All the individuals in the sample knew that they had been at risk. Amongst London gay men today virtually all men know whether they have been at risk and therefore whether they might be seropositive, even if they do not know their status. This does not mean that every gay man will know, as in the cases above where individuals had agreed with partners only to have safer sex with outsiders, but to have unrestricted sex within the relationship.

On the other hand UK heterosexuals are currently unlikely to feel that they have been at risk of HIV.

COUNSELLOR: 'Do you think he knows that he has been at risk of HIV?'
PATIENT: 'I don't think it would ever enter his head. He thinks AIDS is for homosexuals.'
COUNSELLOR: 'There's been a lot of coverage on the TV and in the papers.'
PATIENT: 'Not on the sports pages there hasn't.'

It follows that the first step is to try to work out with the patient who they have had sex with over a reasonable period of time (depending on the incidence of the epidemic in areas in which they have had sex) and to try to work out which partners would definitely have known that they were at risk. It is best to be conservative in the assumptions made.

COUNSELLOR: 'Do you think she knew she had been at risk?'
PATIENT: 'She should have done. She got about a bit. I was one of many.'
COUNSELLOR: 'Do you think she thought you had HIV?'
PATIENT: 'No, obviously not.'
COUNSELLOR: 'What are the chances she thought any of them had HIV?'
PATIENT: 'All right, so she probably thought she was safe. Didn't we all?'

On the other hand there is not much point in chasing every sexual partner anyone has ever had:

PATIENT: 'I met him in a club in Amsterdam. We spent a delirious weekend.'
COUNSELLOR: 'You had unsafe sex?'
PATIENT: 'We had every kind of sex: anal, oral, you name it, we did it. It was great.'
COUNSELLOR: 'Did you discuss safer sex?'
PATIENT: 'No, but he had loads of condoms. We just left them out after the first night.'

If the gay man referred to above had condoms, it is a reasonable bet that he was aware of the risks of unsafe sex. What are the possibilities of tracing across Holland a gay man with whom the patient had a weekend fling three years ago, and with whom the patient has lost touch, just to tell him he may have been at risk of HIV?

It is not just gay men who have multiple partners with whom they are no longer in touch.

COUNSELLOR: 'How many sexual partners have you had?'
PATIENT: 'Since when?'
COUNSELLOR: 'Well, let's start with the last three years.'
PATIENT: 'Twenty, maybe thirty.'
COUNSELLOR: 'Do you remember who they were?'
PATIENT: 'You must be joking.'

Having established partners who can be located and who could not reasonably have realised that they are at risk, the question arises of how to follow those up. Self-notification has advantages. The call on scarce health resources is reduced and the patient knows the individual concerned and therefore may have a better idea of how to approach them. On the other hand it is not easy to tell ex-partners of one's positive HIV status and the patient may, understandably, feel that their confidentiality is compromised. Under those circumstances the patient and the counsellor may decide that contact tracing is the most appropriate approach. This involves the counsellor, or someone else from the clinic, seeking to contact the individual who has had sex with the patient, and informing them that they may have been in contact with someone with HIV infection. The contact is likely to need considerable support themselves under these circumstances and matters have to be handled tactfully.

Telling future sexual partners

Whether a patient should tell future sexual partners that they have HIV infection depends on the sexual activity they intend to have. If the patient intends to engage only in mutual masturbation and body-rubbing, it is difficult to see why they should tell partners about their status unless they want to. However patients do, from time to time, go further than they would like sexually. If a patient intends not to tell future sexual partners, he has to be aware that he must remain entirely in control of what he is doing sexually. If he cannot be sure of remaining in control, he has no option but to discuss the issue with future sexual partners, or to stay celibate. Drink and drugs and not having decided how far to go are the great enemies of staying in control. Most people can decide what they will and will not do and stick to that if the stakes are high enough.

For some people, both gay men and heterosexuals, not telling future partners is not really an option at all. As mentioned earlier, amongst heterosexuals no-risk safer sexual activities tend to be a prelude to penetrative sex, rather than an alternative to it. The young ser-opositive heterosexual haemophiliac boy just starting to take girls out is not going to tell the girls that he is infected if he is only going to take them out or to engage in petting. Eventually, if he finds a girl he wants to form a long-term relationship with, he is going to have to tell her. When he does, he is very likely to end up with a rejection. He may minimise this risk by forming as strong a relationship with her as possible before telling her, but there is no way he can avoid a strong probability of rejection. Also, by telling her he is exposing a personal and socially stigmatising fact about himself. He must be sure, whatever her reaction, that she will not tell others without his agreement. Guiding him through this sort of problem is not likely to be easy.

For the gay man things are likely to be a bit easier, simply because HIV is so common among homosexuals. But telling a partner may be far from smooth sailing, however, particularly if the patient is seeking to form a longer-term partnership.

How to tell partners

Telling sexual partners that one is infected with HIV is stressful. It needs careful attention from both counsellor and patient. Sometimes it is straightforward, and the patient is confident that he can handle the telling. For other patients it is a difficult issue and needs careful thought. In helping patients to be successful in telling others there are several issues worth attention.

- *Helping the patient to pick the right time and occasion.*
When telling a partner it is helpful to choose a time when the partner is unlikely to be stressed to start with, and when there is time to discuss the issue without interruption from other commitments, visitors or telephone calls. Sometimes this is not possible, but it helps a lot if it is.

- *Practising telling.*
It is extremely valuable for the patient and the counsellor to practice together how to tell the other person and what to say. This can be done in the form of role-plays.

  - The counsellor needs to get a clear picture of what the partner is like and how he usually reacts to difficult news. The patient should be able to provide this information.
  - The counsellor can then take on the role of the partner and the patient can practise telling him. In this way the patient can gain confidence in telling and can practise different ways of telling to see which is the best; and the counsellor can help with suggestions as to how the patient can handle the situation better.
  - It also helps if the counsellor and the patient occasionally exchange roles so that the patient can feel what various approaches are like for the person being told. Sometimes it helps to start out this way if you have an unconfident patient. The counsellor can act the role of the patient and work through various possibilities until the best of the options is identified, and then the patient can take over the role.

Where a patient intends to tell a partner it is always wise to ensure that he has fully understood the facts about HIV, since the conversation may well turn to issues of fact at some point.

- *Being available for the partner.*
The counsellor should always make it clear to the seropositive person that he would be only too happy to see the partner or talk to them on the telephone, after they have been told. The partner will often have points that he wants to talk through and he has a right to do so with the counsellor. In this sort of situation the discussion with the partner sometimes turns to issues surrounding the patient. The relationships between counsellor and patient and between partner and counsellor are both confidential ones. It is important to establish with

the patient what aspects of his discussions with the counsellor he is or is not willing to have discussed with the partner.

- *Seeing the couple together.*

When the patient has told his partner it is often helpful for the counsellor to see them together as a couple if they wish. It can be helpful to discuss issues jointly, particularly where there are relationship stresses or where putting safer sex into practice is an issue, but it must be made clear that each person has the right to see the counsellor individually as well. Sometimes it is more useful to find another counsellor for the partner; it depends on the circumstances.

- *Telling the partner for the patient.*

Occasionally patients want the counsellor to tell their partner for them. Some counsellors have strong views about this, feeling that the patient is handing over responsibility. I have never seen it that way. Few things could be so potentially difficult as to tell one's partner that one is infected with HIV, so if the patient really wants me to tell them, I am, ultimately, prepared to do it.

Social support

There is good evidence that the better the social support someone has, the less prone to anxiety and depression they are in the face of HIV infection. People who are more anxious and depressed may, in turn, be less able to harness such social support as is available, but it seems likely that helping people increase and maintain their social support will result in real benefits for their wellbeing and quality of life.

It is very difficult to separate the emotional aspects of social support from the practical ones. The people who provide sympathy, encouragement and advice when things are difficult are likely to be the same people who feed the cat, or the person with HIV, when they are ill.

People differ in the extent to which they want or require social support and this may well change over the course of their HIV disease, particularly as they develop symptoms. Sources of social support differ between people. For the gay man who knows many other people affected by HIV it is often natural to turn to others within the gay community. For the heterosexual in a rural area of Africa it is likely to be the family which is the primary source of social support. However these are only general considerations; people differ according to their particular personal circumstances and they differ in the way that they like to get their social support. Some people are gregarious and get their social support from many different people, while others rely on a few key friends.

In order to get social support in relation to HIV it is necessary for others to know that one has the infection. Where people are unwilling to tell others because of fears of rejection or of adverse reactions, they are less able to recruit social support. People with HIV infection often find that the reactions of others are far more positive and supportive than they expect. However there are sufficient examples of people finding themselves ostracised, dismissed from work or evicted from their homes, to suggest that their fears are not always ill-founded. One patient of mine told over a hundred other people and said every one was sympathetic. However this is probably unusual.

For the newly diagnosed HIV seropositive it is important to consider the likely reactions of those they wish to tell. It is also important for them to consider who else those others may tell. Even if a friend is sympathetic they may tell others who are less so.

Peter was part of a group of people working as a team. He was obliged to take time off work as a result of HIV-related symptoms. He felt that he owed an explanation to those he worked with since his absences caused them to have to work harder. He told three people from his team that he was HIV positive. All of them were extremely supportive. He had an admission into hospital and one of them confided in their immediate manager. He too was supportive but told the personnel department who informed a higher manager who was less supportive. Peter was dismissed from work on a pretext.

Having a serious problem, of whatever sort, leads many people to feel they want to tell someone else about it. It is all too easy to stagger out of a result-giving session and tell the first possibly sympathetic individual. It is for this reason that it is important for the person seeking HIV testing to consider at pre-test counselling who they will want to tell if they turn out to be positive. It is often a matter of balance; people can be told over a period of time and it is important to get the order of this right. Once someone has been told, they can never be un-told.

COUNSELLOR: 'What about telling other people? Are there people you want to tell?'
PATIENT: 'Yes. I've thought about this a lot. I need to tell my friends, or at least some of them. I've always been very up front with my friends. I wouldn't want to think that there was a secret about me that they didn't know. I think it would split me off from them.'
COUNSELLOR: 'Who do you think you would like to tell about your status?'
PATIENT: 'I have several friends with HIV or AIDS and I would like them to know. I think they would be very supportive. I'm still pretty close to David; he was my partner for a while in the early 1980s and we are still good friends. I know that he is negative but we have discussed the risks many times over the years.'
COUNSELLOR: 'Is there any possibility you might have infected him?'
PATIENT: 'No, that was all over long ago. I just want to tell him as a friend.'
COUNSELLOR: 'What about other people?'
PATIENT: 'I have two or three other close friends I want to tell.'
COUNSELLOR: 'How do you think they will react?'
PATIENT: 'I think they'll be very sympathetic.'
COUNSELLOR: 'And discreet? Can you be confident that these people will keep the news to themselves?'
PATIENT: 'I think so. If I ask them to keep it to themselves, they will. That's important, because I want to tell people myself, keep things under control.'
COUNSELLOR: 'Are you going to tell all these people immediately, or are you going to tell some first and others later?'
PATIENT: 'To start off with I'm going to tell David. He came with me here today. He's in the waiting room. Then I'm going to tell other people when I see

them. One or two I'll ring up, the others I'll wait until the moment seems
right.'

COUNSELLOR: 'And you feel comfortable with that?'

PATIENT: 'Yes.'

Friends are often more straightforward than family. You can pick your friends but your
family are an 'act of God'. People differ enormously in whether and when they want to tell
their family about their status, and matters are often complicated by family dynamics.

When Jose knew that he was seropositive he wanted to tell one of his sisters, to whom he
was particularly close. She knew of his past drug-use and she knew that he had not been
well recently. However he did not want his other sister to know because he perceived
her as unsympathetic and 'straight-laced'. The two sisters were close and he was worried
whether his sympathetic sister might pass on the information. He also wanted his mother
to know; she had always supported him when he had been in difficulties. However she
discussed everything with his stepfather who had rigid views and might simply, he
feared, cut him off from the family. If both his sisters knew of his infection, either of
them might tell his mother in any case and if she was to know, then he would rather tell
her himself.

This sort of complicated situation is not uncommon. There is no alternative but for the
counsellor to work through a series of scenarios about the best order in which to tell people
and what to say. One family member can sometimes be used to help inform another family
member.

Elaine had contracted HIV during an affair while working in the Far East. She kept her
status from her family for some years. However when she became ill she wanted her family
to know what was wrong with her. She was not sure what their reaction would be, particularly her mother who was a very religious woman with strong moral views. Eventually
she confided in her sister and they agreed that the sister would discuss the issue with the
mother. The mother was concerned, but not at all censorious as Elaine had expected.

It is unusual for families to reject a person because they have HIV infection. On the other
hand it does happen, and where it does the result can be great emotional distress for the
person with HIV, even if they were not particularly close to their family. Rejection is not
usually because of HIV itself. It tends to come through rejection of behaviour which the
family are unable to come to terms with: the person with HIV being gay, or having used
drugs, or being perceived as 'promiscuous'. The moment when the family discover someone
is HIV infected is sometimes the moment when they discover that their son is gay or their
daughter injects drugs.

When to tell the family is important. One of my patients wanted his mother to know about
his status before anyone else. Indeed for some years only his mother and one other person
knew. However very often people seek to avoid their family knowing of their status while
they remain well. They want to protect their family, particularly their parents, from the
knowledge that they are seropositive, unless it is absolutely necessary – typically when they
develop AIDS or when they become seriously ill. Brothers and sisters are often told before
parents. This is often because parents are perceived as having a greater vested interest in

their child's wellbeing, because they are often old and considered unable to stand the shock, because they may die before the patient and thus can be kept in blissful ignorance, and because many people have the feeling that they have let down their parents in some way by getting infected.

Social support can come from people other than partners, family and friends. In many parts of the world there are voluntary support organisations aimed at helping those with HIV, both in terms of psychological and practical support. They provide sources of support where disclosure is less of an issue, where a sympathetic response is more or less guaranteed and where an individual can meet other people with similar problems in a nonthreatening environment. They also often offer a range of practical help, from legal advice to 'buddying' services where volunteers befriend people with HIV and offer practical and emotional support. It is important for the counsellor to make an HIV positive individual aware of what support organisations are available in the area, and to put them in touch with such organisations if they so wish.

For many people faced with HIV infection such support organisations and support groups provide a key role. Where such support organisations are not in existence the counsellor could consider whether it might be possible to start one up. Several of the UK community support groups originated from groups of individuals attending the same hospital, who were brought together and provided with the facilities to meet regularly.

Support organisations are not a panacea. A sizeable proportion of my patients have not found them helpful or have not wished to use them. There are particular problems with some groups of patients. In London many patients from sub-Saharan Africa are refugees or students from particular countries, and they are worried about meeting people from their own country and word of their status getting out into a small community or even getting back to Africa. In addition, people from different countries within sub-Saharan Africa often have little in common. In some countries there are, or have been, civil wars and two individuals from the same country may find that they have been on opposite sides.

The possibility of making use of support organisations, however, is one that needs to be discussed with every patient, even if they do not avail themselves of the opportunity.

Finally, there are other people who provide social support to people with HIV infection. In a study on carers of those with AIDS (Kocsis *et al.* 1990) a surprising range of carers were involved with people with AIDS, including landladies, neighbours and local church groups. The support provided by hospital staff is also sometimes overlooked. The great advantage of hospital staff is that, hopefully, it is possible to tell them almost anything without having to worry about how they feel about it. With friends, relatives and others, individuals with HIV infection often feel that they have to 'hold back' on sharing their feelings when they feel particularly bad, because they do not want to upset or burden the other person.

Of course it is not only people who know that an individual is infected with HIV who can provide social support. Social life generally is important. Many people neglect their social lives if they are busy. They may actively avoid socialising if their mood is low. The result can be social isolation. Some quite simple steps can often make major improvements in a person's social life generally.

Support groups have been mentioned earlier. Going through back address books and looking up old friends is often a very fruitful way of establishing a better social life. So is meeting with existing friends. Few people are so busy that they will not welcome a suggested evening out from someone they have not seen for a while. Pursuing interests which bring the patient into contact with other people of like mind is also helpful.

George had had an interest in railways as a child. He had retained this over the years. He had a rather narrow social life revolving chiefly around work. He wanted to do something about this and after consideration he joined a local railway preservation society and got involved in their work at weekends. He did not tell them about his HIV status and found that this was, if anything, a relief, although when he became ill many of his new friends visited him in hospital.

While people who are not aware of a patient's HIV status cannot offer direct support on that issue, they can contribute enormously to the patient's wellbeing and enjoyment of life. Increasing and extending social life is a potentially effective anti-depressant.

Keeping well

Most people with HIV infection want to take positive steps to improve and maintain their own health. One of the problems is that we are not always sure what is and is not helpful (Green & Hedge 1992). However the act of taking control of their own health is, in itself, often a useful one for the person with HIV. It is part of the process of taking control over life, which can contribute considerably to the wellbeing of the patient. It is, therefore, worth considering with the patient what they might usefully do in terms of self-help.

Regular medical monitoring

Regular check-ups and even CD4+ counts can be valuable, although there is the risk with the latter that they may be a source of distress. The main benefits of regular monitoring are that it can put the patient's mind at rest if things are going well, and if the patient's immune functioning is declining there is the opportunity to consider the use of antivirals and, probably more importantly, prophylaxis against PCP and, potentially, other opportunist infections. There are some conditions which it is important to catch early, CMV retinitis being one. Exact advice in terms of prophylaxis and antivirals changes over time and it is important for the counsellor to keep abreast of the current advice.

Cutting down or eliminating drugs

There is evidence that smoking can increase vulnerability to chest infections (and hence speed an AIDS diagnosis) and so patients should, if possible, give up smoking. There is no evidence that alcohol in moderation is harmful but heavy drinking should be reduced. There is little convincing evidence that recreational drugs affect the underlying disease process, but patients should be advised against excess use of these. Moderation is important but this is something that the patient can do to help themselves; it is not the basis for a campaign by the counsellor. Having HIV is bad enough, without having to listen to well-meaning moralising about the evils of smoking or whatever.

Avoiding other sexually transmitted infections

Safer sex is important, not just to protect the partner(s) of the infected person but also to protect the patient against sexually transmitted infections which might speed up disease progression. The risk of being infected by a different variant of HIV from another individual is difficult to assess with recent swings in thinking, but to be on the safe side, it is probably better avoided.

Avoiding other infections

Taking care over hygiene is important in anyone who is immunocompromised. It helps to ensure that meat is properly cooked through, not to eat at restaurants or roadside stalls where hygiene is doubtful, particularly when abroad, and to drink bottled water when on holiday if the water supply is doubtful. It also makes sense to wear rubber gloves to deal with cat litter or earth which may have been contaminated with faecal material from animals. In other words, the patient should take the steps which any prudent person would take. There is, however, little point in the patient becoming hypochondriacal about people with colds or going into crowded places. Susceptibility to many everyday infections, particularly upper respiratory tract infections, appears to be little affected and avoiding other people altogether is unlikely to make the seropositive live longer, although it may be miserable enough to make life seem a good deal longer.

Avoiding stress

It is commonly believed by patients and many health professionals that stress affects HIV disease progression, although there is currently no convincing evidence of this. Stress is impossible to avoid and pleasant things like getting married or meeting new people are as stressful or more stressful than many unpleasant things. I have seen patients become more stressed as a result of feeling that they are stressed and that this is making their health worse. This circle needs to be short-circuited. It helps to review with the patient the sources of avoidable stress in their life and how they might cut them out. This is in the interests of their mental wellbeing and enjoyment of life, and patients should be reassured that they are not making their health worse through anxiety.

Exercise/getting fit

There is no evidence that this affects disease progression in the longer term, although it has been the subject of surprisingly little research. However, it cannot do any harm, if done sensibly, and may possibly help. A sensible amount of exercise is good for almost anyone, well or ill. There is increasing evidence that regular exercise is effective in preventing and relieving depression, so it is probably well worth encouraging patients to do it.

Healthy diet

Depressingly, nothing brings out more cranks and fanatics than the subject of diet. Eating a well-balanced diet is important in maintaining health. However there is no evidence that any particular diet is better for those with HIV. Instead, a mixed diet, whether vegetarian or carnivorous, is what is required. Faddy diets based around avoiding long lists of foods or consuming large amounts of some particular food should be avoided, unless there are good medical reasons for them. Even sensible but novel diets can occasionally have unexpected results.

Peter, a seropositive man, came in to say that the had been suffering from excessive frequency of bowel movements for three weeks. He felt sure that he had caught an opportunistic infection, but nothing had been found on tests. Close questioning revealed that he, a lifelong carnivore and junk food enthusiast, had shifted over to a high fibre vegetarian diet recently. He had not made the connection between the two events.

For anyone with problems or concerns about their diet, a meeting with a dietician is important. This is particularly the case where a patient is losing weight. Many HIV patients, particularly those with oral problems, find that their food does not taste as good as it used to, or even that they have partially lost their sense of taste. Planning a more interesting diet packed with the patient's favourite foods, or simply a more spicy diet, can sometimes work wonders. Also worth looking out for is the patient who loses his or her appetite as a result of depression, where treatment of the underlying condition is important.

Alternative therapies

Few alternative therapies have been sufficiently well researched in relation to HIV disease, to be able to say whether they are effective. The term 'alternative therapy' covers a mixed bag of different treatments, from herbal remedies to various massage/manipulation therapies, from aromatherapy through to treatments based on crystals or numerology. Most of these treatments are, at worst, harmless and may help to maintain the patient's morale – something which is worthwhile. While it is possible that some alternative treatments may make a positive contribution to the patient's physical health, there is simply insufficient evidence to be sure.

On the other hand, I have seen patients driven close to the point of bankruptcy by quack practitioners with their cure-all nostrums, and there have been cases of patients being sold useless or potentially harmful 'remedies'. If a patient wants to use alternative treatments, that is entirely their decision. In most cases it will not cause any harm and it may be a positive contribution to health. The counsellor can sometimes play a useful role in talking through any treatment to help ensure that the patient does not come to physical or financial harm, and is not persuaded to give up conventional treatments without proper thought.

Vaccines

There should be no problem with the use of killed vaccines. There is a theoretical risk attached to live vaccines in the immunocompromised individual; however cases of adverse reactions are unusual. Regular advice is published in the main pharmacopoeias on the use of vaccines in adults and children with HIV infection, or hospital pharmacy departments can usually advise. It is worth considering that theoretical risks from vaccines have to be offset against the real risks of infection with wild pathogens.

Overview

No two people are the same, therefore no two counselling processes are the same. Patients react differently to the same situation because their past histories cause them to see things in a different way. Different counsellors approach the same issues in the same way. However all good counselling, in whatever field, is based on trying to find out about the patient, about their objectives and what scope they have for manoeuvre. Then it is a matter of partnership between the patient and the counsellor to achieve a successful outcome. Ironically, the best outcome of any episode of counselling is when the patient does not need to see the counsellor any more because they have matters under control themselves.

References

Dawson, J., Fitzpatrick, R., McLean, J., Hart, G. & Boulton, M. (1991) The HIV test and sexual behaviour in a sample of homosexually active men. *Social Science and Medicine*, **32**, 683–8.

Higgins, D.L., Galovotti, C., O'Reilly, K.R., Scnell, D.J., Moore, M. & Rugg, D.J. Evidence for the effects of HIV antibody counselling and testing on risk behaviours. *Journal of American Medical Association*, **266**, 2419–24.

Green, J. & Hedge, B. (1991) Counselling and stress in HIV infections and AIDS. In: *Cancer and Stress* (eds C. Cooper & M. Watson), Wiley, Chichester.

Green, J. & Kentish, J. (1995) The right to know HIV test results. *Lancet*, **345**, 1508.

Jacobson, N.S. & Margolin, G. (1979) *Marital Therapy*. Brunner/Mazel, New York.

Jadresic, D., Riccio, M., Hawkins, D., Wilson, B. & Thompson, C. (1989) *Impact of HIV diagnosis on mood*. Presented at the Vth International Conference on AIDS, Montreal, June 1989, Abstract WBP 201.

Landis, S.E., Earp, J.L. & Koch, G.G. (1992) Impact of HIV testing and counselling on subsequent sexual behaviour. *AIDS Education and Prevention*, **4**, 61–70.

Otten, M.W. Jr, Zaidi, A.A., Wroten, J.E., Witte, J.J. & Peterman, T.A. (1993) Changes in sexually transmitted disease rates after HIV testing and post-test counselling, Miami, 1988–1989. *American Journal of Public Health*, **83**, 529–33.

Perry, S., Jacobsberg, L.B., Fishman, B., Weiler, P.H., Gold, J.W.M. & Frances, A.J. (1990) Psychological response to serological testing for HIV. *AIDS*, **4**, 145–52.

Stuart, R.B. (1980) *Helping Couples Change*. Guildford Press, New York.

Zenilman, J.M., Erickson, B., Fox, R., Reichart, C.A. & Hook, E.W. (1992) Effect of HIV post-test counselling on STD incidence. *Journal of American Medical Association*, **267**, 843–5.

Chapter 5

Counselling People with AIDS, their Partners, Family and Friends

Barbara Hedge

Introduction

To be told one has AIDS can come as a shock even when a person is prepared for it. The implication of the diagnosis, that HIV has damaged the immune system to such an extent that the person is susceptible to life-threatening diseases, can take away any last hope of living without becoming sick or of a cure being found before it is needed. Now that CD4+ counts (a measure of immunosuppression) are taken regularly, many patients are aware of their decreasing health status and some may already be taking antiviral or prophylactic medication. For others, knowledge of HIV infection and an AIDS diagnosis may occur concurrently, as they only presented for medical investigation when their health started to deteriorate.

The face of AIDS has changed dramatically over the last 10 years. The understanding of opportunistic infections and carcinomas to which people with AIDS are susceptible has increased, and advances have been made in their treatment. However, people are acutely aware of the nastier manifestations of AIDS, such as diarrhoea, disfigurement, neuropathy, loss of weight, loss of sight, cognitive impairment and dementia. The prognosis of death from an HIV related illness is still there. The uncertainty attached to the course of HIV disease and its poor prognosis frequently causes intense emotional reactions, even in those who are clinically well. The CD4+ count is often taken as a measure of health, and as counts continue to drop people with AIDS continue to feel stressed.

There are many parallels between the difficult issues facing people with AIDS and facing those with other potentially terminal illnesses. For people with AIDS and their caregivers additional problems may have to be faced, such as the stigma and discrimination attached to gay sex or drug use, or racial intolerance. For people who only become aware of their HIV infection when they become unwell, and who did not knowingly have any risk of HIV infection, the AIDS diagnosis may be accompanied by distressing revelations about the sexual experiences or drug using behaviours of their partners.

AIDS is most prevalent in young and middle-aged people, with their caregiving partners also being young or middle-aged. Consequently, AIDS is an issue for people while they are still advancing in their careers, establishing relationships and bringing up families.

Emotional reactions to AIDS

Most people with HIV infection expect to receive an AIDS diagnosis one day. But when expectation turns into reality, hopes of continuing good health are shattered. For some, the uncertainty of not knowing whether their symptoms will result in an AIDS defining illness will have caused great distress, and the diagnosis will bring relief, but for most people it also brings new concerns and anxieties. Many people do not know how they will cope with living with AIDS and considerable psychological adjustment may be required. When people experience a serious illness they may begin to look unwell. A long illness away from work in a young, previously healthy person is unlikely to pass without comment. Relatives and employers may begin to query a person's health status and decisions as to whether to tell parents the diagnosis, or whether to remain in employment, may have to be considered.

Such precipitating factors have been shown to contribute to the level of stress experienced. Other stressful events faced by many people with AIDS are dilemmas concerning medication, difficulties in maintaining close relationships, sexual problems, being bereaved, caring for children with HIV disease and explaining to children about HIV or death in the family. As it appears that it is the cumulative stress level which leads to an inability to cope (Hedge *et al.* 1992), it can be seen that an AIDS diagnosis with multiple issues raised simultaneously can frequently be a time of acute distress. Intense, negative psychological reactions such as anxiety, helplessness, hopelessness, depression, guilt, anger and a loss of self-esteem commonly occur.

Shock and denial

When an AIDS diagnosis is confirmed, shock, numbness, disbelief and denial are frequently experienced. Some people show their shock outwardly, losing control, weeping and appearing confused, with expressions of disbelief and anger. Others may appear to freeze, profess that they are fine, then attempt to withdraw from the situation as quickly as possible.

It is not uncommon for some delay to occur before people are able to accept the full significance of having AIDS. Initially, individuals may deny knowledge of the diagnosis, or minimise its undesirable consequences by asserting that they will return to a pre-AIDS stage of disease once better. This can be quite disturbing for carers as it appears that the diagnosis has not been understood. Such initial denial indicates how difficult it can be for people to give up hope of remaining well for ever.

Fears and concerns

Immediate concerns on receiving an AIDS diagnosis are worries about likely prognosis, and the pattern of disease. Common beliefs are that people die immediately they have AIDS, and many fear uncontrollable pain and dying if not death itself. A lack of information and misperceptions about treatment plans or drug regimes all intensify fears of the future and may encourage avoidance behaviour and denial.

People with anxiety are often preoccupied with their concerns. Consequently they may also experience difficulties with concentration, and with remembering what is said to them.

This may exacerbate fears if they misinterpret this as symptoms of HIV organic brain involvement.

Anger and frustration

Many people express their anger at what they see as the unfairness of becoming infected with HIV. Although HIV transmission can be linked with specific, unsafe behaviours, many variables appear to determine whether infection actually occurs. Individuals with AIDS can often feel that their disease is unjust when they see those who led similar lifestyles escaping infection. Anger can be directed towards themselves, their need for drugs, or their sexuality, or towards another whom they think was associated with their infection.

Some popular ideas which suggest that illness progression can be abated by the adoption of a particular diet, or by maintaining a positive approach to living with HIV, can lead to frustration and anger when it becomes apparent that despite following the recommended approach, disease progression has not been averted. The anger may manifest itself as angry outburst towards those who are trusted and reliable such as partners, counsellors and nurses.

Guilt

When the answer to the question 'why me?' cites a personal behaviour such as having unprotected, penetrative sex or injecting drugs with a shared needle, the causation can become interpreted as fault, particularly when there is stigma attached to the behaviour. It is easy then for people with AIDS to attribute their illness as a punishment for past behaviours, to feel guilty at being sick, to feel they are a burden to their loved ones, and that they have let their family down. Guilt can also be attached to the possible infection of others through personal behaviours, even when these were not recognised at the time.

Hopelessness

As well as concerns about what may happen in the future, an AIDS diagnosis is often seen as a turning point when life becomes a progression of illnesses, pain and death. When there appears to be no future and nothing to live for, it is not uncommon for people to think of giving up. It is easy for people with a physical illness to withdraw, and with little social contact or self-direction a long-term depression can occur, with a lack of interest in food, increasing sleeping problems and a fall in libido. These in turn can result in a further loss of interest in the outside world and increase the depression.

Loss of self-esteem

A high self-esteem requires a positive (on balance) self-perception. The more positive attributes there are to find, the easier this is. For a person with AIDS many of these will have disappeared. Illness may have resulted in body wasting or disfigurement; lowered energy levels may mean that the individual has had to give up employment or social activities so can no longer think of himself as a competent professional or as a good sports person. The resulting perception may be of a weak, frail person dependent on others for daily necessities.

A loss in self-esteem can easily lead to a lack of confidence in many areas of life, including vital decision making. People may hesitate to contact friends or family for fear of rejection. They may think that slowness in body or mind precludes them from participating socially, and may withdraw, increasing the chances for a depressive reaction and a further loss in quality of life.

Helplessness and loss of control

The experience of AIDS is different for everyone; no one can predict how it will affect a particular person physically, psychologically, intellectually or socially. People's thoughts may be coloured by the course their illness has taken. When sick, some people will have been dependent on their partners, parents or hospital staff. Increasing dependence on others and loss of independence can be evidence of a loss of control over life and in such circumstances feelings of helplessness can be considered normal. So although some people attempt to fight the disease, aiming to control it, others give up and adopt a 'helpless' role, rather than trying to discover what in their lives is still possible, interesting and enjoyable.

Suicide thoughts and intention

It is not uncommon for people with an AIDS diagnosis to entertain ideas of suicide. This option can be seen as a way of regaining control and as an immediate, painless solution to problems, easier than a life of unpredictable diseases and an uncertain death. Often people report a decision that they will kill themselves at a particular future stage of their disease, for example when they receive the AIDS diagnosis, so they do not have to suffer repeated bouts of illnesses or possible pain with poor quality of life. When people have coped well with asymptomatic HIV disease by deciding to spare themselves the traumas of living with AIDS by ending their life at that point, it can be quite frightening to realise that this day has arrived. Although it is commonplace to have suicidal thoughts, few people have developed suicidal plans. For many patients thoughts of suicide may appear a rational response to the increasing severity of HIV disease; for others suicidal thoughts may accompany clinical depression.

Counselling people with AIDS

Counselling involves more than simply giving information. It is a process which assists individuals in:

- Acquiring an accurate understanding of the facts
- Relating relevant information to their own needs
- Clarifying the nature of the problem or difficulty
- Setting goals for the necessary changes
- Identifying available resources
- Facilitating actions
- Living with the consequences.

Although medical interventions are increasingly successful in reducing the effects of opportunistic infections and malignant disease, there remain many uncertainties in disease progression. Encouraging denial of the diagnosis or giving unsubstantiated reassurance concerning future good health does not assist individuals to live with AIDS; rather it increases the chance that people will experience further shock and distress should their health deteriorate. Counselling needs to address the difficulties of living with no precise prognosis, to provide opportunities for people to develop the necessary coping skills for living with uncertainty, and to explore ways of maximising quality of life.

Aims of counselling

Counselling people with AIDS has two major aims. The first is to help individuals adjust to living with AIDS. The second is to help people maintain behaviours which will minimise the chance of them transmitting HIV. Counselling support is frequently offered to a person's partner, friends and family who may also be distressed. When they are supported, they in turn can provide valuable support to the person with AIDS.

Breaking bad news

Sometimes, when people are critically ill, they ask for reassurance that they will recover and survive. It is important that a counsellor is able to address the uncertainty of prognosis. Although breaking bad news can be difficult, when carers postpone telling a person some vital information, or only partially inform them, the situation is not necessarily eased. Recipients' stress can be increased as they try to determine what the diagnosis is, or whether the prognosis is poor. Even when people are given information they would rather not hear, when it is imparted sensitively and with empathy people generally prefer the truth. After initial sadness or shock they are then able to prepare to cope with the facts. When professionals are overprotective and give false messages of hope, people often feel disempowered and unable to trust them in any future situation.

Counselling interventions

Adequacy of information

A frequent complaint of patients in many medical settings is that they feel inadequately informed about the details of their illness and the treatments they may need. Consequently, they worry about the implications of their symptoms, and the proposed tests and medications. This may occur when doctors have failed to provide the necessary information, or when they have provided so much, or given it when a person was in shock, that few facts were absorbed or retained.

As an accurate understanding of the issues is essential if informed decisions are to be made, a counsellor's first task is to check what understanding a person does have of AIDS and of their own illness. Any misperceptions can then be corrected and important informational gaps filled. It can be useful to back up what is being said with written information. Many leaflets are now produced which can prove beneficial. They describe the various illnesses associated with AIDS, discuss the expected benefits or side effects of medications and drug trials, address the issues involved when considering starting a family or progressing with a pregnancy, and provide useful contact addresses and telephone numbers.

It might appear that such leaflets could provide a cheap alternative to counsellors. However, it has been found that as well as providing information, leaflets frequently raise many new concerns in the readers and so an opportunity needs to be made for people to ask questions and discuss the issues raised. This suggests that leaflets, although very important in providing take away fact sheets, are best used as an adjunct to the counselling process.

Adjusting to an AIDS diagnosis

As well as requiring adequate information about HIV disease, a good adjustment to an AIDS diagnosis needs an insight into its implications for the future. Counselling provides a setting in which individuals can relate their knowledge of the general facts and uncertainties about AIDS to their own situations. Adoption of a problem solving approach in which people recognise their own needs and their resources (social support and coping skills), make their own decisions, put decisions into practice and live with their consequences, can be useful. This approach is described in detail in Chapter 13. It can help people to consider living with inevitable change, rather than focusing on all the losses and the few gains which AIDS has afforded them. This can give the opportunity for people to create a new meaning to life. Often, as people adjust they report an increased capacity to savour the ordinary, such as an array of spring flowers, a piece of music or an interesting discussion, none of which require enormous resources or fantastic good health.

It is important that the philosophy of living positively with AIDS is not misinterpreted as a requirement to express only positive emotions and to deny other feelings. Counselling can help individuals understand their emotions by exploring their feelings and attitudes towards AIDS. This prevents secondary distress, where people are worried that their responses to AIDS are not normal, and that everyone else has coped better than them. Once people are able to understand their emotions and feelings they are in a position to adopt strategies to cope with them.

Coping strategies

The impact of stress on mood and quality of life can be mediated by the coping strategies adopted. The counselling process allows people with AIDS to explore their aspirations, priorities and goals, and assess the coping strategies they use. An active coping approach encourages people to become involved in solving their own problems, for example by requesting more information or clarification when they are unsure, and by making their own decisions rather than passively waiting for dilemmas to be solved by others. Such an approach has been found to decrease psychological distress and increase quality of life. Not only do problems become solved, but with involvement people feel less dependent and more in control over their lives, and have increased self-esteem and feel less depressed.

When people feel guilty about their illness, or are only able to think about death and dying, they may attempt to cope by denying their diagnosis. This is rarely successful; avoidance of the issues usually leads people to become increasingly isolated and depressed, with lower self-esteem and a poorer quality of life.

Social support

There is a wealth of evidence demonstrating the health enhancing effects of social support in those with chronic physical illnesses. Good social support networks have been shown to be associated with an increased quality of life in people with AIDS (Namir *et al.* 1989). In many chronic illnesses the biological family and the spouse provide most of the social support for an ill person. With AIDS this is often not the case; the family may be unaware of the person's HIV status, sexuality or lifestyle. People with AIDS are frequently young, living independently some distance from their family of origin, maybe with a same-sex partner or by themselves. This means that the social support network of people with AIDS is likely to be very different from the traditional pattern, with partners and close friends providing most support. The number of people in the support network does not seem to be of great importance, as simply having many friends and relatives does not mean that help will be forthcoming. The important factor in coping with AIDS appears to be how adequate the available support is perceived. This is generally highest when there is a regular partner or a stable group of close friends.

As there are many people, some of them already bereaved through AIDS, who report no close friends, it can be seen that the psychological effect of having little or no significant support is clearly an issue for many individuals. It is not always easy to access support, even when it is available. For many people with AIDS their partner and many of their friends are also HIV positive. This can result in people not seeking social support in order to avoid burdening others, especially those who may have similar difficulties. In communities where many people have already lost their lives to AIDS, the availability of support is continually decreasing. Consequently, the need for structured social support is increasing.

Two components of social support have been identified: emotional and instrumental. Emotional support requires the availability of someone who will listen, understand and be concerned about an individual's feelings, which can make them feel accepted and loved. Instrumental support entails the provision of specific assistance with day to day tasks. Both appear to be necessary to provide a buffer against the stresses encountered while living with AIDS.

By helping and encouraging people with AIDS to examine their social networks, counselling can assist them to judge and identify the willingness and ability of others to respond to either or both of these needs. For people with sparse social networks, or where support is judged less than adequate, adoption of a problem solving approach can help to extend people's horizons by giving consideration to all possible options.

There are alternatives to close, personal support. In the UK, the Terence Higgins Trust operates a 'buddy' system which will pair a suitable volunteer with a person with AIDS. Many centres run support groups for people with AIDS. These vary in style; some are oriented to helping people explore and share their feelings, while others adopt a more information seeking and problem solving approach. The counsellor can provide the first line of support by guiding people with AIDS towards organisations and networks which will meet their personal needs.

Self-esteem

People derive much of their identity and self-esteem from observing and evaluating how others relate to them. Individuals with physical illnesses such as AIDS frequently bring out protective and caring responses from others. If a person interprets these as an indication that they are incapable of managing an independent life, their identity changes to that of a sick, dependent person, which may diminish their personal dignity and lower their self-esteem.

It is important for an individual to retain the identity of the person they were prior to AIDS. Counselling can help people identify areas in which they remain self-sufficient and those in which they need some help. Assisting people to retain as much independence as possible enables them to retain control of their lives and maintain their former identity, and increases their self-esteem.

Communication and assertiveness skills

People may find it difficult to discuss important issues with their doctors or to prevent others from making decisions for them, because they have poor communication or assertiveness skills. People with AIDS may be unable to voice their fears, concerns or wishes because they do not wish to upset their partners or carers. They need to be able to counter unreasonable demands made by family or friends, to be able to initiate conversations about medication with physicians, and feel able to change their care if they are not satisfied. Training in communication skills teaches people how to state their needs and feelings in a non-challenging manner.

When people are appropriately assertive, not only do they benefit from fulfilling their immediate needs but they also experience secondary gain as they maintain their self-esteem, feel empowered to deal with issues as they arise, and maintain some control over their lives.

Addressing thoughts of suicide

The potential for suicide in people with AIDS is real, as many stressors which are associated with an increased suicide risk – such as multiple life events, depression and social isolation – are found in those with HIV disease. An increase in suicide has been documented in men with AIDS in New York and may well exist in other countries. Although it is quite common for people with AIDS to have suicidal thoughts, few people have developed suicidal plans. For many patients thoughts of suicide may appear a rational response to the increasing severity of HIV disease; for others suicidal thoughts may accompany clinical depression. If the latter, it is important that the person receives adequate treatment for the depression.

To prevent suicidal behaviours it is necessary to turn hopelessness into hope. Consequently, it is important to create opportunities for the negative aspects of HIV disease to be raised and for possible coping strategies to be considered. Frank discussions of what might be gained and what lost if suicide is attempted frequently reveal fears of repeated illnesses or pain, desires to avoid these and remain in control of life, and altruistic wishes such as not to become a burden to loved ones.

Once the reasons for suicidal thoughts have been established, it is possible for counsellors to discuss alternative options for dealing with the feared situations. Some of these will not previously have been considered, such as writing a 'living will', or discussing with doctors in advance the patient's wishes concerning resuscitation or continued medication for an infection should their life have minimal quality. Giving a person the skills to implement such plans can reduce anxiety and allow negative perceptions of the future to be balanced with the remaining positive aspects of life. Chapter 12 gives a detailed description of the management of anxiety and depression.

When the thoughts and feelings of surviving friends and relatives are appraised, together with an exploration of the continuing positive aspects of life despite AIDS, people usually re-evaluate and the appeal of suicide frequently diminishes.

Consideration needs to be given to the possible results of a failed suicide attempt. Many attempts do fail and people may then live with AIDS, brain damage and other physical illnesses.

Procedures can be established which help people deal with sudden suicidal thoughts. Encouraging people to be attentive to their mood shifts and to notice when they are losing control of their emotions or when their behaviour is becoming impulsive, can allow them to recognise when they need outside help. A simple strategy to reduce the likelihood of an impulsive suicidal act is to give people emergency telephone numbers, e.g. The Samaritans, a local HIV helpline, and the address of the local accident and emergency department; and to elicit an undertaking to contact one of these immediately they feel the need Any definite intentions and plans should be taken seriously and the person referred to specialist psychological or psychiatric services if appropriate.

Specific issues and dilemmas

Telling others the diagnosis

Many people with AIDS are reluctant to tell their parents or their work colleagues about HIV infection and ask for advice on how, when or what to tell others. While people are well there may be good reason to tell only close friends about HIV, as little practical support is required and it can be dispiriting to have others fearing the worst every time a minor cold or flu is experienced. In some cases a family or employer may not be aware of a person's sexuality or lifestyle and so telling reveals more than just an illness diagnosis. However, when someone requires hospitalisation, maintaining secrecy about an illness may cause more stress than it prevents. If a person decides to keep their illness a secret until they are terminally ill, a family may have to adjust to the person's sexuality, illness and imminent death simultaneously. This can cause great distress to many parents who, while not necessarily understanding or agreeing with their child's lifestyle, feel hurt that their son or daughter was not sufficiently confident of their continued love and support to tell them sooner.

All families are different so there is no one right way to tell parents things they would rather not hear. However, a few generalities can be made. If parents are told over the telephone that their child is sick, there is nothing to stop them imagining the worst. If the news is broken face to face, when the person is relatively well, parents can adjust more gradually to the situation. With such a revelation parents may well be in shock, so arranging to tell them at the beginning of a visit allows time for them to adjust, ask questions and feel reassured that their offspring is receiving good care. It can be useful to tell a sympathetic sibling or other close relative about the diagnosis before parents, so additional support is available. The counsellor can help a person to evaluate the best time and way in which to break the news. Sometimes a role play, with the counsellor playing a shocked and rejecting parent, can convince a person that his parents would never respond like that, or can inspire confidence that he could cope even if the reaction was negative.

A general rule for assessing when to tell employers or work colleagues is to adopt a 'need to know' principle. While a person is well, HIV infection will probably have little impact on life at work and there may be no reason to tell anyone. If certain tasks at work become impossible because a person is too weak, unable to maintain a full-time job or may spread infection by undertaking certain procedures (for example, infected health care workers), then telling colleagues what they need to know can ease the situation. This might simply mean telling them that the person has a chronic or serious illness and has been advised to cut down on their work load. Counselling can help people plan their own strategies for telling others, if and when necessary. This can reduce the anxiety about what might happen should others find out.

Adjusting to role changes

The onset of illness can frequently be accompanied by changes in role. A person who has played an active part in a relationship may find that their partner has to take over duties and responsibilities. Previously self-reliant people may need to be cared for by others. The independent lifestyle of a young, fit adult may change to that of a dependent, infirm person. Establishing new roles within a relationship can be difficult; frequently both partners would prefer to maintain original roles.

What can be even more difficult is the effect that a variable illness pattern can have on such roles. Partners who have adapted to caring for sick people may find it difficult to revert to previous roles when periods of good health are experienced. Frequent readjustment to how much care people with AIDS need, and how much they will accept, can emphasise the course of HIV disease progression.

Relationship and sexual difficulties

Sexual dysfunction has been widely reported in people with AIDS. For some it is a consequence of severe illness and accompanying low libido; for others who are, physically, relatively well it can be associated with a fear of infecting sexual partners. When first diagnosed, sex is often far from people's thoughts and abstinence may seem a reasonable option. However, as adjustment to AIDS increases, sexual desire can return. Counsellors can ensure that people are aware of this and are prepared to negotiate and practise safer sex whenever necessary.

People with AIDS are usually very keen to protect sexual partners from acquiring HIV. Even with a regular partner who knows of the infection, discussing safer sex can be difficult as it is a reminder of the risks of infection, illness and death. Such thoughts may reduce sexual desire and induce fears of sexual expression. This can lead to the avoidance of any physical contact in case it leads to a sexual encounter. Signs of love and affection such as touching, hugging and kissing are all boosts to a person's self-esteem. The withdrawal of such signs may leave a person feeling that they are worthless, and may result in lowered mood and diminished quality of life.

Encouraging a person to explore safer sexual issues with a partner is usually beneficial. Often only a simple statement of sexual desires and concerns, which indicates that a person would like to have sex but is scared of infecting the partner, is necessary for a couple to start discussing their feelings and safer sex options, and to renew their sexual life.

A common concern for people with AIDS is that they will never again have a sexual relationship. They fear that asking a new sexual partner for safer sex will be an admission of their HIV status and that telling will result in rejection. Counselling can help a person adopt a self-confident approach in which they indicate to a prospective partner that these days unsafe sex is not an option for anyone, regardless of HIV status. It can be difficult to decide when to first broach safer sex. If people hesitate too long an unsafe sexual encounter may occur simply through embarrassment. Once it is clear that a sexual relationship is being offered, the earlier that safer sex is mentioned, the easier it is for any partner unwilling to practise safer sex to leave without losing face. Frequently prospective partners express relief that the topic has been addressed and they are happy to keep sexual practices safe (see Chapter 15).

Medication issues

Although there is no cure for HIV disease, there have been many advances in the treatments for opportunistic infections and tumours and increasing availability of antiviral medications. People with AIDS are frequently offered the opportunity to take complex cocktails of drugs and to participate in clinical drug trials.

The suggestion that a person might benefit from taking antiviral medication can become a negative marker of health status, as it implies that the immune system is damaged. Ensuring that a person is able to make an informed decision by providing accurate information about the proposed drug, its possible side effects and the medication procedure, can help to minimise the emotional impact of the decision making process.

Similarly, the offer to participate in a trial of a new drug may be interpreted by a person with AIDS as their last chance, particularly when they have previously experienced a number of adverse drug reactions. Counselling support allows an exploration of the interpretation attached to treatment offers.

In order to prevent the development of opportunistic infections, people with AIDS are usually offered a variety of prophylactic medications and may be advised to continue them for the rest of their lives. Long-term adherence to medication regimes is difficult to maintain in any chronic illness, particularly when the treatment is unpleasant or the regime time consuming or complicated. A common co-infection in those who are severely immuno-compromised is cytomegalovirus (CMV) which can cause eye disease and may lead to blindness. Following a CMV eye infection, maintenance therapy involving intravenous drug administration three or more times a week through an in-dwelling catheter is usually necessary. If the in-dwelling line is not kept clean infection can occur which may lead to septicaemia and if the treatment regime is not maintained there is an increased chance of further eye disease.

Helping a person to establish a lifestyle which can cope with the recommended treatment regime can increase their compliance. This might involve the support of a partner or the involvement of a district nurse on a regular basis. Compliance is also improved when the person has adequate emotional support. When a partner, close friend or counsellor is available to help a person adjust to the stage of HIV disease which necessitates such intense, continuous medication, it appears that their motivation for living increases and with it, increased compliance with medication regimes.

Child bearing issues

The rates of transmission of HIV from mother to child vary widely, with higher rates in those with advanced disease. The decision to become pregnant, continue with a pregnancy or father a child may be difficult to make. Not everyone decides to remain childless; for some bearing a child avoids negative, cultural reactions directed towards childless men and women, and for others children provide a reason for living. The desirability of people with HIV disease having children is often questioned. The counsellor's role is not to judge the decision but to ensure it is made with adequate, accurate information and with all possible options explored. Although most of the literature addresses childbearing as a woman's issue, many men experience lowered self-esteem and depressed mood when taking a decision not to have children or when realising the possibility of having infected a child (see Chapter 9).

Death and dying

Issues about death and dying may cause great distress for people with AIDS, yet they may be reluctant to voice them, fearing that once mentioned their thoughts will become reality. Counsellors can become worried when people appear to be avoiding issues which are causing them concern, but efforts to force a topic into the open are rarely rewarding. If counsellors give opportunities for an issue such as death to be discussed, people are free to respond to these openings when they are ready.

People with AIDS often find it easier to discuss death and dying fairly early on in their illness, while they are relatively well, when they can realistically address these as issues for future concern. Many people want to put their affairs in order before they die and seek answers as to when this should be done. Exploring the possible benefits or difficulties associated with leaving affairs unsorted until people are very ill, can foster an understanding that doing what is necessary – e.g. writing a will or discussing funeral arrangements – while they are well, rather than waiting until the last moment, will allow them time to focus on the important issues in their lives and to express important messages such as love, concern and gratitude.

With the realisation that life may be curtailed by an AIDS related death, it is not uncommon to find an increased interest in mortality and spiritual issues even in those who have previously ignored religion. Counsellors are often chosen as suitable people with whom to air these topics as they are not professionally aligned to any particular belief system. On occasion this may require, with an individual's consent, a referral to a spiritual leader.

As the immune system deteriorates there may come a time when no treatment regimes are able to stop the progression of disease. This can be a difficult time for physicians who would like to continue trying every permutation of possible medications, and for the person who is not sure whether it is beneficial to continue treatment, particularly if it has nasty side effects. Some patients may have given this issue great thought whilst they were well and have left advanced directives. These can either be written, in the form of a living will, or verbal, having told a partner, relative or carer of their wishes concerning active treatment or palliative care in various scenarios. Although it is always important to check with people that their latest directive still stands, the existence of such arrangements can diminish people's anxieties that their wishes might not be respected should they be too ill to communicate them. A living will can also assist a partner by removing from them a decision to stop active treatment.

Grief and bereavement

Bereavement in the context of HIV infection presents some unique features. It is not unusual for people who themselves have AIDS to be already bereaved through AIDS. When partners have already died people have an intimate knowledge of an AIDS related death. This can then be viewed as a model for their own death, with the added realisation that they will probably face the experience alone.

Another facet of AIDS related deaths is the multiple bereavement experienced by people living in communities where many friends or family members have already died from AIDS. Support networks become damaged by multiple bereavements and available social support decreases. For those surviving with AIDS this can easily lead to increased isolation and complicated patterns of bereavement.

The counsellor may be involved in various ways. First, direct support may be needed by a person in dealing with the many losses associated with HIV disease: relationships, sex, employment, control, health, hope, and a future. Secondly, counselling can address the intense grief which may be experienced at the loss of a partner or a child. Thirdly, the person may need help in grieving with the community loss experienced. The counsellor may also be instrumental in developing community-wide programmes aimed at providing new, supportive, social networks.

Partners, families and friends

Many people with AIDS fear telling others of their diagnosis. Not only do they wish to spare those close to them the upset and distress that the diagnosis of a potentially life-threatening disease provokes, but many dread being rejected by their partners, family and friends. The fear of being avoided or abandoned is not completely unreasonable. Most people with AIDS notice that certain relationships with colleagues and friends seem to disappear after HIV or AIDS is diagnosed.

People may avoid someone with AIDS for fear of becoming infected through proximity or touch. A more common reason for avoidance is that it can be deeply distressing to see the physical or emotional changes which AIDS may bring about in a person one cares about. The distress can be particularly intense for people who are themselves HIV positive, or who believe they might be and are attempting to avoid the issue. Although such emotional distancing helps people to maintain denial in the short term, it can lead to complicated bereavements after a person has died, when people find it difficult to accept the way they have behaved.

As adequate social support is vital in maintaining a high quality of life in people with AIDS, it is crucial that others have the opportunity of counselling support to help them understand their emotional reactions and develop the skills necessary to cope. People with AIDS benefit when those close to them are able to provide companionship, emotional support, information, and advice (Hays *et al.* 1994; Folkman *et al.* 1994). With supportive partners, family and friends people can often live longer in their home surroundings and may be able to achieve their preference of dying at home.

The support of carers also has a secondary gain. It can help alleviate the demands on the formal health care system, whose resources may be stretched by the increasing numbers of people with AIDS. Although caring for carers requires resources, it can prove more cost-effective than providing extra primary care.

Partners

Being the partner of a person with AIDS can be onerous. One task is to help the person deal with the everyday practicalities of having AIDS, such as ensuring they take the recommended medication or assisting them with complicated treatment regimes. Another task is to maximise the patient's quality of life by maintaining their motivation and encouraging them to adopt active coping strategies. Partners also have to cope with the reality of their own losses as they see their relationships changing and the people they love deteriorating physically and maybe mentally. They have to deal with anticipated grief as they recognise that the death of their loved ones is inevitable. Counsellors can support the partners of people with AIDS in much the same way as they support the people themselves – enabling them to express and understand their emotions, develop the necessary coping skills, utilise available social support and elicit further support when necessary.

Unexpected emotions can be disconcerting. Partners may find they are unreasonably irritable or angry. Given time to explore their feelings they may find that daily occurrences, such as always being the provider of the meal or always cleaning and ironing, are all reinforcers of the message that their loved one has limited energy because he is ill. Although reactions may initially seem out of proportion to the behaviour which elicited them, once people realise that they are reacting to the impact of the underlying message they can focus their coping appropriately.

An unexpectedly difficult time for partners can be when an improvement occurs in the health of the person with AIDS. At this time it is easy for relationships to become strained. Most relationships involve some role diversification, even if not along traditional lines. It can be difficult to alter these, but in times of immediate need, such as severe illness, people adjust their roles quite quickly. It can be more difficult to reverse roles later, particularly in an illness such as AIDS where the long term prognosis is poor. Once the emotional adjustment to a person being ill has been made, partners cannot easily reverse their feelings when people are physically well.

The uncertainty attached to the course of disease can also cause practical difficulties for partners. If they are considering becoming full-time carers, it is not immediately clear when this might be necessary. Many partners have to continue working to support the couple financially and not all employers are willing or able to accept long term absences from workers, particularly when these cannot be planned in advance. This can place a partner in the invidious position of having to decide whether to continue working and leave the care to another, or to abandon financial independence and maybe a career in order to care for a partner. Counselling can give couples an opportunity to address such issues in advance of decisions being required. This allows time for a problem solving approach to be adopted and all feasible options to be considered.

If both the patient and the partner are offered counselling support, joint couple therapy can be offered. When both partners are confident that this will meet their needs it can be advantageous as it enables a counsellor to observe any communication difficulties between individuals, and avoids pathologising either person. Rather it suggests that living with AIDS can be difficult and indicates that a co-operative approach to evolving coping strategies can be beneficial.

This may not always be the best solution. In some partnerships there are secrets which an individual may not wish to express in front of a partner but which may require support. For example, it is not unusual for a person to wonder whether they contributed to their partner's infection, either by advocating a sexually open relationship or by being unfaithful them-selves. Others may experience difficulty in expressing their concerns, anxieties and distress that their partner is dying. Such problems can best be dealt with by individual counselling.

Although good, open communication is generally beneficial to a relationship, there is the danger that when one person has AIDS this can become the sole focus of the relationship. Not only does 24 hour problem solving become wearing, it is unlikely to be more productive than frequent, well spaced, shorter sessions. Counselling can help people restrict the time they spend discussing illness and AIDS. For many couples, deciding to review the diffi-culties and dilemmas weekly, or daily, for a limited period frees them to spend more time on activities which make life enjoyable and which support the relationship.

Another dilemma for couples can be in deciding how much time to devote to each other. People can feel that because there may be little time left they must spend every minute together. However, it is important for partners to continue to give their own life some meaning. This might be achieved by giving themselves a regular slot in which to pursue an interest, such as going to the gym, or simply by allowing themselves an evening with no responsibilities while friends support the patient. If longer breaks are required, regular, formal respite from caring can be organised with the provision of professional care support.

In order to create a pleasant environment for patients, partners may avoid expressing their feelings about AIDS. However, when the emotional impact of a person's illness is not acknowledged, the patient may summise that it is absent, indicating a lack of love or con-cern. Consequently, partners need to be aware of the balance which needs to be struck between the amount of concern they show for themselves and the amount of support they deliver.

Although friends may provide a first line support for a partner at stressful times, they too may be emotionally involved and unable to deliver the necessary support without becoming more distressed themselves. Many centres provide support groups for partners which provide a safe forum in which problems can be addressed objectively, as other group members are not personally or emotionally involved.

The HIV positive carer

Unlike most potentially terminal illnesses, partners of people with AIDS are also often infected with HIV. It is quite common to see the less ill partners neglecting their own health and effectively denying their own needs, in order to support their sick partners. Although some bias in care may well be inevitable, counselling both partners can help each to recognise the other's needs and a balance in care to be adopted. Surviving partners frequently see their lover's death as a model for their own. They may fear that they will not be as brave as their partners were. Support in helping people evaluate their own needs and feel confident with their own preferred coping skills is often required.

Families

Families may only be told of a person's HIV disease after they have AIDS and are ill. Seeing a relative sick can have a significant emotional impact on those close; parents may feel guilty for not having accepted a gay relationship, or feel responsible for their child's sexuality or drug use. Looking for a just world, many parents need an explanation as to why their son or daughter has a potentially terminal illness. They may think they have failed, or blame a partner or friend who leads the same lifestyle.

An initial reaction can be a suggestion that they remove their offspring from their current situation, take them home and care for them. This may not always be appropriate. Many people with AIDS have an adult partner or a network of supporting friends who may welcome support but wish to remain involved. Caring for a sick child, even when they are adult, may raise many emotive issues for a parent. Parents frequently remark that it is not 'natural'; children should be burying their parents, not vice versa.

Occasionally partners and parents can come to blows, both fearing that the other is not caring sufficiently well for their loved one. If counsellors can help both parties to recognise that their aims are the same – to give the best life possible to the person with AIDS – then a co-operative rather than competitive approach to caring can be adopted, to the patient's benefit.

Even when people with AIDS have no partner the thought of becoming dependent on their parents again after having established themselves as independent adults, can be quite dispiriting and can lower people's self-esteem. Counselling parents can help them to acknowledge that their offspring is no longer a child, to respect and encourage the offspring's independence and control over their own life, and to communicate their willingness to assist when asked. Once an understanding of the person's needs is established, many parents become important assets to a patient.

A difficulty can arise when people have made it clear that they do not wish their family to know their diagnosis, and when parents or relatives are closely questioning carers. It is important for counsellors to stress the principle of confidentiality, helping parents to accept that it is the right of any person not to divulge their diagnosis. If they also help the patient and the family to communicate their thoughts and feelings more, this may well improve the relationship sufficiently for them to address the previously banned topics. Breaking confidentiality is not justified and is likely to result in neither patient nor family feeling confident in the counsellor.

Friends

Anxieties about interacting with someone who is seriously ill, and uncertainty as to what behaviours are most helpful or appropriate, sometimes cause friends to remain distant or to behave in ways which are perceived by the ill person as unsympathetic, insensitive or rejecting.

Friends may ask how to help a person with AIDS. The general advice is to maintain the friendship on the previous basis, not avoiding interactions (physical or more usually emotional), and to act naturally, expressing love and concern, providing a shoulder to cry on and being someone who will listen. As people with AIDS need to access as many of the pleasures of their previous life as possible, friends can be of enormous support, providing companionship and the opportunity for enjoyment and discussion. They can help people participate, mentally if not physically, by introducing interesting topics of conversation and by arranging activities which the person can still enjoy. If an opportunity for reciprocity can be created, it helps to give meaning to the patient's life and increases their self-esteem. It is important that friends find a way of being supportive without taking over a person's life. The person with AIDS should be encouraged to do as much as possible and be in control of his or her life.

Sometimes people with AIDS choose to confide in one close friend and ask for confidentiality to be maintained. This can put considerable burden on the chosen friend who may be distressed with the news and who may need support himself. Many breaches in confidentiality can be traced to such a need rather than to spurious gossip. It can be easier to maintain confidentiality within a small group of friends who can mutually provide support for each other. Counselling can help a person with AIDS to consider how important the maintenance of confidentiality is for them, and how it is best addressed.

Overview

Counselling people with AIDS may not be able to solve the many difficulties they face. However, it can provide a forum for the expression of emotions, and can equip people with useful strategies for coping with AIDS. All those close to a person with AIDS may be emotionally affected by the illness. Extending support to such people can enhance not only their quality of life but also the life and death of the patient. This suggests that provision of adequate counselling services is of paramount importance.

References

Folkman, S., Chesney, M. & Christopher-Richards, A. (1994) Stress and coping in care-giving partners of men with AIDS. *Psychiatric Manifestations of HIV Disease*, 17, 35–53.

Hays, R.B., Magee, R.H. & Chauncey, S. (1994) Identifying helpful and unhelpful behaviours of loved ones; the PWA's perspective. *AIDS Care*, 6, 379–92.

Hedge, B., Petrak, J., Sherr, L., Sichel, T., Glover, L. & Slaughter, J. (1992) *Psychological crises in HIV infection*. VIII International Conference on AIDS, Amsterdam. Abstract PoB 3803.

Namir, S., Alumbaugh M.J., Fawzy, F.I., & Walcott, D.L. (1989) The relationship of social support to physical and psychological aspects of AIDS. *Psychology and Health*, 3, 77–86.

Chapter 6

AIDS Dementia – Counselling Issues

Agnes Kocsis

Introduction

This chapter concentrates primarily on the effects of the human immunodeficiency virus (HIV) on the brain and the consequent effects on the lives of the people concerned, their partners, lovers, friends and family. It covers in less detail the opportunist infections which can affect the brain when someone is HIV positive. Such infections are due to the immunodeficiency caused by the presence of HIV in the body, which leaves it prey to a range of different infections. The brain is one of the potential sites of such infections and they can have their own effects on mental functioning and the everyday life of the patient.

The brain can be a direct target of HIV in a way which was not recognised in the early stages of our knowledge about the disease. Over the last 12 years our understanding of the effects of HIV on the brain has increased, although much is still unclear. At its most extreme, HIV infection of the brain can result in very significantly impaired functioning – socially, at work and in everyday life. This is known as dementia. This manifestation of HIV infection is currently not treatable or reversible in the way that many of the brain opportunistic infections are. Health professionals and others involved in the patient's care have the responsibility therefore of ensuring good management in terms of practical and emotional support as the only, but much needed, intervention.

In order to counsel effectively those who are experiencing the effects of HIV in the brain, and those around them, the counsellor needs to have a reasonable knowledge of the causes of the changes observed and the likely course of disease. The first section of this chapter is therefore devoted to an explanation of the causes of HIV related brain disorder, its diagnosis and presentation. The second section describes ways in which counselling may assist those facing this difficulty, including a summary of the implications for counselling of what we know about the causation of AIDS dementia.

The chapter does not attempt to describe the complex process of assessment for the presence of HIV in the brain, or to give exact criteria for diagnosis. For this it is suggested that the reader consult Price and Perry (1994).

Background

Many terms are used to refer to the effects of HIV on the brain. Among the most commonly used are:

- AIDS dementia complex
- HIV/AIDS (related) dementia
- HIV/AIDS (related) brain impairment
- HIV/AIDS encephalitis
- HIV/AIDS encephalopathy
- HIV/AIDS cognitive impairment
- HIV related cognitive/motor complex.

It is important at the outset to distinguish between dementia and encephalopathy. Dementia refers to observable changes in behaviour, personality and cognition and, formally, is defined as 'significant effects on social and occupational functioning'. Encephalopathy refers not to behaviour but to the underlying state of the brain, meaning literally 'disease of or damage to the brain'. If someone is dementing there is obviously an underlying state of encephalopathy, although it may not be detectable by currently available methods.

The term AIDS Dementia Complex was coined by Navia and Price from the Sloan-Kettering Centre in New York. They called it a complex because in AIDS the dementia can manifest itself as a complex trio of changes in cognition, personality and motor function.

Encephalitis means 'inflammation of the brain'. In describing the direct effects of HIV on the brain this term is not appropriate for everyday clinical use. The presence of HIV in the brain may or may not cause encephalitis. While examination of the brains of people who have died of AIDS and also had dementia indicates that encephalitis is sometimes present, it is by no means always so. Encephalitis can also be a consequence of one of the opportunist infections of the brain, as in herpes encephalitis.

HIV (related) cognitive impairment refers to impoverishment of any or all aspects of the 'output' of the brain concerned with our mental processes – attention, concentration, memory and so on. It is due to the activity of HIV in the brain. HIV related cognitive impairment may be mild, moderate or severe. If it is severe, the person will be diagnosed as having AIDS dementia. In this case the person will have great difficulty in managing everyday affairs and will be obviously unusual in his or her interactions with others. If it is only mild or moderate, the diagnosis is likely to be one of HIV related cognitive/motor complex. Individuals in this category will still be able to function effectively in their daily lives, even perhaps at work, but will not be as mentally efficient as previously. They are likely to deteriorate eventually, but since other opportunist infections may intervene and the time course of the activity of HIV in the brain is highly unpredictable, someone with mild HIV related cognitive impairment may never dement.

The term HIV related brain impairment is a catch-all phrase for all consequences of HIV on the brain, whether due to opportunist brain infections or as a direct result of HIV in the brain itself. However, it may be used also as a way of avoiding the term dementia. For many patients and carers the term dementia can be frightening, with connotations of madness and loss of identity. This issue is addressed in more detail below.

This chapter is primarily concerned with those who, as a direct result of HIV in the brain, have either dementia or a milder form of cognitive impairment which is still significant enough to impact on their everyday functioning.

Stress, anxiety and depression

There is sometimes a degree of confusion about the possible role of stress factors in the development of changes in behaviour and cognitive functioning in someone with HIV. There is often a reluctance in health professionals to consider the fact that both stress and organic factors can at the same time influence the behaviour of an individual. Attempts to reach an either/or decision between the two alternatives can lead to absurdities. Quite extreme difficulties may be attributed to stress without an attempt to consider possible organic causation, that is to say physical rather than psychological reasons for the difficulties the patient is having.

In the real world, either/or distinctions may not always be appropriate. Interactions between stress reactions and organic problems can be complicated and varied. It is entirely possible that someone with HIV could be under stress and consequently anxious and/or depressed, but also have HIV active in the brain. In other words the two problems can occur at the same time in the same individual but be unlinked. On the other hand the difficulties experienced by the individual due to brain changes can themselves cause anxiety. In some cases the presence of HIV can in itself cause brain changes resulting in altered mood and even, occasionally, psychotic episodes.

How HIV attacks the brain

The exact mechanisms responsible for the significant changes in behaviour and thinking observed in some people with HIV infection are not well understood. There are many apparent paradoxes even in the better understood aspects. This section deals with the basics of the overall process inasmuch as these are directly relevant to the process of counselling and managing someone with HIV infection. The underlying mechanisms are covered in more detail in Price and Perry (1994).

As explained in Chapter 1, HIV can easily attack those cells in the body which carry the CD4 receptor. It uses the CD4 receptor to gain access to the cell. The commonest cell type to carry the CD4 receptor is the CD4+ T-cells. These are cells which 'switch on' a large part of the body's defences against disease. The attack by HIV on them is the main underlying element in the development of the immunodeficiency which is the most striking element of AIDS. However, T-cells are not the only group of cells attacked by HIV. Cells of the brain are also directly attacked. These are the macrophages and microglial cells, which have their origins in the bone marrow and then migrate into the brain. As they do so, they can carry HIV into the brain. It is possible that there may be other points of entry to the brain for HIV, but this seems to be the main one.

The brain is essentially composed of two types of cell: white cells (the supporting network, called glial or glue cells) and grey cells (the neurons), which are the cells which do our thinking. The microglia and macrophage cells have various roles in the brain but, among other things, they form part of the white matter. The neurons are a different cell line and the virus is not able to enter, or at least to replicate within, these cells. However, it seems that the presence of the virus in the brain has an indirect effect on neurons as well. The number of neurons in the brain of HIV positive individuals as a group is on average lower than in uninfected individuals and it is clear that in those who show HIV-related dementia, the thinking processes mediated by the neurons are impaired.

There has been much speculation about the nature of the effects on the neurons which cause these changes. Two main types of explanation have been put forward:

(1)   Part of the virus, its outer coat known as gp120, is toxic for neurons. Therefore gp120 which is present as the virus replicates in the brain could itself produce damage to the neuronal network.

(2)   The body's own response to HIV infection may in itself cause damage. For instance it has been suggested that cytokines – chemicals produced by immune cells in the brain in an attempt to fight against the invading virus – may either damage neurons or set off other processes which result in their damage.

The areas of the brain which have the highest populations of cells susceptible to HIV infection are the so-called sub-cortical areas, in the lower areas of the brain. These areas govern a whole range of processes such as balance, arousal, emotion, speed and motivation. However it would be unreasonable to suppose that the effects of HIV on the brain would be limited to these areas. The brain has complex pathways linking its various areas and damage to one area tends to affect the functioning of quite different areas. The neurons of the cortex are also, as explained above, indirectly affected by HIV. The changes in brain processes and therefore in thinking, behaviour and even motor skills which result from the activity of HIV in the brain are wide-ranging and can be profound, and are not limited to those activities usually thought of as sub-cortical. However, quite often these are the earliest functions to be affected.

When HIV infection occurs

From early on, HIV can be found in the cerebro-spinal fluid (CSF, the fluid surrounding the brain and spinal cord) of many individuals with HIV infection. The extent to which this reflects actual viral replication in the brain is unknown. Finding HIV virus in the CSF at this stage does not, in itself, predict the development of dementia later. It is probable that, in these early stages of disease, the body's immune defences are sufficiently intact to be able to limit the replication of the virus within the brain. The majority of HIV seropositives who have HIV in the CSF at this early stage do not develop either dementia or any cognitive impairment associated with its presence there, even when they progress to AIDS.

It is known from autopsies that many individuals who are HIV infected have HIV within their brains even at a point where they do not seem to show any overt changes in mental functioning. It is not yet understood why HIV causes no apparent effect on brain functioning in one individual, while causing extensive effects in others. One possibility is that the difference is at least partly a function of the exact strain of HIV with which the individual is infected. HIV is a highly changeable virus with many variants. It appears that some strains of the virus are more likely than others to infect macrophages. Other factors, such as the person's age, previous health and any previous injury or damage to the brain (e.g. through head injury or heavy drug or alcohol misuse) may also influence the later course of HIV in the brain.

Rates of HIV-related brain impairment

In the early 1980s there were fears that the majority of people with AIDS would develop cognitive impairment to some degree, if not dementia. While we cannot yet predict on an individual basis who will or will not develop HIV related encephalopathy, current estimates suggest that no more than 16% of HIV seropositive individuals develop HIV related dementia as one of the features of their infection with HIV. It is uncertain whether this figure is set to change as the life expectancy of people living with HIV increases as a result of better treatment of opportunistic infections.

Up to a third of people with AIDS may have mild cognitive impairment related to activity of HIV in the brain. In many cases the impairment is too mild to have much impact on everyday functioning. It is, however, worth considering that up to 70% of individuals with AIDS may, at one time or another, have some kind of brain involvement if one includes the effects of other opportunist brain infections. So CSF problems in AIDS are more common than might be expected from a consideration of the direct effects of HIV alone.

Effects of HIV activity on the brain

In order to understand the effects of HIV in the central nervous system, it is important to remember that not only our thinking or cognition but many aspects of our behaviour, mood and personality are dependent on brain states. An altered or disrupted brain will therefore potentially cause a range of effects from sudden and violent changes in mood to confusion, disorientation and disinhibited behaviour. It is convenient to divide up the effects into those on personality, as seen through behaviour, and those on cognition. The list below is not exhaustive but is a guide to the presentations one might expect. It is crucial to remember that the diagnosis will be made primarily on the basis of formal neuropsychological assessment and/or extreme observable signs. Moreover the diagnosis will depend on the presentation of a panoply or pattern of changes which cannot be explained otherwise.

In terms of behaviour and mood, possible signs will be abnormal (i.e. abnormal for that individual given the circumstances):

- Talkativeness, sociability
- Emphasis on immediately reinforcing behaviours (e.g. spending money on luxury items, ordering enormous amounts from catalogues)
- Agitation and inability to concentrate
- Exaggerated and impractical plans
- Lack of care with personal hygiene/appearance
- Inappropriate social behaviour (e.g. inappropriate sexual advances, rude personal remarks, excessive and exaggerated complaints or demands)

Other signs sometimes occurring are:

- Lack of motivation

- 'Flat' affect without expression of sadness, guilt or fear of the future which would indicate depressed mood
- Reduced speech output
- Lack of concern about personal affairs

The cognitive effects are likely to be primarily:

- Difficulty with the process of planning and deciding
- Slowing of thought
- Vacancy
- Confusion
- Vagueness
- Unusual distractibility
- Inability to concentrate and consequent absent-mindedness and memory difficulties.

The impact of these on daily living are discussed further below.

It cannot be emphasised too strongly that in the matter of assessment and diagnosis, every care must be made to consider other, or additional, possible reasons for perceived changes. Neuropsychological assessment should be used to test out the possibility of HIV related brain impairment. The assessment should also be made in the broader context of the individual's history and cultural context.

Counselling

As in other aspects of HIV, the emotional support of a patient and the surrounding carers is not the sole province of the professional counsellor. It is hoped that the suggestions in this section will be helpful to a range of professionals involved in the care of a person with HIV in the brain. Indeed, unless the patient has a previously established relationship with a professional therapist or counsellor, it is only with mild cognitive impairment that the offer of sessions is likely to be greeted in positive fashion. Especially in more advanced stages, the patient may well (although not necessarily) prefer to maintain contact with familiar professionals who may then find counselling inherent in their role. Carers, however, may be happy to see someone who is not involved in the day to day care of the patient. Effective counselling, whoever may be doing it, requires that the individual should have thought through some of the issues.

Dementia

Dementia is a term with which many people will be familiar, albeit more from the colloquial meaning, usually used in a pejorative sense. Also people may well have experience of someone, perhaps an elderly relative, with dementia. If they have known someone with dementia of the Alzheimer's type, for example, they may have quite a frightening image of the demented individual.

Before considering how to help others cope with dementia, it may be useful to consider your personal reactions to the news that you had a progressive condition that could lead to dementia. When I have discussed this with groups of professionals, these are some of the thoughts and fears that were expressed:

- I would be so afraid of humiliating myself, of doing embarrassing things
- I would be afraid of being a burden on others
- I would think of killing myself
- I wouldn't want to embarrass others
- I would be afraid of being dumped in an institution
- I would hate the idea of looking revolting – not thinking of cleaning myself up
- I would be afraid of losing my memories – everything that makes me 'me'
- I would be afraid of losing my spirit
- Other people would make all my decisions for me – I would hate that.

On the other hand, others have suggested that there might also be positive aspects: that there would be a sense of floating, of not having to deal with reality, of abandonment – in a positive sense.

Often, too, the question of insight arises. Would I know what was happening to me? What would it really feel like? This is a useful question. A person with dementia should not be treated as someone lacking feeling as well as mental capacity. A central idea of counselling in this area is that people with HIV related dementia do feel – contentment as well as fear, comfort as well as confusion and anxiety. Even someone with 'flat' affect, who is in many ways not motivated, can feel resentful at an infringement of independence or delighted with the visit of a friend, but they may not be able to express their feelings in easily comprehensible ways. The task of the professional is to observe as well as to ask and, from an understanding of the condition, attempt to predict the factors most likely to maximise the person's sense of well-being.

The reason for thinking through these personal responses is that professionals' attitudes towards the patient and their carers will be coloured by their own view of the situation. Health professionals and care managers are only human. If someone in a counselling role genuinely feels that dementia is the worst thing that can happen to anyone and that there is no way to ameliorate this terrible situation, then it is unlikely that either patient or carers will glean much comfort from the counselling interaction. Moreover, a counsellor with such a strong feeling of doom in relation to dementia, who notices changes in someone's behaviour or cognition suggestive of HIV in the brain, might be unable to mention this possibility or even to refer the patient for neuropsychological testing or other investigations.

There was a time when sex, death and suicide were taboo topics. Many health professionals are now adept at conversing about these issues. Dementia, however, is still in many ways taboo and it may be part of the counsellor's task to lift some of the mystery and fear.

As a first step it is important for the counsellor to be familiar with the actual presentation of HIV dementia, which is in many ways less extreme and distressing than some other comparable conditions, for example dementia of the Alzheimer type. While the personality of the individual does change, and atypical behaviours occur as described elsewhere in this chapter, the person almost invariably maintains their essential characteristics in a reassuring way. One way of describing the changes is that the previous characteristics become more extreme and magnified. Alongside this there is the kind of vulnerability which a small child has, in terms of a short attention span, the need for immediate gratification and also the need for predictability, familiarity, structure and a level of independence matched to their skills.

As with a child, it is skill and application rather than intelligence which are lacking, and interest and appropriate activities are required. The adult with HIV dementia will retain much learned knowledge and will sometimes surprise those around, for example by detailing all the medication being taken or reeling off long telephone numbers. Of course it is important to remember that they are an adult and not a child, but it is a useful way to think about some of the sorts of mental changes which happen, as long as the analogy is not taken too far.

It is useful therefore to bear in mind the specific cognitive difficulties involved and how they may impact on daily life. By doing this, the global fear of the blanket term dementia may be dissipated and made more normal and manageable.

Effects of HIV in the brain

The counsellor, along with all others involved in the support of the person with HIV in the brain, has to bear in mind the specific difficulties in thinking that the individual has, if they are to provide support and communicate appropriately. Some of the difficulties which will affect the process of counselling are problems in concentration and attention, for instance:

- Poor attention and concentration (e.g. reading forms, receiving information, carrying out tasks which require sustained attention)
- Difficulty in planning ahead (e.g. tasks for the day)
- Difficulty in thinking of more than one thing at a time
- Difficulty in attending to more than one person talking
- Particular difficulties in dealing with unfamiliar items and tasks
- Problems in following through on actions with several parts (e.g. cooking, housework, letter writing, keeping track of financial affairs).

Problems with memory can occur, for instance:

- Problems with behaviours linked to particular dates or times of day (appointments, taking medication, birthdays)
- Difficulties with losing track during chains of actions (e.g. 'why am I in this room?' 'what have I been doing for the last while?')
- Problems in following more recent complex events without much personal relevance (books, plays, other people's doings)
- In more severe cases, memory for personal history (the events of one's life) may also deteriorate.

Implications of cognitive changes

Attentional difficulties mean that it may be wise to:

(1) Keep counselling sessions short
(2) Summarise frequently
(3) Refer back to the overall aim of the sessions frequently
(4) Keep notes or a tape of the session which the client may keep.

Planning difficulties mean that:

(1) Goals and decisions will need to be discussed in detail
(2) Notes or a taped record should be kept of the steps involved.

Confusion and disorientation mean that:

(1) References to concrete places, people and times may helpfully be incorporated
(2) Reference to previous conversations can be useful for reinforcing the relationship.

Helping the patient

Decisions, independence and control

The central points to bear in mind when helping the person with brain impairment are that:

(1) The emotions experienced by the individual should be assumed to be as powerful and complex as previously, unless shown to be otherwise
(2) The style more than the content of counselling must take into account that the individual's capacity for previously used problem-solving strategies, and for expressing emotional needs, is reduced
(3) The counsellor is likely to have to take an active role in addressing issues and suggesting solutions.

The third point touches upon one of the many difficult ethical issues surrounding HIV related brain impairment. How can we accommodate our philosophy of empowering patients? In order to allow patients choice in relation to their physical care and social needs we generally try to meet expressed need rather than to impose solutions. We are also concerned to avoid unduly influencing patients in their decision-making. Thus, normally, if a care manager offers a patient alternative accommodation and the offer is refused, the matter is likely to rest there. Similarly we are not usually likely to pass comment on a patient's lifestyle or habits, even if these appear bizarre to us. Nor are we likely to go against the patient's expressed wishes concerning information to relatives or treatment. In the case of someone whose decision-making abilities are impaired, should we change our style of interacting with the patient or do we need to modify it?

I would suggest that the answer lies not in being any more dogmatic or forceful with individuals than we otherwise might be, but in affording them more time and giving them more assistance in the decision-making process. It is frequently reported, sometimes with puzzlement, sometimes with frustration, that a person with HIV related brain impairment has refused a number of offers of 'help' – home care of various kinds, arrangements for day or respite care, alternative accommodation, etc. This is particularly the case when the suggestions concern unfamiliar people or places. This, on reflection, is not so surprising. A person with a reduced capacity to understand and make sense of the world will naturally have a great wish for certainty, predictability and familiarity. Strangers and new surroundings are slightly stressful, even for the best adjusted and functioning individual because they demand new understanding and new choices of behaviour. Familiar people and predictable timetables on the other hand are relaxing in that they allow us to respond from our existing repertoire of behaviours. This is more comfortable, if only because it avoids the need to learn new names, faces and rules.

Ironically, the need of a person with HIV related brain impairment to maintain the status quo may be most acute just at the very time when professionals, relatives and partners are urgently attempting to meet care needs. This in itself may involve them in asking the patient many questions, suggesting an array of options in quick succession and possibly introducing a number of new workers as well as new places to visit. How can this apparent impasse be dealt with? Once it is understood that reluctance or even apparent stubbornness may be due to the nature of the cognitive difficulty itself, a number of solutions present themselves.

The first consideration is to try and channel the discussions with the patient through someone who is already familiar to them and trusted by them. This again highlights the enormous advantages of having identified the existence of HIV related brain impairment in its early stages. Early assessment allows a relationship with a care manager, counsellor or clinician to be cemented so that planning can take place calmly. Later, if urgent steps regarding safety or hygiene are required, the familiar professional can have a central role in facilitating the decision-making. It may also be possible to involve a friend or family member. It is sometimes the case that the person most closely involved with the patient finds it too painful and intrusive to the relationship to negotiate professional care issues. There may however be someone else in the patient's social network who would be willing to help.

> A patient's aunt went along with him to see a potential residential placement which the patient himself had previously refused. Her presence seemed to help him to relax enough to enjoy his visit and he decided to move in after all.

Once a trusted person has been identified, it is usually best to prioritise decisions and tackle the most essential first. There can be a tendency to try and solve a number of issues all at once, e.g. should the patient live at home or go for convalescence, should the children be looked after at home or should they stay with a relative, how much home care should be provided, does the person need a bath aid, etc. Trying to solve all problems at the same time leaves not only the patient, but everyone else, confused. Identifying the most important and most pressing decisions is vital. Once the most important decisions have been made and set into place, it is likely that the patient will feel more secure and willing to consider other more minor necessary changes.

It is important to see that these recommendations are not put forward as elements of a receipt for manipulating patients into accepting what professionals have decided for them. The spirit is rather that the person's specific cognitive vulnerability has to be recognised and allowed for in the decision-making process. However, after all our best efforts the person with cognitive impairment may still choose to say no in the end!

Discussing HIV related brain impairment with the patient

As discussed above, few of us find it easy to talk about dementia with a patient because of the images that this term evokes. That is not, however, a reason for side-stepping the issue. It is best to seek to be truthful but undramatic. For example, in the case of someone who has presented with subjective concerns about memory and concentration changes, and who has recently been neuropsychologically assessed showing impairment, it may be possible to go through some of the following points.

COUNSELLOR: 'You have told me that you are concerned about your concentration and memory, that you find you have to rely more than before on your diary. When you went for testing recently you found some of the tasks quite difficult and you were slower than you probably would have been before. It is likely that this is because of HIV in your brain. That is making it harder for you to remember/concentrate. You have to put more effort into things that you did before without thinking. It would be sensible for us to think about how you might make things easier for yourself at this stage.'

This is not intended as a set script, but an illustration of some of the points that need to be made. It may not be possible to go through these points all at once. It may perhaps be necessary to go through them over a period of a few meetings, depending on the person's level and responsiveness. The counsellor might then discuss things like using a diary, relying on a partner or friend for prompting about appointments etc. You could also say something like: 'It might also be useful to think about how you could allow yourself space to concentrate on the important things without worrying too much about the everyday things.'

At this point the counsellor could consider what tasks the person finds difficult or frustrating in terms of activities of daily living, in order to try and remove those tasks which could be carried out by someone else. This is helpful because an overloaded brain is less efficient and the threshold for being overloaded is lower in someone with brain impairment. Just removing some of the tasks can make the individual more efficient at the remainder.

As an example, the business of shopping and cooking will require considerable mental effort for someone with at least moderate HIV related brain impairment. This is because it involves planning (what shall I eat, what ingredients do I need), possibly writing (making a list), remembering (the list, if not the items) and then orchestrating the different elements of food preparation. Computer shopping will make the task easier, but meanwhile other ways of facilitating the task will have to be found. Options may include assistance to carry out the tasks from a professional home carer, friend or other carer, or someone taking over the task entirely. The actual tasks to be removed and the individual solutions will depend on the circumstances. The aim is:

● To simplify the number of things the individual has to attend to
● To consider the elements which the individual finds rewarding and try to preserve these while eliminating others
● To put in just enough support for the task (JEST) to restore the manageability of the task
● To ensure that the patient feels, as far as they wish, that they are taking active steps to improve their well-being.

Throughout it is important to emphasise the extent to which the patient has control over a whole range of issues. Few people relish the idea of losing control over their affairs and most particularly over their behaviour. The counsellor or whoever is in the counselling role can ensure in many ways that the patient is given the message that control and decisions are possible and in fact expected. Even giving thought to the appointment times that are offered can be part of the overall approach, for example allowing the patient to choose between different times or whether the appointment will be in outpatients or at home.

Emotional issues

The patient may need to discuss feelings of frustration, anxiety, loss, boredom etc. The first need, however, for patients and their carers alike will almost certainly be to understand what the diagnosis means, i.e. what the implications are for the immediate as well as for the long term future. Until there is a clearer understanding of this, they will not know what they are trying to adjust to, either emotionally or practically.

The counsellor must therefore be prepared to give information, practical advice and suggestions on how to proceed – to patient and carer alike. This in itself will provide emotional support and will pave the way for dealing with the deeper feelings subsequently.

Dealing with uncertainty

In the case of HIV related brain impairment, as with so many aspects of HIV, we all have to deal with a large element of uncertainty. While uncertainty is itself a psychologically difficult state because of the need to hold a number of potentially different scenarios in mind, someone with HIV related brain impairment is, by the nature of the condition, rather less likely to be troubled about visions of the future, except in mild or early stages. This then is the time when, if the person is aware of the possible prognosis, plans can be made for arranging enduring power of attorney, drawing up a will, and making any other arrangements which the person wishes to make while able to do so.

> COUNSELLOR: 'It is very difficult to know whether or not you are going to deteriorate in terms of finding it harder to plan and make decisions. It could be that in the future you will feel less interested in your financial affairs or your possessions, although, again, we cannot assume this. It seems sensible though for you to make sure that you make any arrangements that really matter to you now, so that you can rest in the certainty that the important things will be looked after. It also means that you are in control and that you can decide how you would like things to be.'

Parents with HIV related impairment

It can be distressing to see a child of a patient with HIV related brain impairment try to puzzle out the change in their parent. There are likely to be a number of issues to deal with, and there is general guidance on dealing with families in Chapter 10. It is most important to ensure that any child involved is helped to understand that the parental withdrawal or unusual behaviour is due, not to something the child has done, but to the illness. The child's age and general maturity will dictate how this is explained, but avoiding the topic will almost certainly cause more distress than a sensitive acknowledgment of the changes. Just as for any close adult, there can be a sense in which there is an early bereavement – an apparent loss of the well-known and loved person, to be replaced by someone who looks the same but who behaves differently.

In line with the different styles of presentation described above, the parent may be either very variable, chaotic, unpredictable and perhaps agitated, or else very unresponsive and apparently without interest in the child and his or her activities. The latter represents a more advanced stage of decline. In both cases, the child's emotional and physical well-being may be questioned. In the case of very young children, it will obviously be unsafe for them to be in the sole charge of a parent diagnosed with HIV related brain impairment unless it is very mild, and even then the situation will need to be very closely monitored. It is quite possible for a deeply caring and responsible parent with brain impairment to decline in the space of a few months to the stage where a small child is left alone locked in the house with the gas left on.

The parent will also have to be supported during this time to ensure that additional care for the child where necessary is perceived as helpful rather than intrusive or threatening.

Cross-cultural considerations

A Ugandan patient with diagnosed HIV dementia was concerned to send her son back to relations in Uganda. She kept insisting that she needed to send him together with a Xerox. The workers concerned puzzled over this and decided it was another manifestation of the bizarre thought processes and behaviour which had led to the woman leaving her child in highly dangerous circumstances. It was finally clarified by a Ugandan care organisation that with a Xerox machine a family in Uganda could earn a considerable amount. The plan was therefore entirely rational, taking into account the son's future well-being.

The above is a small example of the need to clear one's mind of assumptions and pre-conceptions in relation to a patient or carer, and to be as well informed as possible. While this is most acute in the case of people who come from a culture clearly different from the counsellor's own, factors such as age, class, occupation, religion, education and sexuality are all areas on which counsellor and patient may differ and where, therefore, the counsellor may have to take care to ensure that misunderstandings are avoided.

There is a strong argument for the counsellor developing links with the cultures and groups which patients and their carers represent. This will make it more likely not only that potential sources of misunderstanding can be clarified, but also that the counsellor may be able, even if only indirectly, to reach those patients who do not use services in the conventional way because of unfamiliarity, distrust or active fear of alien doctors and an alien style of medicine. Most of our hospitals and services are still designed essentially for those comfortable (if not entirely content) with western medicine. This can manifest itself in relation to the understanding of illness or death or even in relation to the presentation of hospital food.

The counsellor who is trying to convey an understanding of the implications of HIV in the brain for a particular patient or family may need to stop and wonder about basic ways of thinking. Do you, for example, think of the heart or the brain as the origin of thoughts? Your answer to that question is in itself likely to be culturally determined. In western Europe at least, it is common for the heart and the head to represent two different styles of responding to the world, with the brain responsible more for the rational, and the heart for the irrational. However, the involvement of the heart is seen as more symbolic than real. Most people believe that it is the brain which feels emotions and which thinks. It is accepted that damage to the brain will be responsible for a person finding it difficult to function in a number of different ways.

In other cultures, for instance in parts of East Africa, it seems that the heart is seen, in everyday terms, as being the seat of thinking in general; in everyday parlance and thinking, the heart is seen as more central to an individual's mental life than the head. This may be important in considering a person's beliefs when they are told that there are changes in the brain.

If a counsellor is using an interpreter, care must be taken that she is well briefed beforehand; for instance, in some languages dementia would be translated as madness, with implications not only for the soul or essence of a person, but even for their mortality.

Other considerations are the different types of impact which the dementia will have in different families and relationships. Some of these are considered in the next section.

Helping the carer

Partners, lovers, family and friends are likely to feel the impact of HIV dementia acutely, often even more so than the patient and, certainly, in the later stages of dementia the carer is often the counsellor's primary client. It is essential that at least the main carer involved should be offered ongoing support from the time that the diagnosis is made. Often the whole family will need some intervention. Initially the main need will be for facts and information about prognosis which will allow a fuller understanding of the implications for the immediate and long-term future. Without this, the carer may persist in beliefs such as:

- 'It will get better – they just have to find out what it is'
- 'It's all my fault that he's not talking to me'
- 'Those drugs they were giving her for PCP have really affected her'
- 'The doctors are not trying any more – all she needs is proper stimulation'.

It is numbing to discover that months after health professionals and care managers have been speaking of a patient as having diagnosed HIV dementia, the carer still has not been informed of the diagnosis or what it means. Sometimes this can occur simply because it has been assumed that the carer will hear from the patient. A moment's thought will confirm that a patient with memory impairment, a poor attention span and lack of interest in the outside world may not be a reliable informant. On the other hand, the clinician may be reluctant to start involving the carer where the patient has always been very much in control of treatment decisions and has never involved anyone else. This is perhaps the first of many shifts in emphasis and the first of many dilemmas which the professional dealing with HIV dementia is likely to face.

While every individual will react differently to the situation, there are some categories of response which are likely to recur in clinical practice and these are described below. The nature of these examples is to caricature complex responses, but they may be helpful in highlighting some of the possible issues to be dealt with.

The anxious carer

A patient with HIV dementia will not be able to function normally in everyday life and will therefore need a degree of help and supervision. Establishing the correct level of help is, however, quite difficult for a number of reasons. First of all, as explained above, an intelligent person pre-HIV dementia does not become unintelligent due to HIV. The difficulty is rather with maintaining concentration, keeping to the task in hand and remembering what one is doing and why. The ability to do these things can vary with time of day, fatigue and the number of demands on attention at any one time, and therefore lapses and times of good functioning may be variable and difficult to predict.

The natural response of a concerned and loving partner is to want to keep the patient in sight at all times. This may happen gradually in response to changes in the patient, or the carer may suddenly become much more concerned once he or she understands the reason for the patient requiring supervision. The patient, however, may perceive the situation rather differently and feel restricted, intruded upon and humiliated by a new level of 'interference' with personal issues such as financial transactions. Depending also on the level of insight of the patient, there may be a high level of frustration and a desperate attempt to maintain control. For someone with poor insight, there may appear to be no reason for concern – say about road safety or reliability when preparing food. In this case the counsellor's role is often to discuss what might be considered an acceptable level of risk for the carer on the one hand and for the patient on the other, and to negotiate an agreement if possible.

One tack may be to separate the feelings of concern and anxiety for the well-being of the patient, the sense of responsibility for that well-being that the carer may be carrying, and the actual need for the patient to maintain as much autonomy as possible. The situation may be seen by the participants as either total 'restraint' or total supervision; in many cases there can be a solution acceptable to both. For example, the patient may enjoy the preparation of food but could have a buddy or home care assistant visiting during those times if the carer is out at work. The patient may agree to keep excursions short and local and the carer may have to accept a certain level of risk for these excursions.

The ambivalent carer

There may be many reasons for a carer's ambivalence. The professional may have to take time to discover the nature of the relationship between the carer and the patient before the advent of HIV dementia. Most relationships have their weak spots. The carer may feel that the changed situation is the last straw, may see it as an opportunity for escape, or may be trying to resign herself to battling through. A mother caring for her adult son, for example, may be distressed and disturbed to find herself again treating him like a child, when she had learnt to look to him for support.

A carer who is also HIV seropositive may be afraid of the dementia as presenting a spectre of their own future, but a future which may be experienced alone without anyone to take the caring role. Whilst previously the couple may have shared their diagnosis as well as the rest of their lives, now the carer may be left not only 'alone' emotionally, with an unresponsive or unsupportive partner, but alone with many of the burdens of everyday living that were previously shared. It is understandable under those circumstances that the carer may feel loving but at the same time resentful and over-stretched.

Whatever the reason for the ambivalence, it is helpful if the counsellor can allow the carer to express the difficulties frankly without fear of censure. Humans seem capable of feeling a range of apparently incompatible emotions towards the same person. Accepting this as normal can be reassuring. There is no one perfect model of caring to which people should be expected to adhere. However, each individual in that role may have a range of demanding self-expectations which need to be examined.

The guilty carer

Guilt may be a by-product of the ambivalence described above, or it may be the response of a carer who feels the need to keep the patient entirely happy and satisfied but is naturally unable to achieve this. The expression of guilt can disguise another set of feelings – perhaps a difficulty in accepting the reality and the irreversibility of the changes in the partner and blaming the failure to improve on some more personal failure.

Guilt and frustration in the carer will need to be explored carefully so that both the counsellor and the carer can go beyond these feelings to maximise the potential in the relationship left between the patient and carer.

The belligerent carer

Not all carers will welcome professionals of any sort and particularly those bearing bad news. There may be hostility towards the professionals as representative of a service, or the professional may simply be in the line of fire for the carer expressing a general level of anger and frustration.

> The wife in one African family was furious with her husband who had HIV dementia for having stopped going to work and for failing to carry out his duties of care towards her and her family. Her perception of him was that he had become lazy and thoughtless and probably had another woman because of his apathy towards her. (This despite the fact that he hardly ever left the house.) The couple had recently lost a child who had died of AIDS and there was considerable residual anger towards the hospital for having administered AZT which they felt had prompted the child's demise.

Dealing with the couple's joint sadness over their child and taking some of the household burdens off the wife so that she was less stretched, allowed her to listen and accept the nature of her husband's difficulties and to turn to other family members for the emotional support she needed.

The dissatisfied carer

Sometimes frustration and anger may emerge less obviously than in the above case, by a constant nit-picking about elements of the service received. This may present itself as a series of phone calls to various professionals complaining about services or difficulties encountered. While it could be that these are genuine and need to be tackled, carers sometimes feel that they can only really get access to professionals by talking about practical, rather than emotional, concerns. Complaining about others may also relieve a sense of helplessness or being out of control which the onset of dementia in a partner or family member may provoke.

In addition to keeping an eye on the actual grievances, a tactful acknowledgment that the carer is over-burdened and needs some personal space to talk about the impact of HIV dementia may relieve the pressure on other hospital services.

The over-active carer

Staff looking after patients with dementia sometimes say something like: 'I can never get a reply out of Johnny; Bill always answers for him. Bill's never off the ward and he's always monitoring what we try to do . . .'

Carers can gradually start to compensate for the increasing passivity, verbal slowness and confusion in their partner or relative by becoming their spokesperson. This may be motivated by the wish to avoid the person being humiliated or to conceal the difficulties from others, or even by the need to deny the existence of any problems. It can also be a way of trying to keep others out of a private relationship, of not letting the patient get 'taken over' by professionals and thus taken away from the carer. In addition, of course, not all medical services are equally sensitive or equally willing to acknowledge the central role of carers, and the over-activity may be a bid for attention.

The over-active carer is almost bound to come to a crisis point when it is no longer possible to prevent others noticing and challenging the attempt to keep professionals from communicating direct with the patient. The counsellor can help by offering support to the carer, acknowledging the caring role and seeking further information from the carer about the patient and their relationship.

In the case of one very vociferous and over-active carer, it emerged that staff had correctly surmised that there was quite an abusive relationship between carer and patient and that the patient was quite afraid of his partner. Once the intensity of feeling in the carer had been acknowledged in the couple, the difficulties around the medical care were dissipated. With therapy the couple were able to discuss some of the pressures around them and the patient was also given a 'voice' in spite of his difficulties in self-expression.

The role change carer

Carers who are forced into a change of role within the relationship may find the adjustment particularly difficult, although occasionally it can also be a liberation. It is useful to explore with carers the extent to which there has been a role shift for them in relation to the patient, and the implications of this.

It is also important to be alert for over-identification with the caring role. Although not always the case, it is likely that the patient will die first. The carer will then be stripped of that role and will revert to the person he or she was before. Emphasising the need to care for oneself and to maintain the threads of one's previous pre-carer life, can allow the person to deal with bereavement more easily.

The unbelieving carer

CARER: 'He's always been like that – he never kept a diary. I always had to do the practical things anyway. He's not interested in organising himself. I don't know what you mean about this HIV in the brain. He's going through a hard time and he doesn't want to talk to anyone at the moment.'

CARER: 'I think you're wrong about this psychotic episode. He's experiencing an emotional re-birth. This has been a long time coming and I'm so pleased. He's been under a lot of stress and this will make it all better so long as you don't try to write him off with this HIV in the brain idea.'

The first point to remember is that the carer may be right, depending on the evidence to hand. If the carer is having difficulty in coming to terms with the situation, the easiest way forward may be to accept the carer's perception as one alternative explanation and to keep the 'HIV in the brain' as another. The counsellor and the carer can hopefully then join forces in trying to support the patient, whichever explanation holds good. There is never any point in trying to convince or argue, only in trying to ensure that no-one suffers as the result of any perceptions involved.

The wonderful carer

Some of the above sections may suggest that carers are demanding or problematic as a group. On the contrary, many appear to find resources in themselves and in the relationship with the patient which allow them not only to manage, but to intensify their closeness and to experience the meaning of their love through the demands made on them.

Carers have said that what they most need is:

- Accurate information
- Practical help
- Someone central to communicate with
- The opportunity to discuss problems as they arise, rather than from week to week
- Time for setting aside the day to day difficulties to consider their own emotional needs as they change
- To be allowed to laugh and enjoy things with the patient without being expected to be downhearted all the time.

Groups for carers

We have set up a group for the carers of people with HIV dementia, which allows experiences and information to be shared and passed on. The group is focused on the idea of preparing others for the task and this helps to give some perspective to the situation in which they find themselves.

One of the main issues to emerge is the sense of emotional loneliness in cases where the patient with HIV dementia is withdrawn and therefore no longer offers 'cuddles and concern'. The shell of the relationship seems to be there, without the 'pearl' as it were. There then has to be new exploration of the emotional aspects of the relationship, but knowing that this can often be achieved by a shifting of style and expectation is reassuring. Spending time together in pleasant places, listening to music looking at photographs, touching, being with friends – all these can continue and hold the thread of relationship.

However, many carers agree on the importance of acknowledging the existence of a 'pre-bereavement' process. There is a sense in which they 'lose' the relationship they had before its due time and this can lead to intense feelings of regret and anger towards the patient. This is natural, and expression of these feelings often allows more room to the more positive feelings.

One carer, however, said: 'I think of her as gradually slipping away from me, of becoming enveloped in a fog, like floating away into the distance. I feel sad but it allows me to feel the sadness of losing her little by little. One day I know she won't be there but maybe then I will be able to think that she is just invisible through the mist.'

Counselling professional carers

As discussed earlier, the brain impairment aspect of HIV infection is one which can evoke strong emotional responses from patients and carers alike. Staff can feel helpless, over-stretched and consequently irritable with a brain impaired patient who is constantly wandering off the ward or making demands for a constant flow of sandwiches and tea – as though under the illusion that the ward is some luxury hotel. If at all possible a behaviourally disturbed patient with HIV related brain impairment should be 'special-ed' on a medical ward, either by a psychiatric nurse or by a nurse with some appropriate experience. Concomitant psychotropic medication is likely to help any extreme behavioural disturbance within the space of a few days, although occasionally a few weeks may be required.

Staff can gain a great deal of support through, for example:

- Good understanding of the causes of the behaviour, personality and cognitive changes
- Occupational therapy support to prevent the patient getting bored and wandering
- Guidelines for communicating with the patient, with emphasis on simplifying communications, writing down any instructions and trying to keep ward procedures as predictable as the patient's condition permits
- The availability of a counsellor who will see the patient and the informal carers
- Some discussion of the feelings raised by individual patients and how this can influence the staff's interaction with them.

Overview

While HIV dementia and its related problems pose a real challenge to our services, there appears to be increasing impetus to acknowledging the difficulties posed by this aspect of HIV and offering a human and thoughtful response. As we become more able to talk openly about the issues with patients and carers, we are likely to dissolve yet another taboo.

Acknowledgments

Much of the material in this chapter has been put forward by patients and carers themselves, clear about separating the useful from the merely well-meaning. Other issues have arisen through discussions with colleagues and other professionals through the courses I have run at the National AIDS Counselling Training Unit. Particular acknowledgment is due to Matthew Shaw, Janet White, Ulrike Schmidt and Kirstin Aginkgube who are members of the Neuropsychiatric Working Party at St Mary's Hospital, London, to Betty Feldman who gives carers a voice, and to my colleagues Graham Frize and Paul Chadwick. Last but not least the charity AVERT provided funding for research which was the foundation stone for all the work described here.

References

HIV, AIDS and the Brain Price, R.W. & Perry, S.W. (eds) (1994). Raven Press, New York.

Chapter 7

The Counselling of HIV Antibody Positive Haemophiliacs

Peter Jones

By the end of July 1992, a decade into the HIV epidemic, the majority of people with haemophilia or a related bleeding disorder who were infected with the human immunodeficiency virus (HIV) as a direct result of their treatment in the UK, were alive. The need for counselling them, and their relatives and friends, remains. There is also a continuing need for the care of those who have been bereaved. The counselling required is time consuming, often repetitive and sometimes emotionally draining. It requires a long-term commitment to the person and to his or her family. As Mark Winter has pointed out (Winter 1991), such a commitment needs to recognise that each family is 'a unique collection of individuals who happen to be related, all of them responding in a different way to the same crisis'.

The full extent of HIV infection in the haemophilic population of industrialised countries only became apparent in 1985. In that year antibody testing revealed that the majority of people treated with multi-donor clotting factor concentrates within the preceding five years had been infected. Paradoxically, most people with haemophilia living in developing countries without recourse to modern therapy had escaped this iatrogenic infection. What was not known in 1985 was the likely extent of overt disease in those testing positive for HIV antibody. As time passed early optimism that the majority of those infected would remain well had to be tempered, from estimates that only one in a thousand would eventually develop overt disease to realisation that a majority would eventually progress to AIDS. The increasingly gloomy prognosis meant that the foundation of counselling, reliant as it is on factual information, shifted rapidly, with the speed of change adding to uncertainty in the case of both counsellors and counselled. Most people can accept and adapt to bad news quickly and remarkably well, but uncertainty increases the likelihood of failure to come to terms with adversity. Uncertainty was increased by difficulties in being able to give a realistic prognosis, ill-founded arguments about casual spread, and disagreements about testing and management within the health care professions made public by unprecedented media hyperbole. In consequence, effective counselling of individuals, their partners and their families had to be continually adapted to the changing picture of the epidemic.

In that respect infected people with haemophilia are no different from others carrying the virus. In other respects there are differences, often profound, which had to be recognised if haemophilic families were to be given adequate help. Most differences hinged on the underlying coagulation disorder, but some reflected feelings about the lifestyles of other groups of people primarily involved in the early stages of the epidemic in western society. Susman-Shaw (1991) has remarked that 'families with haemophilia and HIV infection have two life threatening disorders to contend with simultaneously'. In order to exercise control over the first they are reliant on the goodwill of blood donors, many of whom are paid. In the early stages of the epidemic the media focused on these donors, and emphasised the links that then existed between payment and intravenous drug abuse, and between altruism and homosexuality. Small wonder that the initial anger of some of those with haemophilia was focused on these groups, which were simultaneously being labelled as having a very high risk of transmitting HIV infection, and thus AIDS.

The background of haemophilia

In order to understand why the counselling of people with haemophilia is so often different from the counselling of others, it is necessary to understand the profound effect that the clotting disorder alone can have on individual and family health.

Haemophilia is an inherited disorder of blood coagulation. The genetic defect is present on one of the X chromosomes and it is this sex-linked recessive mode of inheritance that results in females (XX) being carriers, and males (XY) having haemophilia. There is thus an immediate analogy to HIV infection, which may be carried unknowingly in the cells of people who are otherwise healthy, and who look and feel perfectly well.

Among haemophiliacs 70% have a family history of the disorder but in 30% it arises *de novo*, the most celebrated example being Queen Victoria who passed the defective gene to her daughters Alice and Beatrice, who were carriers like her, and to her son Leopold who had severe haemophilia. Like other carriers of genetic disease Victoria suffered the guilt of knowing that some of her descendants, notably those in the Russian and Spanish royal families, had been burdened by a defect passed on to them directly from herself. At least she was spared the remorse of many of today's carrier mothers who feel that their haemophilic sons also became infected with HIV as a direct result of their actions in giving them treatment for their bleeding episodes.

Clinically haemophilia presents as recurrent bleeds into joints and muscles. These closed bleeds, which account for over 95% of all bleeding episodes, continue until the pressure exerted by the tissues surrounding the bleeding site equals the pressure of escaping blood. This means that joints become swollen, tense and exquisitely painful. Eventually the bleed stops and the blood within the joint is slowly reabsorbed, iron and other breakdown products passing into the synovial membrane which responds to the irritation by becoming hypertrophic. The function of the healthy synovium is to secrete an oily fluid into the major joints of the body, helping to provide friction-free movement. As with all secretory tissue this membrane is richly endowed with blood vessels and it is these that rupture and haemorrhage. Hypertrophic disruption of the membrane not only increases the likelihood of repeated bleeds but also prevents secretion of synovial fluid, and friction-free movement is lost. Thus the long-term sequela of the underlying disorder of coagulation is a chronic, painful arthropathy.

The fact that the great majority of bleeds in haemophilia are internal is of fundamental importance when assessing the risk of spread of a blood-borne disease like HIV infection.

Contrary to popular belief, haemophiliacs do not bleed uncontrollably from scratches, small cuts or pin-pricks; the body's protective mechanisms for these are intact. Nor do they bleed externally any more than other people, nose bleeds or blood in the urine being the most usual manifestations. The chances of contamination of the environment and therefore of other people from someone with haemophilia are therefore negligible.

Frequency of bleeding varies with age, being commoner in childhood and adolescence. On average the severely affected haemophiliac has 35 spontaneous bleeding episodes a year. Most of these are recognised within a few minutes of starting, the patient experiencing an 'aura' of unease in the joint. Treatment at this time aborts the bleed and allows an immediate return to normal activity.

Because early treatment prevents disability and because it must be given before the appearance of any physical signs, the foundation of modern haemophilia therapy is one of trust between doctor and patient, and the patient's family. In the early days of the HIV epidemic, AIDS had a profound effect on that trust and a great deal of time and repetitive counselling were needed to restore rapport with the families. In some cases this was made especially difficult because of continuing litigation.

Treatment as the source of infection

There are two types of haemophilia: A and B. Haemophilia B is five times less common than A and in Britain is also known as Christmas disease after the first patient to be found affected. In haemophilia A the biological activity of the clotting protein factor VIII is absent or reduced. In haemophilia B factor IX is affected. Treatment of both conditions is usually relatively straightforward, the defect being corrected by injection of the relevant factor into a vein.

The source material for both factor VIII and factor IX is human blood. In the 1950s and 1960s haemophiliacs needing treatment had to be admitted to hospital to have their factor VIII or IX dripped into them in the form of whole fresh blood or plasma which had been frozen shortly after donation and thawed just before use. The materials had to be freshly prepared because the factors have a short life at body temperature, half the administered dose disappearing within 12 hours. The logistics of therapy were therefore difficult and patients missed much of their education and subsequently their employment prospects because they were in hospital so often. Their alternative was not to treat the majority of bleeds, but inevitably this led to severe crippling within a few years. As a result, many of the older generation of haemophiliacs were already disadvantaged, both socially and physically, before the advent of AIDS. The depth of the handicap imposed by inadequately treated severe haemophilia is revealed by the judgement of many adult patients, who have said that HIV infection has been a worthwhile penalty for the decade or so of good therapy they have been able to enjoy since the introduction of clotting factor concentrates, home treatment and comprehensive care.

In the 1960s it became possible to separate factor VIII from most other plasma components with ease. The resultant material, cryoprecipitate, was of small volume and could be given by syringe or fast-running drip, so bleeds could be treated without having to admit patients to hospital. Unfortunately cryoprecipitate has to be stored in a deep-frozen state in order to preserve its factor VIII content and once thawed several packs have to be pooled together to make up the correct dose. The answer to this problem lay in freeze drying, and the era of commercially viable concentrate production began. Using plasma, or cryoprecipitate derived from it as source material, factor VIII and factor IX are fractionated into highly concentrated, low volume doses. Freeze drying stabilises each dose in a single vial which can then be stored at room temperature and mixed with sterile water to reconstitute biologically active material.

In the 1970s the ease of storage, preparation and use of concentrate revolutionised haemophilia care. Patients (or their parents) were taught how to treat themselves at home and the bonds which had previously tied families to hospitals were severed. Haemophiliacs on home therapy with factor VIII or IX are similar to diabetics on self-administered insulin and, like diabetics, some were soon using their injections to prevent bleeding episodes, a form of management called prophylaxis. This, and the early treatment of bleeds before any significant damage had occurred, resulted in the normal physical and social growth of affected children. The incidence of severe arthritis declined and haemophiliacs began to compete as equals with their non-affected peers at school and work, and in many sports.

In order to achieve this remarkable advance in medical care and improved quality of life, the blood plasma of many donors was required. Factor VIII in particular is a labile protein, each step in fractionation lowering the yield of biologically active material in the end product. Therefore, unlike single-donor cryoprecipitate which, when pooled, might expose the adult patients to 10 or 15 donations, the concentrates required multiple donations, and a prerequisite of the development of the fractionation plants was the supply of large volumes of source material, up to 30 000 donations fuelling one run of concentrate production. Volunteer donor systems, like that serving the UK, could not then compete with the commercial sector which could draw on the plasma of paid donors chiefly living in the US, and in 1973 the importation of factor VIII concentrates into the UK was approved by government.

Prior to the introduction of measures designed to exclude viral contamination of finished product, exposure to multi-donor concentrates inevitably increased the risk of disease transmission. As the incidence of hepatitis B and hepatitis C in the haemophiliac population rose, it became clear that viruses could survive both fractionation and freeze drying. Vaccination against hepatitis B gave some protection, but surrogate testing by performing liver function tests on donor blood was only partially successful in the elimination of risk from hepatitis C. However, although the price of such treatment could be chronic liver disease, the balance was still tipped very much in the haemophiliac's favour. Prior to the modern era of therapy afforded by concentrates, early disability and premature death were commonplace, and before HIV infection the majority of those with severe haemophilia could expect to live a good quality life of normal longevity.

Specific problems relating to HIV positive haemophiliacs

To date the majority of those infected with HIV in the population have been either sexually active adults or children born to infected mothers. In contrast, those infected as a result of contaminated blood or blood product transfusions may be of any age, and in the UK the highest prevalence of infection in haemophilia was in adolescence. This meant that counselling had to be tailored to age and to the wishes of parents, as well as to the circumstances and understanding of older patients and their partners. Because infected haemophilic youngsters faced a bleak future it is not surprising that many parents did not want to burden them with knowledge of their infection. However, the advent of anti-viral and other therapy changed this very understandable attitude earlier than most of us would perhaps like.

Ironically, when parents have eventually plucked up sufficient courage to tell their youngster the truth, they have often found he or she knew already. One boy said that he had not wanted to frighten his parents by telling them he knew (Jones 1991). Whether or not secrecy is preserved, those caring for young people must be alert to the strengths and weaknesses of the family as well as to the needs of the infected children. Above all else this means time: time spent just listening, time spent answering questions, time spent sorting out the vagaries of childhood illnesses and fads from the more sinister manifestations of AIDS related disease, time spent in homes as well as hospitals and, increasingly, time involving family doctors and their staff.

Most haemophilia centres adopted an open-door policy for their families before the HIV epidemic. Haemophiliacs could phone or call in for immediate help with bleeds or other problems at any time. This service had to be hospital-based because this was where the therapeutic materials for haemophilia were stored and dispensed, with prescription often requiring laboratory investigation and guidance. However, the treatment of acute episodes in hospital is only one facet of a haemophiliac's life, and as a result many haemophilia centres try to bring together all the facets by providing comprehensive care. With the active participation of doctors, dentists, nurses, physiotherapists, social workers and members of other professional groups and the lay Haemophilia Society, the aim of this approach is to anticipate and hopefully solve problems relating to subjects as diverse as joint replacement surgery, bullying at school, careers guidance and genetic counselling.

This multidisciplinary approach has served the families well, and has been suggested as the template for the care of others with AIDS in the community (Jones 1987). One of the great strengths of this approach is that the core team with direct responsibility for patient care remains the same, and whatever the circumstances there is always a familiar face for the patient and his or her family to respond to. This is particularly important when admission to hospital becomes necessary, especially if the patient is already confused, in early dementia or is terminally ill. The worst place for anybody with AIDS-related disease to be nursed is in isolation in a small white room in an unfamiliar hospital by staff they do not already know and without immediate access to a telephone to enable them to talk to their family or friends at any time.

A shortcoming of the haemophilia model, partly because of the bias to hospital care and partly because of the rarity of the disorder, has been the lack of involvement of most general practitioners. With HIV infection this is beginning to change – a welcome advance given the crucial and pivotal role the family doctors will have in the management of the epidemic as it continues to spread from the high risk groups into the general community.

It is unfortunate that the pattern of the AIDS epidemic in the west has had such a profound influence on our response. The close link between AIDS, male homosexuality and intravenous drug abuse has led naturally to the disease becoming the prerogative of the units for sexually transmitted disease and drug addiction. The strict confidentiality that has to operate in these clinics, coupled with the prejudice felt and reacted to by these minority groups, has tended to remove AIDS from the remit of many doctors and to reduce the effectiveness of health education within the community. It has also resulted in the isolation of infected individuals, sometimes unable to confide in their families about their sexuality, or in those most equipped to help them. Infected people living in large cities may have recourse to one of the voluntary organisations or to local hospital staff used to coping with the problems of HIV infection; those in other areas often suffer in silence. For them AIDS is a sad, lonely and secret disease.

These attitudes colour the lives and thus the counselling of haemophiliacs and their families. Those living in small communities may not want their family doctor, previously trusted with their medical record, to be aware of their infection in case that record is seen and commented on by someone else working in the surgery. Young men may not disclose their haemophilia to girlfriends or to employers because of public awareness of the association between haemophilia and AIDS. Parents are still wary of enlisting the help of school teachers to keep an eye on infected children who may be experiencing difficulties in learning or behaviour. Even uninfected, HIV antibody negative children have suffered because it has been difficult to reveal their status without implying that other children are positive.

Anticipating some of the problems

Although counselling or social work intervention may be needed at any time, the stress of HIV infection or AIDS increases at certain stages in the life of the haemophiliac. Anticipating these stages and gently guiding people before the associated problems arise helps them to cope more effectively.

The schoolboy

Before the advent of specific therapy it was our experience that it was rare for younger boys to be told by their parents about their HIV infection. Although this situation is changing in families it does not mean that parents are yet ready to share the information with others. However, because both school teachers and peers know about their haemophilia, assumptions may be made and the child harmed by segregation or bullying. Much of this is readily preventable and parents should be counselled to consult their child's haemophilia centre doctor immediately a problem they cannot deal with arises.

Among the difficulties which may present in school as a result of HIV infection are delayed cognitive development and failure to thrive. As immune competence fails in these children, live vaccines may be contra-indicated and prophylactic immunoglobulin may be needed, given either intravenously in order to prevent infections in general or as specific immune globulin. Other difficulties which are more easily resolved by talking to and reassuring staff have been fear of casual contact, and concern about sports and trips abroad. Bullying has affected some children but most haemophilic boys are remarkably robust and taunts of 'Aidsy' are met with the physical retaliation they deserve. However, despite this resilience, it is the norm for young people to conceal both their haemophilia and their infection believing, quite rightly, that it is their business. In the settings of general practice or hospital consultation this attitude disappears. Like most adults, youngsters need the confidence of knowing that their doctors and nurses are being straight with them, and sharing information. In general, children should be active partners in all decisions made about themselves.

Adolescence

Boys maturing to be at ease with their bodies, their sexuality and their relationships with other people in the context of their haemophilia now have the additional burden imposed by the threat of AIDS. Abrupt or insensitive counselling of young men who are beginning to 'feel different' from their peers because of their inherited disorder adds to their alienation. It can be avoided by the gradual establishment of trust afforded by seeing each boy informally and in privacy on several occasions without parents or siblings, and by careful physical examination without paraphernalia of gloves or other protective clothing. This both demonstrates his normality and helps to reassure him that his doctor is not frightened by the infection.

Additional reassurance should come from talk about planning for a future career. HIV infection does not preclude adolescents from taking competitive exams and entering higher education or long term employment. At the present stage of our knowledge it is not possible to suggest individual prognoses and the introduction of antiviral agents may well halt or at least slow down the progression of the disease. What we can say is that there appear to be long term survivors of HIV infection. This good news helps keep hope alive and helps underline the determination of most families that their youngsters' lives be allowed to proceed as normally as possible.

We have always counselled haemophilic adolescents about the inheritance of their disorder so that they and their future wives can make up their own minds about starting a family. This counselling has included advice about contraception and informal and free access to condoms. AIDS has meant that this help has had to be extended to encompass safer sex, a term of ominous significance which intimidates youngsters not yet aware of the joys of 'ordinary' sex. In this respect a booklet from the Haemophilia Society (1990) in the UK has been most welcome.

We do not yet know what effect the knowledge that they may infect girlfriends or wives and their babies is going to have on the long term psychological and social health of haemophiliacs. Our limited experience is that youngsters seem to cope remarkably well with the news, at least in the short term. Some have decided to marry and have children despite long, detailed and repeated explanations of risk from staff often more worried about the future for their patients than the patients are themselves. One rather worrying aspect of these decisions is that the young couple may become isolated from parents opposed to the marriage. This is especially tragic in extended families with a long history of haemophilia and in which several relatives are infected with HIV, because the disruption caused adds to the uncertainty of the disease. It also creates additional work for the haemophilia centre team, who may have to assume responsibility for the follow-up and treatment of the wives and children of their original patient.

The adult

Infected haemophiliacs who were already married at the start of the epidemic have had to work their way through a very frightening and often bewildering series of questions and doubts. Had they already infected their wives? Were the children safe? What were the chances of spread of infection in the future, and were these increased by continuing treatment for their haemophilia? How would knowledge of HIV infection affect employment? Could they still get insurance cover and plan for the future stability of the family and the family home? Was travel abroad still possible, in particular to the US where the need to apply for special permission by waiver was, and still is, seen as an invasion of privacy and an affront to human rights.

These and many other questions relating to the health and financial security of the family were often posed by men feeling the remorse of 'having let the wife and children down' by exposing them both to infection and to an uncertain future. This guilt had been recognised early and talked over openly in counselling because it was leading to increasing isolation of the patient within his own family. Typically an initial reaction was to withdraw from having sexual intercourse, and to be fearful of handling young children. Repeated reassurance was needed, and was helped by seeing the whole family together in a relaxed and informal atmosphere, reserving more formal counselling sessions for husband and wife alone. The hereditary nature of haemophilia meant that affected fathers with carrier daughters were fearful for the health of grandchildren whom they may not live to see. They needed reassurance, both from the point of view of the safety of current and future treatment, and its effectiveness in alleviating or even curing the haemostatic disorder.

Despite the reassurance afforded by government statements on security of employment for infected people, knowledge of HIV infection presents a threat to some jobs. The problem arises most frequently in jobs involving contact with the general public, caterers, publicans, teachers and health care workers perceiving especial difficulty. Whilst the public remain unconvinced of the absence of casual spread of AIDS, their preference may be to drink in the pub not owned or run by a severely affected haemophiliac. This, of course, provides another reason to conceal the underlying disorder and, yet again, isolates the individual from his community.

Everyday health and activities

As a result of their chronic arthritis pain, most severely affected haemophiliacs have relatively easy access to analgesic drugs. Some have become reliant on alcohol or hypnotics in order to ease the pain, particularly at night, while others react to their stress by resorting to heavy smoking. In the context of HIV infection two factors are important. First, the addition of stress imposed by the knowledge of HIV positivity can result in further reliance on drugs, and secondly there is general agreement that most, if not all, of these substances taken in excess may be co-factors in helping to tip antibody positive people into overt disease.

In common with the counselling given to other groups about lifestyle, haemophiliacs should be encouraged to lead healthy and active lives. Whilst advice about good diet, plenty of exercise, and sound sleep might appeal to the younger generations, it is easier said than done for older people. In particular, families already suffering financial hardship because of loss of work simply cannot afford the recommended high protein diets unless they are lucky enough to obtain state assistance. Voluntary organisations like the Haemophilia Society are of immense importance in helping to cope with this aspect of HIV infection, as indeed they are in helping with many other aspects of individual and family support.

Group, behavioural and relaxation therapy have a part to play but sometimes the depression commonly associated with HIV becomes so profound that only medication can help and it is important that anti-depressant therapy is considered early in the course of the disease. Some patients are helped by techniques considered by many as alternative medicine, despite the lack of benefit revealed by formal clinical trial. If relaxation tapes, reflexology or aromatherapy help the individual they are to be encouraged; at the very least they can do no harm. Acupuncture is safe in those with haemophilia, although it is my practice to recommend haemostatic cover.

In the case of infected haemophiliacs, government compensation has helped, and the Macfarlane Trust, which administers a sum of public money set aside to relieve identified hardship, has been of tremendous help to many families with infected relatives.

We have seen particular benefit to the health and happiness of HIV infected people who have participated in a friendship scheme offering confidential support on a one-to-one basis. In our case the scheme has flourished because of the commitment and enthusiasm of a group of students, helped by their tutors and the centre social workers. Similar schemes exist in many parts of the world, notably in the Shanti Project in California.

Some observations on HIV and sex

A fascinating aspect of the epidemic has been to see some of the reactions of both individuals and couples to the HIV public health education on sex. The lower than expected incidence of infection in the general population, together with the extending interval between infection and disease, have resulted in a situation in which it is not unusual for people to put AIDS low on their list of factors to take into account in their decision making. When this happens the drive to have unprotected intercourse, perhaps reinforced by alcohol and sometimes with the aim of achieving pregnancy, overcomes doubts about possible disease transmission. This is especially evident in late adolescence and early adulthood, and should not be confused with denial. Rather it is a normal reaction to a threat that is perceived as remote and with little immediate relevance to getting on with life.

Conventional medicine is concerned with disease and its treatment. It has a long way to go to catch up with life. Most of this chapter is concerned with convention, with a little flavouring added by the experience of families who are withstanding the holocaust created by a small, previously insignificant, retrovirus. I say 'withstanding', not 'withstood', deliberately, because HIV infection and all it means to us and those we treat is not static. To begin to understand one must sense movement, the dynamics of how people respond to threat. Until we do, the essentials of the pandemic will elude us. People do not live by statistics and the advice of experts. They live by intuition, by feeling, by family, and by trust. Denial and anger are very much second class citizens to the zest for life, and to the procreation of that life.

Other effects of HIV infection on an individual's psychosexual life are self evident and are covered elsewhere in this book. One effect we have noted in the couples attending the haemophilia centre is the gradually changing role of the wives. Usually uninfected themselves, their relationship with their husbands changes from the equality of active sexual partnership to the provision of tender loving care. Often sexual contact ceases altogether and the woman adopts the role of mother to her ailing partner.

Fear of death

Some of the most frequent questions asked by infected people relate to the nature of death from AIDS. One of the effects of all the publicity, and of the secrecy surrounding the disease, appears to be a perception by some patients that HIV related death is in some way horribly different from death from other causes. Patients express their fears by asking if they will 'look different' or 'go mad'. They are curious to know what happens at and immediately after death. Will their relatives be allowed in the room and be able to touch and hold them? Does there have to be an autopsy and a public inquest with all the resultant publicity and harassment of widow and other relatives? Will they have to be cremated?

The answers are, of course, that death from AIDS is as quiet and dignified as any non-accidental death, that patients look no different, that they will not be left alone to die and that they can be held and comforted by their relatives, that they can be buried and that there is no need for autopsy or inquest in the normal course of events. The only difference from the majority of deaths is that the body is sealed in a cadaver bag soon after the event (as with other infectious diseases like hepatitis B) so that the family must take their leave of their relative at the bedside, and will not be able to view him later (see Chapter 14).

The concern about 'going mad' is linked to earlier predictions of a high incidence of dementia associated with AIDS. People need to be reassured that AIDS encephalopathy and dementia usually result in a quiet decline in mental faculties rather than in disruption or violence (see Chapter 6). However, it is the neurological and psychiatric manifestations of AIDS that present one of the major difficulties in health and social care. Incontinence, occasional aberrant behaviour which requires sedation, and an increasing need for constant supervision, mean that some families are unable to cope with relatives dying at home.

Finally, patients need to be reassured that strenuous efforts at resuscitation will not be undertaken if death within a few weeks seems inevitable.

Bereavement counsellor

The care of the haemophilic family does not cease on the death of the index patient. Firstly, the hereditary nature of haemophilia dictates long term follow-up of obligatory or putative carriers. Secondly, most (but not all) families will be dependent on help from haemophilia centre staff for at least the first six months of bereavement.

The intricacies of the UK social security system mean that very detailed counselling and practical help should be available for widows and other dependants. Benefits previously available to the patient, and therefore enjoyed by his family, will be withdrawn. As these often include provision both of transport and of a telephone, remaining members of the family who cannot afford their replacement may be isolated at just the time they need to communicate with and seek the solace of others.

We have found informal group meetings of widows, and occasionally of widowers or bereaved fathers, especially helpful. This group, like one run for the mothers of infected children, meets regularly with a social worker to compare experiences and provide individual comfort. Although most meetings take place in the evening in the hospital, the occasional foray into the nearest wine bar or pizzeria is not unheard of. It is salutary to find that it is the sense of humour and friendship of those who have lost relatives because of contamination of treatment, that helps support the staff who prescribed it.

The staff

Staff health is of paramount importance if patients and their families are to be helped. Members of staff in haemophilia centres will have known their patients for many years, and may have been present at the births and marriages of people now dying of AIDS. In this context, which is unique in the epidemic, teamwork is essential and administrators must be made aware of the need for adequate levels of staffing and accommodation, and adequate provision for holidays, sport and relaxation.

As well as treating HIV related illness, staff remain responsible for the full gamut of haemophilia care. Home therapy programmes must be maintained, regular follow-up assessments including musculoskeletal measurement kept, and major reconstructive and dental surgery undertaken. In common with other teams we have easy access to the help of psychiatric or psychological colleagues, but for the most part have relied on the resources already present within the centre prior to AIDS.

In the early days of the epidemic, staff members were tested for HIV antibody because no one had accurate knowledge about casual spread. It has been very reassuring to find that everyone was, and has remained, seronegative within the context of an informal medical setting in which simple common sense and hygiene provide the only protection. Staff wash their hands with soap and water after examining or attending to an infected patient, they wear gloves when taking or administering blood, and they wipe contaminated surfaces down with sodium hypochlorite. Dentists are encouraged to wear eye and mouth protection as well as gloves, and patients are warned about this in advance. In the operating theatre or delivery suite those staff immediately concerned with the procedure wear disposable theatre clothing, plastic aprons and eye protection. Infected people requiring inpatient care are nursed in the open ward unless cubicle or barrier nursing is required because of their preference or because of their presenting illness.

The medical and nursing care of people with AIDS and their families is straightforward, safe and rewarding. The sooner HIV related illness is approached and treated as a disease within the mainstream of medical practice, the better it will be for everyone involved, especially our patients.

References

Haemophilia Society (1990) *Haemophilia, HIV and safer sex – the choice is here.* Haemophilia Society, 123 Westminster Bridge Road, London SE1 7HR.

Jones, P. (1987) AIDS – planning for our future. *Social Work Today*, 9 Feb, pp 10–12.

Jones, P. (1991) HIV and AIDS. In: *Living with Haemophilia*. Oxford University Press, Oxford.

Susman-Shaw, A. (1991) Nursing care of children with haemophilia and HIV infection. In: *Caring for Children with HIV and AIDS* (eds R. Claxton & T. Harrison). Edward Arnold, London.

Winter, M. (1991) The care and management of children with haemophilia and HIV infection. In *Caring for Children with HIV and AIDS* (eds R. Claxton & T. Harrison). Edward Arnold, London.

Chapter 8

Drug Users and HIV Infection

Brian Whitehead

'We must be prepared to work with those who continue to use drugs, to help them reduce the risk involved in doing so, above all the risk of acquiring or spreading HIV. Reaching this less motivated group will necessitate a more proactive approach and a readiness to work initially towards goals that fall short of abstinence ... there are however no master strokes which will deliver the achievement of these goals ... the greatest benefit is more likely to accrue from the sum of multiple small gains derived from an integrated and responsive strategy than from any one single approach.'

Advisory Council on the Misuse of Drugs (1988)

Background

It has now been slightly over ten years since the first report of AIDS among injecting drug users in Edinburgh and London. In those years much has been learnt about HIV and AIDS among this group. Evidence from many countries indicates that long term drug injectors have high rates of AIDS and are changing their behaviour to avoid the risk of HIV infection and transmission. Time trend data from several sources indicate that there have been major reductions in self-reported syringe sharing since 1987, and that the adoption of HIV-protective strategies reflects changes in the social etiquette of drug injecting (Des Jarlais & Friedman 1988, 1990; Robertson *et al.* 1988).

However, risk reduction is not necessarily risk elimination (Strang & Stimson 1990). While risk reduction among injectors has been achieved, risky behaviour leading to transmission still occurs. It is questionable whether the changes which have occurred among drug users are sufficient in time or scale to prevent further epidemic spread, although they may slow it. Gaps still remain between HIV knowledge among drug users and their willingness or ability to implement necessary behavioural change. Many drug users clearly try to avoid risk but still find themselves ending up in risky situations (Stimson *et al.* 1988a). These considerations suggest that there is still a great need to develop and implement behavioural interventions which help people achieve and sustain change.

Not all populations of drug users appear to have changed their behaviour. Much of the available data is from urban regular users of heroin. There is much less evidence for behavioural change in occasional injectors, amphetamine injectors, those living in rural areas, and younger injectors. Most significantly, the changes that have occurred tend to be in the area of drug usage, while there is little evidence of changes in sexual risk behaviours in injecting drug users.

Most of the existing studies are of individuals who are already in contact with treatment agencies. However, it is thought that up to 80% of injecting drug users are not in contact with traditional hospital or community based agencies at any given moment. There is a need to reach these users and there must be concerns about whether the behavioural changes seen in other groups of users are reflected in the behaviour of those not in contact with services.

HIV has spread rapidly among drug injectors in many areas, most notably in the UK in Edinburgh (Robertson 1990). The rapid spread makes the city interesting as a model for the sorts of issues that may influence spread elsewhere. Although the reasons for such rapid spread in Edinburgh have not been fully determined, the two most frequently identified factors appear to be:

(1) *A lack of AIDS awareness amongst injectors.*
    If drug users do not see HIV infection as an immediate threat to them, they are not likely to practise any risk reduction. Evidence suggests that many of the naturally occurring social circumstances among drug injectors prior to HIV infection may facilitate the sharing of drug injection equipment and the transmission of blood-borne viruses. Injection equipment may be shared because of limited availability of sterile equipment at places where drug injectors may congregate to obtain drugs or share information, or sometimes during friendship rituals (Stimson *et al.* 1988b).
(2) *Highly efficient mixing within the drug injecting population.*
    Where drug users are sharing injection equipment only within friendships, or within specific age or ethnic groups, these social boundaries act as limitations on the efficiency of mixing within the total at risk population. Patterns of behaviour which break across such boundaries are likely to increase spread. Drug dealers often keep an extra set of 'works' to be lent serially to their customers, many of whom may want to inject as soon as they have procured their drugs. The sharing of dealers' works appears to have been an important factor in the rapid spread of HIV among injectors in Edinburgh (Robertson *et al.* 1988). There are other possible ways in which boundaries can be broken down. Prisons, for example, may function as a setting for increased risk taking, and therefore of HIV transmission, among diverse groups of drug users and injectors. Different geographical areas may have different micro-cultural patterns in terms of the extent and nature of sharing which increase or reduce the risk of transmission.

Changed behaviours

One of the most significant findings of research into HIV and drug injectors' behaviours has been the sheer extent to which drug injectors have changed their behaviours. There is much evidence that not only have they responded positively to a wide variety of behavioural interventions as a strategic imperative of HIV infection, but many have changed their behaviour prior to entering treatment services in the first instance. Even so, the evidence is clear that many injectors in contact with services do change their HIV and associated risk behaviours more substantially than those not in contact with helping agencies (Stimson *et al.* 1988b).

Studies of methadone maintenance patients in New York have shown that drug injectors who entered treatment early in the HIV epidemic were substantially less likely to become infected with HIV than drug injectors who entered drug treatment later (Des Jarlais & Friedman 1990). The treatment of drug dependency itself has a major advantage as a method of promoting HIV prevention, in that, if successful, it not only prevents HIV infection but also reduces the other individual and social problems associated with illicit drug use. However, the Advisory Council on the Misuse of Drugs (1988) concluded that drug misuse treatment alone was insufficient as a public health measure for preventing the spread of HIV. In part this reflects the fact that treatment of drug misuse fails in many drug users.

Prior to the advent of HIV, abstinence was usually the main criteria by which the outcome of the treatment of drug misuse was judged. Research on specific treatments showed a low rate of success, with high rates of post treatment relapse. Long term follow-up studies showed that approximately 40% of chronic heroin users became abstinent over a period of 10 years. However a large amount of this change could not be attributed directly to treatment. Alongside the data from treatment trials and follow-up studies, the evidence indicated that many chronic drug users became abstinent through other means than enrolment in treatment. There was also evidence that the pattern of usage of drug users was complicated and difficult to predict. Many chronic drug users showed considerable variation in their drug use in the short and medium term, and a considerable proportion of drug users who embarked on drug use did not become chronic users.

All of this makes the longer term outcome of drug treatment difficult to assess, and few controlled trials have more than a short follow-up period. However it is clear that, in any one year, treatment of drug usage itself will cause only a small proportion of users to become permanently abstinent and it would, therefore, be unwise to rely on it as the sole approach to reducing HIV transmission.

On top of these considerations, it is evident that many drug users prefer not to enter into drug treatment, and many others who do enter treatment leave before making any lasting changes in their illicit drug use. Further studies have suggested that drug users make clear cognitive and rational decisions about when, how and for what reasons they wish to contact and make use of services (Miller 1980, 1989). It would be a mistake to assume that the failure of many users to utilise drug treatment services is simply a result of a lack of awareness of such services or what they can offer.

The available evidence suggests two interesting features of drug use; first, that there is considerable adaptability of drug taking behaviour with many routes in and out of drug use, and secondly that there exists a great variety of different patterns of drug use behaviour. This understanding has led to a widening of the goals of drug programmes. There is now a greater variety of goals than simply abstinence. Crucially, there is an understanding that abstinence alone is not the only way of preventing the spread of HIV, and other blood-borne infections, in injecting drug users.

Preventing HIV infection among drug injectors does not require that they completely stop injecting illicit drugs. HIV is spread through quite specific and intimate social behaviours.

HIV positivity correlates with syringe and needle sharing, with the frequency of injecting with used needles, with sharing needles with strangers, with the frequency of injection, with length of drug use, with past imprisonment, with the number of sexual partners injecting drugs, and with travel to HIV epicentres.

The individual risk of infection is related to a combination of personal risk behaviours and the prevalence of HIV infection in the local drug injecting population. This understanding has led to a number of strategies around harm minimisation and reduction, aimed at helping the individual to reduce HIV risks and to keep the incidence of the infection as low as possible in the population of an area. Strategies have included needle and syringe exchange schemes based either in special services or in pharmacies, bleach distribution programmes, programmes aimed at encouraging reduction in injecting, or outreach programmes offering clean works and advice to injectors. In the UK, most cities which have experienced HIV infection among drug users are likely to be using one or more of these methods. Indeed the trend seems to be towards utilising as many different harm-minimisation approaches as is financially and strategically possible. These interventions appear to be well utilised by drug users, which has resulted in the majority of drug injectors in particular cities reducing, though not necessarily eliminating, their sharing of drug-using equipment.

The driving force behind harm minimisation strategies has undoubtedly been HIV. However the move to large scale safer injecting has been linked to decline in the incidence of hepatitis B and other blood-borne infections among drug users.

In parallel with the practical programmes aimed at providing clean works, counselling and educational programmes have been implemented. Indeed, it is often difficult to separate the two elements of harm minimisation. Most clinic-based syringe exchange schemes also offer counselling and education and the provision of such services is probably the main advantage such systems hold over pharmacy-based schemes. Counselling and education programmes include voluntary testing, although there is conflicting evidence regarding the effect of HIV testing on risk behaviour (Mitchell *et al.* 1990), information campaigns, the provision of advice and information, counselling about risk behaviours and protective strategies, offering accelerated access to treatment, adopting new goals for treatment, adapting existing treatment to maximise the possibility of HIV prevention, and developing outreach programmes for hard to reach populations. Underpinning most of these strategies is the need to improve access to drug injecting populations by redefining services so as to make them more attractive to users. There is no way to force users to change, they can only be encouraged and helped to change.

Implementing harm minimisation

The first stage in implementing harm minimisation with a drug user is to assess what their current risk behaviours are. However, it is necessary to go beyond the bare bones of risk behaviours to build up some idea of the context within which those risk behaviours occur. As well as covering the client's drug use and sexual behaviour, the broader issues of harm minimisation can only be addressed by looking at the broader aspects of the client's lifestyle, for instance their relationships, their housing, their legal situation and so on. Current risks, and the wider context in which they occur, serve to provide a profile of the unique pattern of risks and motivators of that individual.

This profile can then be reassessed by the client to identify areas where positive change is possible. It is important to encourage *the client* to undertake this reassessment. Most drug users are used to being told what to do, and resisting it.

Often, the changes which reduce risk can be quite simple. However there are, for any individual, many different possibilities. Table 8.1 illustrates the many changes which may reduce risk in an individual. Which change is appropriate can only be worked out by considering the unique situation of that individual. It is simply unrealistic to set out with a formula for one particular change which all users can undertake, and hope that this will be successful.

Table 8.1 Some possible strategies for reducing risks of HIV transmission.

Risk	Strategy
Borrowing needles/syringes	Getting own needles/syringes
Using unsafe injecting techniques	Using safer injecting techniques
Injecting drugs	Smoking or oral drugs
Chaotic drug use	Controlled drug use
Illicit drug use	Methadone
Regular use	Using infrequently
Intermittent use	Abstinence
Unsafe sexual practices	Safer sexual practices

Inherent in the process of harm reduction and harm minimisation is an acknowledgement of the importance of intermediate goals with drug users. A gain which reduces, but does not eliminate, risk is valuable in itself and is a step on the pathway to further risk reduction. Thus ceasing to share injecting equipment or moving away from injectable to oral drug use becomes a highly significant step forward, even though dependence on the drug might continue. By identifying these sub or intermediate goals, it becomes possible to work towards certain key points in treatment. Change should be recognised as a process of adaptation rather than simply a one-off event. It follows that there will be factors which increase or decrease the likelihood of movement through a process. The benefit of intervention is not intrinsic, but is only understandable when considered for an individual drug user and when the extent to which it assists or hinders movement through the process of change is taken into account.

The prescribing of drugs, most often methadone, by treatment services fills an interesting role in this model. Prescribing can only be considered to be a tool in change rather than treatment in itself. For all individuals the value of prescribing needs to be gauged by the extent to which it may promote further change. It can be seen as one of a range of possible options. Prescribing might best be regarded as an agent that enables other changes to take place.

Prochaska and DiClemente (1984, 1986) have described a theoretical model for understanding change, based on the idea of stages in an individual changing their behaviour. Understanding the point an individual has reached will affect the strategies the counsellor adopts in order to help him. The model suggests that the precontemplative drug user – who has not yet really started to address the issues of change – may be prompted to consider the benefits and costs of their present behaviour compared to some altered circumstances. These considerations may include the identification of benefit associated with a change, or they may be the realisation of the adverse consequences of the present behaviour.

In the stage of contemplation the drug user – who is actively considering change – will conduct in effect a cost-benefit analysis, and this may include separate consideration of the short and long term benefits and costs of change. The counsellor can help to encourage, guide, and make explicit, this process. The movement to the stage of change may be influenced by the availability of help to bring about the changes. Assistance in problem solving is clearly important in this process.

Having effected a change the drug user will again conduct a sort of cost-benefit analysis of the present situation, this time relative to the perceived costs and benefits of a return to previous behaviours. The outcome of such an analysis will be a major determinant of whether relapse occurs.

While the model is an apparently simple one, it shows the importance of change as a process rather than as a single event, and it acts as a reminder that the strategy of the counsellor needs to change with the position of the client in that process. Some of the benefits of using such a model can be seen by considering what it tells us about the role of prescribing.

It is clear from the model that prescribing does not in itself directly bring about change. Change is a process of decision making within the individual. The model acts, in many cases, as an extremely important catalyst and enabler to the process of change. Many drug treatment services use a fixed regime of prescribing. Clearly where there are arbitrary limits or perceived restrictions on levels and choice of drugs, rather than individually defined regimes, there is much more potential for conflict between the worker and the drug user. After all, one of the most important issues for the drug user is the type and amount of drugs available to him or her, and this is historically a point of conflict between users and carers. Of course this is not an argument for prescribing whatever the user wants in whatever amounts, but for seeking to establish a prescribing regime, where appropriate, which matches the needs of the individual rather than a preset policy.

With the rising incidence of HIV infection among drug users, policies on drug management need to be reviewed. In the same way that HIV has required a review of issues such as confidentiality and sexuality in drug treatment services, there is a need to consider the broader treatment issues. Failure to prescribe adequate maintenance levels leads to tensions between patients and staff. Where a patient is unable to cope on a particular regime they will usually seek a way out. They can withdraw from treatment, try to obtain drugs from other legal sources – for instance in the form of pain control – or to try to top up prescriptions with street drugs. The latter is an interesting strategy. Many drug treatment services know, or suspect, that users in treatment are supplementing prescribed drugs with street drugs – thus undermining the purpose of prescribing – and yet they appear to prefer this to reconsidering the prescribing regime a patient is on.

There is a need for a means of managing drug dependence that reduces, as far as is reasonably practicable, psychological or physical discomfort for patients. This is particularly important where they are an in-patient or are recovering from infections associated with HIV. Obviously it is impossible to avoid these things altogether, but as with other areas of health care, reducing suffering is a sensible and ethical objective. The problem is, of course, to reduce discomfort while not overmedicating to the point where this in itself starts to cause problems or to hinder the change process. It is a matter of balance and the process to achieve that balance needs to be a negotiation with the users.

The drug user with HIV infection

Despite some specific problems in the management of drug users with HIV, in most respects they are just the same as anyone else. They need the same counselling approach as outlined elsewhere in this book. Drug users *are* the seropositive man, the pregnant woman with AIDS worried about her baby, the man worried about infecting his partner or concerned about how to tell friends or family about his status. Just because they are drug users, it does not mean that they do not have the same concerns and responses as anyone else. However, there are some specific differences which need to be picked up.

Drug users have historically had poor access to general health care facilities. They are widely regarded as a chaotic, poorly compliant group of patients who have 'brought their troubles on themselves'. Many health care staff have also viewed them with suspicion, concerned that the user may be seeking to manipulate them in some way. There has always been a high morbidity associated with injecting drug use. Abscesses, cellulitis, septicaemia, endocarditis and hepatitis were common problems before HIV, and remain so. The morbidity associated with HIV has been superimposed on this pattern of ill-health. With time the number of drug users who become symptomatic with HIV disease will increase. There is also likely to be an increasing incidence of interactions between HIV disease and other common infections of drug users, given the greater susceptibility and the greater difficulties of treatment in the immunocompromised individual.

Drug use in itself can complicate the recognition and treatment of other health problems. For example, the opiate user may have night sweats and diarrhoea associated with withdrawal, and is also quite likely to have lost weight due to drug induced appetite loss and poor diet. Helping a drug user with symptoms of HIV disease to gain weight may be difficult because of the poor appetite.

Table 8.2 picks out a few of the possible overlaps in symptoms.

Wherever possible it is helpful to promote abstinence from opiates and other such drugs in the HIV infected individual. This is not always readily achievable, at least in the short term, but it is important to try to help the patient avoid injecting drugs. A willingness to use levels of methadone which make this process as easy as possible is obviously important. At the very least it is important to seek to avoid the patient sharing 'works'. The risks to others are obvious, but the risks to the user are considerable.

There is evidence that continued injecting of street drugs increases the rate of decline of CD4+ lymphocytes, possibly as a result of the injection of impure material into the circulation, which stimulates the immune system and so promotes HIV replication. In addition the use of unsterile equipment leaves the patient open to further bacterial and viral infections.

Finally, it is important not to concentrate only on risks associated with drugs and to forget other HIV risks (Schoenbaum *et al.* 1989). Drug users have the same sexual risks as anyone else; indeed, they are usually at higher sexual risk because they are more likely to have

Table 8.2 Overlap of HIV infection and drug use.

Symptom	HIV explanation	Drug explanation
Shortness of breath	PCP, TB	TB, heroin asthma
Cough	PCP, TB, bacterial infections	TB heroin asthma, opiate withdrawal
Fever	PCP or other opportunist infection	Injection abscesses, pneumonia, dirty hit
Sore mouth	Herpes	Poor diet, ulcers
Weight loss	TB, other infections	Poor diet, effect of cocaine or amphetamines
Fatigue	HIV	Withdrawal
Vomiting	Cryptosporidiosis, gut	Opiate withdrawal
Confusion	Toxoplasmosis	Sedative drug use, overdose

partners who also inject. If they are uninfected they may acquire the virus from a sexual partner; if they are infected they may pass it on to a partner. Many drug users engage in prostitution or near-prostitution, exchanging sex for money or drugs. They may not only be prostitutes but also they may be the 'client' of other drug users who are prostituting, particularly where drugs are the medium of exchange. As was noted earlier, achieving changes in injecting practice has proved easier than achieving changes in sexual behaviour in drug users. In the same way, many drug users are young fertile women or the sexual partners of young fertile women, and the possibility of pregnancy and vertical transmission of HIV infection is present.

References

Advisory Council on the Misuse of Drugs (1988) *AIDS and Drug Misuse*, Part 1. HMSO, London.

Des Jarlais, D. & Friedman, S.R. (1988) HIV and intravenous drug use. *AIDS*, 2 (Suppl. 1), S65–69.

Des Jarlais, D. & Friedman, S.R. (1990) The epidemic of HIV infection among injecting drug users in New York City, the first decade and possible future directions. In: *AIDS and Drug Misuse* (eds J. Strang & G.V. Stimson). Routledge, London.

Green, J. & Hedge, B. (1991) Counselling and Stress in HIV Infection and AIDS. In: *Cancer and Stress* (eds C. Cooper & M. Watson). Wiley, London.

Miller, W.R. (ed) (1980) *The Addictive Behaviours: Treatment of Alcoholism, Drug Abuse, Smoking, and Obesity*. Pergamon Press, New York.

Miller, W.R. (1989) Increasing motivation for change. In: *Handbook of Alcoholism Treatment Approaches: Effective Alternatives* (eds R.K. Hester & W.R. Miller). Pergamon Press, New York.

Prochaska, J.O. & DiClemente, C.C. (1984) *The Transtheoretical Approach: Crossing Traditional Boundaries of Therapy*. Dow Jones/Irwin, Homewood, Illinois.

Prochaska, J.O. & DiClemente, C.C. (1986) Towards a comprehensive model of change. In: *Treating Addictive Behaviours, Processes of Change* (eds W.R. Miller & N. Heather), pp 3–27. Plenum Press, New York.

Robertson, R. (1990) The Edinburgh epidemic, a case study. In: *AIDS and Drug Misuse* (eds J. Strang & G.V. Stimson). Routledge, London.

Robertson, R., Skidmore, C.A. & Roberts, J.J. (1988) HIV Infection in intravenous drug users: a follow up study indicating changes in risk taking behaviour. *British Journal of Addiction*, **83**, 387–91.

Satterthwaite, H. (1990) Presentation at National Association of Nurses on Substance Abuse, Chester College.

Schoenbaum, E., Hartel, D., Selwyn, P.A. *et al.* (1989) Risk factors for HIV infection in intravenous drug users. *The New England Journal of Medicine*, **321**, 874–9.

Stimson, G.V., Alldritt, L., Dolan, K. & Donoghoe, M.C. (1988a) HIV risk of clients attending syringe exchange schemes in England and Scotland. *British Journal of Addiction*, **83**, 1449–1454.

Stimson, G., Aldritt, L., Dolan, K. & Donoghoe, M.C. (1988b) Syringe exchange schemes in England and Scotland. *British Medical Journal*, **296**, 17.

Strang, J. & Stimson, G.V. (1990) *AIDS and Drug Misuse*. Routledge, London.

Chapter 9

Counselling in Pregnancy

John Green

Perhaps no area has been more affected by new research findings in the field of HIV counselling than that of counselling the pregnant woman. Because the current information about HIV affects the counselling provided and the counselling strategy to be adopted, it is important to look briefly at what is known currently about HIV and pregnancy. In view of the rate at which we are learning more in this area, it is vital that anyone working with pregnant women (or young women likely to get pregnant) should make sure that they are aware of the latest information. It can be a formidable task. At the time of writing this chapter over 6000 articles and books have addressed the issue, if only in passing.

Background

Mothers are able to pass on the HIV virus to their children – called vertical transmission. It has been estimated that in the US between one and two thousand HIV infected children are born every year (CDC 1994). Chin (1994) estimated that by 1992, 4 million infected children would have been born worldwide. Like all estimates this figure is an educated guess, but no-one doubts that the number is large and growing rapidly.

Infection of the child appears to happen at one of three stags: *in utero*, at birth or through breast-feeding. The relative importance of these three routes is difficult to assess but transmission at all three times may be substantial. It is not possible for an infected father to pass on the virus to the foetus without the mother becoming infected first. There is no evidence that the health of an HIV-infected mother is adversely affected by pregnancy.

The rate of transmission of HIV from mother to child varies widely from study to study. The rate is somewhere in the 14% to 39% range (Peckham 1994), with most studies reporting figures in the 14% to 25% range. Rates appear to be higher for children in developing countries, higher for mothers who are producing more virus, higher if the child is exposed to more maternal blood at birth, higher if the child is premature and higher where the mother has more advanced disease and where her CD4+ count is lower (Boyer *et al.* 1994; Erb *et al.* 1994; European Collaborative Study Group 1992; Peckham 1994). Viral characteristics, particularly tropism for particular cell types, may play a part in determining whether transmission occurs (Levy 1993). Injecting drug use does not appear to affect transmission rates. Interestingly the rate of vertical transmission of HIV-2 appears to be much lower than that for HIV-1, perhaps as low as 1% (Adjorlolo *et al.* 1994).

There appear to be a number of actions which may reduce the rate of vertical transmission. It is thought possible that caesarean section may do so, by reducing the exposure of the child to maternal body fluids during the birth. Evidence for this is equivocal at the time of writing, although trials are taking place. There can be problems in assessing this issue from published data. Many caesarean sections are done as emergencies rather than as elective procedures so that women having caesareans may not be strictly comparable to women with vaginal deliveries.

The European Collaborative Study Group (1992, 1994) found that women who had emergency caesarean sections had a lower rate of infection among their babies than those who had a vaginal delivery, but there appeared to be no difference between elective caesarean and vaginal delivery. However, correcting the data for health of the mother suggested that caesarean section did, in fact, offer some protection. Vaginal deliveries involving scalp electrodes, episiotomy and instrumental deliveries carried a higher risk only in clinics where they were not routine, possibly reflecting their use in more difficult deliveries. It has been suggested that cleansing the birth canal may also influence the risks of transmission.

The most recent area of interest has been the administration of zidovudine (AZT) to mothers in order to prevent transmission. In one study women were given zidovudine in the second and third trimesters, and intravenous zidovudine during the birth, and zidovudine was given to the infant for a period after the birth. The infection rate among children whose mothers were on zidovudine was 8.3% and that of mothers on placebo was 25% (CDC 1994). The women in the study had mild to moderate immunosuppression and had never taken zidovudine; the effectiveness of the drug in other groups is unknown, although in a small non-randomised study Boyer *et al.* (1994) reported a protective effect in women, with lower CD4+ counts than in the first trial.

Although there is no evidence that zidovudine causes any ill-effects in the infant or increases the rate of birth defects, there must always be a concern about the theoretical possibility of problems developing later, perhaps many years afterwards. This is particularly important because, of course, the majority of children born to infected mothers in the absence of zidovudine will not be infected, so many children will receive the drug unnecessarily. The exposure of the infant to zidovudine might be reduced if it was clear where the effective action of the drug was occurring, for instance it might be that using the drug only during the birth, or at the end of the pregnancy and at birth, might be as effective as longer-term administration. Other concerns include whether the drug would have similar effects in women who had already been taking zidovudine for a period, and who therefore might have drug-resistant HIV strains. Also, there is a potential concern that administering zidovudine to women who are otherwise well might produce drug-resistance and therefore reduce the effectiveness of the drug when they do become ill.

This is an area where new data will fill in the gaps in our knowledge, but the best estimate of the situation at the moment would seem to be:

- Women who become pregnant early in their infection, while they remain well and virus levels in the blood remain low, are less likely to give their infant HIV. Therefore if a woman wishes to become pregnant in spite of the risks, she would be better doing it early rather than late, when transmission may be more likely. However, even early in the course of infection the risks of infecting the child are substantial.

- There are actions which can be taken to reduce the risks of transmission once it is known that a woman is pregnant, including administration of AZT, avoidance of breast feeding (Dunn *et al.* 1992; Palasanthiran *et al.* 1993) and, possibly, caesarean section and cleaning of the birth canal. But note that some of these may not be practicable in a developing country where drugs and other resources are scarce.
- Most babies born to infected mothers, even where the mother is in advanced disease, will be uninfected.

HIV testing in pregnancy

There are clear potential benefits for a woman having an HIV test during pregnancy. She can take actions which may reduce the risk of her child being infected, and if a child is known to be HIV infected, or may be so, it might be possible to provide more detailed medical follow-up than would otherwise be provided. There are other implications, like the effectiveness, and possibly the safety, of vaccinations. It is also possible to put into action some of the counselling steps outlined in Chapter 10.

On the other hand there are stresses for the mother. Few occasions could be as distressing to a woman as waiting to see whether her child has a disease which will probably kill it, and which she herself has passed on to it. Some women may have a reasonable fear that, if they are tested for HIV, they may be rejected by their partner or subject to physical violence (Green & Kentish 1995; Temmerman *et al.* 1995). While the reason for testing the mother is primarily to affect transmission and care for the child, it is the mother who is tested. In other words, HIV testing in pregnant women raises exactly the same problems and issues as it does in women who are not pregnant. The specific issues around pregnancy are additional.

It is easy to lose sight of the fact that HIV testing in pregnancy is for the benefit of the mother (and the child), and to see it as having some vague additional benefit over and above the welfare of either. There must be doubts whether, for instance, testing of pregnant women is of value if only strict grounds of financial cost-benefit are considered (Blaxhult *et al.* 1993). The costs of testing programmes with pregnant women are high and can strain the resources of even relatively well-resourced services (Chrystie *et al.* 1995). There are no grounds for thinking that the testing of pregnant women is going to make much impact on the spread of the disease in the population generally, even in countries where rates among pregnant women are high (Heyward *et al.* 1993). Indeed there are grounds for suspecting that pregnancy may be a poor time to pick to try to influence someone's sexual behaviour, since their behaviour is likely to be different while pregnant and immediately after the birth, especially if they usually have multiple partners. It is probable that the longer the gap between encouraging someone to change their behaviour and their actually having the opportunity to try putting change into practice, the less likely they are to do so.

In view of these considerations, most countries have taken the view that mandatory testing of pregnant women is not justified. However, the question of whether to offer the test to all women or whether to seek to identify women at high risk ('case-finding') is rather more difficult. It is important to keep in mind the fact that the objective is to identify as many women as possible who are pregnant and HIV positive (and want to know) rather than to test as many women as possible. A programme which tests 95% of pregnant women but all the high risk women are in the 5% which refuse, is not very useful. This is far from an academic possibility. There is evidence from other areas of HIV testing that individuals at higher risk may be less likely to be tested (Mansson 1990). The picture is clouded by numerous studies of the acceptability of HIV testing to women, many of which utilise samples of women who believe themselves to be (and are) at low risk.

There are advantages and disadvantages to both approaches – offering the test routinely and 'case-finding' – and these are discussed here.

Offering the test routinely

Offering the test to all pregnant women is expensive. Within the UK the experience has usually been that there is a high refusal rate among pregnant women (Howard *et al.* 1989; Meadows & Catalan 1992). Rates of uptake are much higher elsewhere in Europe, possibly because less stress is placed on the importance of informed consent and perhaps because of different attitudes among health care workers and patients about who should take decisions about clinical tests and on what basis (Chrystie *et al.* 1995).

In part, variations in test uptake may reflect the attitudes of the person offering the HIV test – how keen they are to persuade the woman of its benefits – as well as perhaps personal characteristics of the counsellor (Meadows *et al.* 1990). It is also worth bearing in mind that it is not necessarily a sign of bad counselling to have a low uptake of the HIV test. In most areas of the UK at least, the majority of women attending antenatal clinics have probably been at very low risk of HIV infection. If a woman goes through pre-test counselling and decides rationally that she does not wish to be tested because she has been at very low risk or no risk, that decision cannot be seen as a 'failure' for the counsellor.

It is also worth considering that most of the data referred to above dates from before the information on the possible value of AZT in pregnancy, and some of it from before the possible benefits of caesareans became known. At the time these studies were being carried out, a women who would not consider a termination and did not intend to breast-feed could do little to affect the probability of having an infected child. Of course if a child is known to have, or to be likely to have HIV, paediatric surveillance can be more intensive and this may benefit the child to some extent. However, the test might have been seen by many pregnant women, not entirely irrationally, as of marginal value to them.

In the UK the approach has been to offer the test routinely to women in high prevalence areas. Providing the approach is one of offering the test, and not coercing women into having a test they do not want, it is difficult to see any clinical reason why this should not be a good approach. Indeed, it offers the beneficial opportunity to talk to women about HIV and other sexual risks. For the overwhelming majority of women – who will turn out to be seronegative – this is likely to be the only tangible benefit they get from the testing system.

The great concern with this approach is that it is expensive. There is always going to be a temptation to minimise the pre-test counselling of women to vanishing point in order to keep down the cost. Clearly pre-test counselling with someone at lower risk is not likely to take as long as that with someone at higher risk because there is less to talk about, but it will still take a significant amount of time if it is done properly. There is no way around this; if counselling is to be done properly, it needs resources.

Case finding

Case finding is identifying individuals who are at high risk and offering the test to them, rather than routinely offering it to every pregnant woman. It should always be accompanied by a 'testing-on-demand' system, i.e. if women are not routinely being offered the test it makes sense to ensure that they are aware they can have one if they want to ask for one.

The great advantage of case finding is the lower cost. Fewer women are identified, therefore fewer women have to be counselled and tested. Scarce clinical time can be concentrated where it is needed and there is much less chance of counselling being skimped.

The approach is only likely to be effective if two criteria are fulfilled:

(1) It must be possible to identify, reasonably readily and reliably, characteristics of individuals at higher risk of HIV infection
(2) Health care staff must be assiduous in searching out individuals with characteristics which put them at increased risk.

With regard to the first criterion, case finding is less likely to succeed in areas of high heterosexual spread where it is difficult to identify clear characteristics of those at risk. On a purely practical level, the amount of questioning required to identify risk levels in areas of high spread can sometimes be so great that savings in resources over routinely offering the test may be negligible.

In the UK, the vast majority of cases of HIV infection in pregnant women occur in one of two groups (Ades *et al.* 1993). One group is women who are either current or former injecting drug users, or the sexual partners of such individuals. The second group is women who have been sexually active in areas of high heterosexual spread or who have had sexual partners from such areas. It happens that, because of the pattern of links between the UK and other countries, a large proportion of women in the UK with HIV infection are from sub-Saharan Africa. With a case finding approach, such women may see that they are being offered the test and not others. They may feel that they are being 'picked out' on the basis of being African, and it would be understandable if some women felt rather aggrieved about this. There is some evidence that women at increased risk of HIV infection may be more likely to have a test if it is offered routinely rather than being targeted (Barbacci *et al.* 1991).

With regard to criterion (2) above, there are problems. The system depends on the clinical team making an assessment of who is likely to be at risk in their area, drawing up a list of criteria for who will be counselled and offered the test, and then ensuring that the criteria are actively searched for in every case. There are worrying reports of women-at-risk, with characteristics which show that they are at-risk, being missed by case-finding systems. On the other hand the approach should work and can work, if it is properly applied.

It is worth stressing that elsewhere in the world the situation is by no means as clear as in the UK in terms of individuals at risk, and even in the UK, case finding will miss some individuals who are infected. On the other hand, so will offering the test to everyone, since some women at risk will refuse the test.

Deciding on a system

In the UK the standard approach at the time of writing is to offer the test routinely to all women in areas of high prevalence, and to case-find in areas of low prevalence. The use of anonymous seroprevalence surveys allows an analysis of the underlying rate of infection in an area and how many individuals with HIV are probably not having HIV tests. This appears a rational approach, although changes in epidemiology in the future might change the balance of advantage. However, the decision on how to approach the issue of testing will partly depend on the level of resources available and on the identification of suitable criteria on which to base case finding. If the test is to be offered routinely, resources must be available to offer appropriate counselling, and if case finding is to be adopted, it is essential that it is effectively and systematically put into practice.

Identifying those at risk

Identifying those at risk is important if a case finding approach is to be used. This is addressed in more detail in Chapter 18. While that chapter focuses on developing countries, the principles apply equally to developed countries. The important approach in case finding is to make sure that every case is compared against the case finding criteria. It is not always possible to assess the relative risk of an individual on the basis of their obvious characteristics and it is usually necessary to ask some questions. These can be drawn up into a standardised protocol. They then need to be asked of every woman, preferably when the woman is first being booked for antenatal appointments.

In areas outside major conurbations in the UK the main risks to women are likely to be having injected drugs or having had unprotected sex with someone who did so, having had sex with an individual who was infected through blood or blood products, or having sex with a partner from an area of high heterosexual spread whether in the UK or abroad. Each of these possibilities needs to be asked about in turn:

COUNSELLOR: 'Have you ever injected drugs?'
PATIENT: 'No.'
COUNSELLOR: 'Have you ever had a sexual partner who injected drugs or who might have injected drugs?'
PATIENT: 'No.'
COUNSELLOR: 'Have you ever had sex with a partner from overseas?'
PATIENT: 'Well, yes, about five years ago. I was working abroad at the time.'
COUNSELLOR   'Tell me about it . . .'

Antenatal staff sometimes have problems about people's sexual histories as it has not, in the past, been a usual part of antenatal care. However it is essential that they should feel able to do this if a case finding approach is to be taken. It helps if it is explained to women why these questions are being asked and is stressed that they are routine. Providing written information about HIV and about who is at greatest risk also helps. Any woman, whether she fits the picture of someone at increased risk or not, needs to be informed that she can have a test.

Offering the test

It is important when offering the test to a woman – whether as a result of case finding or as part of a policy of offering the test routinely – to explain why the test is being offered.

> COUNSELLOR: 'We are asking every pregnant woman here whether they want an HIV test, as a matter of course. Let me explain why...'

The explanation will be in terms of the perceived advantages of the test to the woman. It is important to stress that the test is voluntary:

> COUNSELLOR: 'This test is for your benefit, not ours. If you don't want to have it, that is entirely up to you.'

It is, perhaps, easier to handle this situation with a policy of routine testing than with a policy of case finding, where it is important not to appear to be judging the woman in any way.

> COUNSELLOR: 'OK, so you have injected drugs in the past. We are asking anyone who has injected drugs in the past whether they want to have an HIV test; it's up to you whether to have one, of course. The reason we are offering the test is that people who have injected drugs, if they have shared 'works', are more likely to have picked up the virus.'

In other words, the best approach with case finding is to be frank and straightforward about why one thinks that a particular woman has been at increased risk. There is little point in hedging round the issue and trying to express it in an easy way. A woman who is clear why she is being offered the test is able to evaluate for herself whether she has really been at risk. In the above example, if the woman has never shared works she is able to evaluate that that aspect of her behaviour has not, in fact, put her at risk.

Pre-test counselling

If the woman declines to have a test and declines to think about the issue further, the most that can be done is to provide written information on HIV – if this has not already been done – and then move on to the rest of the antenatal work.

Some women will not want the test but may be receptive to more information about HIV infection. This is a useful moment to provide some basic health education information, whether the woman has been at increased risk or not. If time can be taken to consider with the woman whether she has been at risk, this can be extremely useful. Discussion of risk may lead her to change her mind about being tested. More importantly, there is some advice which a woman who has been at increased risk can usefully adopt whether she wants to know her status or not. For instance, choosing not to breast feed reduces the risk of transmission and is not dependent on knowing one's status. In the west such an approach is entirely practicable, but in developing countries with poor access to safe alternative nutrition such an approach is not practicable. The baby of a mother at increased risk can also be particularly closely monitored post-natally.

If possible, all women need to be encouraged to consider not just past risks but also current risks of HIV infection. While I am not aware of any conclusive evidence on the subject, there would seem to be good reason to suppose that women who became infected with HIV while they were pregnant might be at particularly high risk of transmitting the virus. The period just after infection is associated with a burst of antigenaemia and with a lack of protective immune response in the infected person.

Where a woman wishes to consider the test, it is appropriate to offer pre-test counselling. Pre-test counselling for pregnant women is much the same as pre-test counselling for anyone else (Chapter 3). It is a time to:

- Provide information about HIV infection and specifically about the transmission of HIV *in utero*, at birth and through breast-feeding
- Explore the level of past and current risk of HIV infection of that particular woman
- Consider with the woman the advantages and disadvantages of being tested for HIV infection in her own particular case
- Consider what changes in risk behaviour might be helpful for the woman during her pregnancy and in the future
- Ensure that she has begun to think through what the consequences might be if she is either positive or negative
- Ensure that she has thought through who she will tell about being tested and about the result, and that she has appropriate social support
- Ensure that she is aware that she can take time to assess whether she wants the test; she does not have to take a decision there and then.

There are three special problems with this approach in antenatal. The first is that it takes time, and ante-natal clinics tend to be short of time. On the other hand it is worthwhile, given the problems of telling an inadequately prepared pregnant woman that she is infected with HIV and may have infected her unborn child. Of course the time taken for pre-test counselling for a woman who has been at low risk is less than that for a woman at high risk, simply because there is less to discuss.

If the test is to be offered to every woman routinely, additional resources will need to be deployed or work restructured to allow for the extra work. It is the time required to deliver appropriate pre-test counselling to every woman which has led many health agencies to decide on a case finding approach since the time overheads are likely to be much less.

The second problem is that there are the various complicated issues about transmission and our uncertainties about these. Most patients want straight answers from health care staff. Where there are no straight answers things can get difficult.

COUNSELLOR: 'If a woman has HIV she can pass that on to her child through breast-feeding. So it is important if you are infected, or if you may have been at risk, not to breast feed.'

PATIENT: 'Yes.'

COUNSELLOR: 'If we know a pregnant woman is infected we may be able to reduce her risk of passing on the virus to her child by giving her a drug called AZT. It is important to say that it only reduces the risk, it doesn't take the risk away entirely.'

PATIENT: 'How big is the risk?'

COUNSELLOR: 'As I said before, it depends a bit on the health of the mother and when she picked up the virus. The best guess at the moment is that a woman who is not actually sick has a one in four or one in six chance of passing on the virus. Taking AZT maybe reduces that to half, perhaps a bit more, perhaps a bit less. We don't have as much information just at the moment as we would like . . .'

The information at the beginning of this chapter provides an overview of the current state of play. However it is important that anyone counselling in this field should be up to date about what is going on, and there is certain to be new information, even in the time between this chapter being completed and the book coming out. The principles of counselling in this area remain the same, but the details of the information can change enormously and have an enormous impact on the decisions women take about whether to have a test and what steps to take if they find they are infected.

What can be offered to a women will differ from country to country. Many developing countries will simply be unable to afford the costs of giving AZT to every pregnant infected woman, or to perform caesarean sections simply on the basis of the serostatus of the mother. In these circumstances the potential benefits to the mother of being tested are much less and one might expect, were all other things equal, to see less uptake of the test.

Finally, it is worth considering that in almost every counselling and testing programme in the world aimed at pregnant women, whether in high or low prevalence areas, the vast majority of women will be uninfected. More than that, the vast majority of women who have been at increased risk will be negative. One of the key purposes of counselling programmes is to stop women getting infected. They may be negative at this pregnancy, but they may become infected before they get pregnant again in the future, or while they are bringing up their child. Providing to women at risk of HIV infection counselling which prevents them from getting infected in the first place, is more important even than trying to intervene with women who are already infected. It is important not to end up with a system purely aimed at identifying and testing women who are already infected. A successful programme needs to go beyond that.

Post-test counselling the pregnant woman

Most HIV test results in pregnant women will be negative. It is important to discuss with seronegative women who have been at risk, and who may be at risk in the future, ways of reducing those risks. It is very tempting just to reassure on the basis of the test result and then move on to something else.

The starting point for post-test counselling of a seropositive pregnant woman is to remember that it is similar to post-test counselling any other seropositive woman. It is easy to get preoccupied with the fact that the woman is pregnant and to attend only to that. The pregnant woman with HIV infection has exactly the same needs and problems as any other woman who finds that she is infected. The problems surrounding pregnancy are additional. The other side of the coin also applies. Although the woman may be HIV positive, it does not mean that she does not have exactly the same problems, fears and difficulties as every other pregnant woman. For the woman who finds herself pregnant and HIV infected there are, however, very specific problems, described here.

Uncertainty about whether her baby will be infected

Every mother wants a healthy baby. The thought that her baby might be infected with HIV is a source of great heartache to many infected women. There is, usually, no way of telling whether her baby will be infected or not prior to birth. The use of newer laboratory techniques can now often tell whether a child is infected quite soon after birth, certainly before the child would normally serorevert. Even in the west these techniques are not available everywhere and they are unlikely to be available in most developing countries. Explaining clearly to the mother what can and cannot be done to establish the infection status of the child, and that most women do not have infected children, can be of immense value. Otherwise there is little that can be done other than to encourage the mother to express her feelings and to ensure that she has adequate support, both professional and informal.

Guilt

Concerns about possible infection are often made worse by feelings of guilt about the fact that the mother has, in some way, put her baby at risk. These feelings are common even when, say, the mother has been monogamous but infected by her partner; in other words they go beyond the strictly rational. Again, there is little that can be done practically other than to offer support, encouragement to express these feelings and the provision of a little gentle common sense. No woman deliberately sets out to give her baby HIV; it is essentially an accident.

Fears for herself

The mother's fears for herself are often amplified by fears about what will happen to the baby if and when she becomes sick. Forward planning is vital and the more effective the contingency plans that can be made the more likely it is that the mother's level of anxiety can be reduced. This issue is one of essentially bringing forward a process which needs to be carried out after the birth in any case (see Chapter 10).

Concerns about birth defects

There is no evidence that birth defects are more common in children born to mothers with HIV infection, and it is important to stress this to women. Many women do not understand the difference between the viral infection and physical abnormalities in children.

Problems with partners and family

These are not at all uncommon and can be very acute. The issues involved are no different from those covered elsewhere in this book (Chapters 4, 5 and 10). The following example illustrates the sort of problems seen.

Margaret was a 32 year-old woman who had settled in Britain from Africa. Her husband was also African. She had two previous children, aged two and five. When she was three months pregnant she found out that she was HIV positive. She dare not tell her husband, even though she suspected that she had caught the virus from him. She was concerned that he would leave her, or even be violent towards her. At the same time she was concerned about the possibility that one or both of her other children might have been infected, although they both seemed well.

Margaret was left essentially unable to tell her husband that she was infected and uncertain about the status of her children. It is hard to think of a more wretched situation.

It is important to work with both members of the couple and sometimes even with other family members, where this is appropriate, practicable and wanted by the patient.

Deciding what to do

The woman who finds that she is seropositive has to take a number of decisions in a hurry. As treatments change the decisions change, but at the moment one decision to be taken is whether to have a termination. There is little evidence to suggest that being seropositive encourages many women to have a termination (Selwyn *et al.* 1989; Johnstone *et al.* 1990). Rates of termination of pregnancy are reported in many studies to be higher in women with HIV infection than in other women, but this may simply reflect other differences between the groups. For instance, unmarried drug users with no steady income are over-represented among infected women and may already, whether infected or not, have a higher than usual rate of termination of pregnancy.

Our own experience has been that few women have chosen to have a termination solely on the grounds that they have HIV infection. To most women there seems little sense in terminating a pregnancy simply in order to avoid one's child being sick. Where pregnancies have been terminated the grounds have usually been the mother's feeling that she could not cope both with looking after the child and having HIV. It is our impression, supported by anecdotal evidence from colleagues, that seropositive women who terminate often become pregnant again fairly rapidly.

Raising the issue of termination, as always, has to be done very tactfully. It is important not to make a woman feel that she is being encouraged to terminate. It is an option for her, not one suggested to her. Women often have very powerful reasons for wanting to become pregnant or continue a pregnancy even when they are aware of the risks.

Mary was a 29 year-old drug user. She was symptomatic but did not have AIDS. Her partner, Alan, was very ill with AIDS. She was aware that she had HIV infection but still became 'accidentally' pregnant when she forgot to take her pill regularly. On discussion she was adamant, defensively so, that she wanted to continue with the pregnancy, even though there was no pressure to do otherwise. She told the counsellor, 'Alan's going to die, I'll be dead soon. This baby is the only thing we've ever done in this world that's worth anything. At least there'll be a little bit of us left, and I hope it does better than we ever could.'

Another decision the seropositive pregnant woman has to take is whether to take AZT during the pregnancy, and whether to have a caesarean or other procedure aimed at reducing the risk of transmission. Current information about this is mentioned earlier in the chapter. It is important to inform the woman what is known and what is unknown. Hopefully a start on this will be made at pre-test counselling, but some decisions will have to be made post-test.

Preparing for the birth

Almost every woman worries about whether her unborn child is all right. Where there are legitimate concerns about HIV this can easily spill over into other concerns about the child. It helps to reassure about those aspects of the child's development where reassurance is possible. For instance, where the results of other tests are normal or where results from examinations or scans are available, particular attention needs to be paid to reporting these back to the woman.

The procedure for the birth also needs to be explained to the woman. If staff are to take any particular precautions, these and their purpose need to be explained to the woman. This is particularly important if the woman has given birth before and will see differences in procedure aimed at infection control. It is important to normalise the birth as much as possible, to avoid unnecessary additional precautions and to remember that additional infection control procedures do not preclude staff being friendly and encouraging to the patient. Of course it might be argued rationally that all births ought to be carried out with the same levels of infection control; however human nature being what it is, there is always going to be a temptation to apply stricter control procedures where the mother is known to be seropositive. It is essential not to add to the woman's troubles by making her feel like a dangerous outcast.

Overview

Few areas of counselling in HIV disease are as difficult and as stressful for all concerned as counselling pregnant women at risk of HIV disease. It is important to have clear procedures at every stage to make sure that the test is offered appropriately, that women are supported appropriately whether they decide to be tested or not, and that they are offered the most up-to-date information possible. As with any other patient, the pregnant woman will not always decide on a course of action which seems the wisest to the counsellor or other staff. However it is her life, her baby and her choice. The best we can do is to inform the mother as much as possible, and once she has made a choice, to support that choice.

References

Ades, A.E., Davison, C.F. & Gibb, D.G. (1993) Vertically transmitted HIV infection in the British Isles. *British Medical Journal*, **306**, 1296–1299.

Adjorlolo, G., DeCock, K.M., Ekpini, E. *et al.* (1994) Prospective comparison of mother-to-child transmission of HIV-1 and HIV-2 in Abidjan, Ivory Coast. *Journal of the American Medical Association*, **272**, 462–6.

Anon. (1994) Immunological and virological clues for mother to child transmission of HIV-1 and HIV-2. Editorial in *Journal of the American Medical Association*, **272**, 487.

Barbacci, M., Repke, J.T. & Chaisson, R.E. (1991) Routine prenatal screening for HIV infection. *Lancet*, **337**, 709–11.

Blaxhult, A., Cain, A. & Arneborn, M. (1993) Evaluation of HIV testing in Sweden. *AIDS*, **7**, 1625–31.

Boyer, P.J., Dillon, M. & Navaie, M. (1994) Factors predictive of materno-foetal transmission of HIV-1, preliminary analysis of zidovudine given during pregnancy and/or during delivery. *Journal of American Medical Association*, **271**, 1925.

CDC (Centers for Disease Control) (1994) Effectiveness in disease and injury prevention. Zidovudine for the prevention of HIV transmission from mother to infant. *Morbidity and Mortality Weekly Review*, **43**, 285–7.

Chin, J. (1994) The growing impact of the HIV/AIDS pandemic on children born to HIV-infected women. *Clinical Perinatology*, **21**, 1–14.

Chrystie, I.L., Zander, L., Tilzey, A. *et al.* (1995). Is HIV testing in antenatal clinics worthwhile? Can we afford it? *AIDS Care*, **7**, 135–42.

Dunn, D.T., Newell, M.L., Ades, A.E. & Peckham, C.S. (1992) Risk of human immunodeficiency virus type 1 transmission through breast feeding. *Lancet*, **340**, 585–8.

Erb, P., Krauchi, S. & Burgin, D. (1994) Quantitative anti-p24 determinations can predict the risk of vertical transmission. *Journal of Acquired Immune Deficiency Syndrome*, **7**, 261–4.

European Collaborative Study Group (1992) Risk factors for mother-to-child transmission of HIV-1. *Lancet*, **339**, 1007–12.

European Collaborative Study Group (1994) Caesarean section and risk of vertical transmission of HIV-1 infection. *Lancet*, **343**, 1464–7.

Green, J. & Kentish, J. (1995) The right not to know HIV-test results. *Lancet*, **345**, 1508.

Heyward, W.L., Batter, V.L., Malulu, M. *et al.* (1993) Impact of HIV counselling and testing among child-bearing women in Kinshasa, Zaire. *AIDS*, **7**, 1633–37.

Howard, L.C., Hawkins, D.A., Marwood, R. *et al.* (1989) Transmission of human immunodeficiency virus by heterosexual contact with reference to antenatal screening. *British Journal of Obstetrics & Gynaecology*, **96**, 135–9.

Johnstone, F.D., Brettle, R.R. & MacCallum, L.R. (1990) Women's knowledge of their HIV antibody status: its effect on their decision whether to continue the pregnancy. *British Medical Journal*, **300**, 23–4.

Mansson, S.A. (1990) Psychosocial aspects of HIV testing – the Swedish experience. *AIDS Care*, **2**, 5–16.

Meadows, J. & Catalan, J. (1992) HIV seroprevalence and antenatal clinics. *Lancet*, **339**, 622–3.

Meadows, J., Catalan, J., Sherr, L., Stone, Y. & Gazzard, B. (1992) Testing for HIV in the ante-natal clinic: the views of midwives. *AIDS Care*, **4**, 157–64.

Palasanthiran, D., Ziegler, J.B. & Stewart, G.J. (1993) Breast feeding during primary maternal Human Immune Deficiency Virus infection and risk of transmission from mother to infant. *Journal of Infectious Diseases*, **167**, 441–4.

Peckham, C.S. (1994) Human immunodeficiency virus and pregnancy. *Sexually Transmitted Diseases*, **21** (suppl), S28–S31.

Selwyn, M.D., Carter, R.J. & Schoenbaum, E.E. (1989) Knowledge of HIV antibody status and decisions to continue or terminate pregnancy among IV drug users. *Journal of American Medical Association*, **261**, 3567–71.

Temmerman, M., Ndinya-Achola, A., Ambani, J., Piot, P. (1995) The right not to know HIV test results. *Lancet*, **345**, 969–71.

Chapter 10

Counselling Issues for Children and Families Living with HIV Infection

Diane Melvin

In the UK and other European countries, the early 1990s saw a substantial increase in the number of HIV positive adults who became infected through heterosexual contact. The number of women known to be HIV infected showed the greatest increase and at the time of writing there are well over 3000 women known to be HIV positive or to have AIDS in the UK. However, figures obtained from anonymous screening programmes indicate that the number of women known to be infected is a considerable underestimate of the actual number of HIV positive women. The majority of women will be of child bearing age so an increase in the number of infected women will be accompanied by a parallel but smaller rise in the number of children who are HIV positive. Vertical transmission, i.e. from mother to child, is the route of infection for almost all new paediatric HIV cases in the UK and other countries which now screen blood products for the presence of the virus. However, all the children living in families where someone is HIV positive will be affected by the presence of HIV whether or not they themselves are infected.

Much of our knowledge about the emotional and psychological needs of HIV infected persons is based on situations where homosexual or bisexual experiences and/or drug use have featured in the life experiences of the infected person. There is also an increasing body of knowledge built up around children, young persons and adults who have acquired HIV infection through contaminated blood products – in particular the haemophiliac population. In most of the situations described here, there is usually only one family member who is infected. In contrast, where there is a child who acquired HIV infection via vertical transmission, there will be at least one other family member – the mother and also maybe the father and/or other siblings or relations – who are also HIV infected. Thus the focus of care in these situations extends from the individual and their partner to the needs of the whole family (Fig. 10.1).

It is the impact of HIV infection on family structures and functioning, together with the complexity of change and loss within such families, which will be the central theme for this chapter. Identifying particular stress points for individuals within these families will be discussed, as well as a consideration of the needs of wider affected family members as well as those directly infected by this disease.

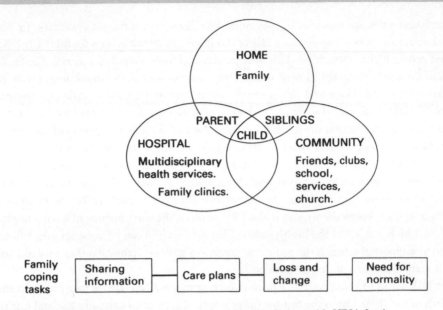

Fig. 10.1   Interlinking systems in the care of families living with HIV infection.

Background to paediatric HIV infection

Whilst present knowledge about the natural history of HIV infection in children is much less extensive than that known for infected adults, it is an area of rapid learning and research (Pizzo & Wilfert 1994). Some caution needs to be exercised in extrapolating directly from data available from other populations which may differ significantly in demographic characteristics to that with which the counsellor is working. Familial and cultural factors, health and social provision, treatments and interventions may differ significantly both across countries and within communities and this makes it difficult to be clear about the effects of HIV separate from other factors. For example, in many of the paediatric populations reported from US centres there will be a high incidence of IV drug use in the parents of those children. The presence of such drugs in the system of the developing child, together with the lifestyle in which their parents and families live, may have a significant influence, particularly on measures of developmental outcome.

Vertical transmission

Virus transmission from an HIV infected woman to her baby can occur at three different times:

(1) Pre natal via placental exchanges whilst the baby is in the uterus
(2) At the time of delivery as the baby moves through the birth canal and may be exposed to body fluids
(3) Post natal – mainly via breastfeeding which has been shown to increase the risk of transmission by about 15% to 16%.

Transmission rates are reported to vary quite significantly in different countries. In European centres an average transmission rate of about 15% to 20% has been found (ECS 1992). Studies report higher rates from African countries and from some US centres. The health status of the mother, the drugs used during pregnancy as well as the medication given, the standards of antenatal care and the mode of delivery are all thought to influence the possibility of transmission of the virus. In those countries reporting a higher rate of vertical transmission, it may be that the mother has been infected for a longer period of time or her own health status is poor and these contribute to higher levels of transmission.

Research and clinical management policies try to identify both the times at which transmission is more likely to occur and those factors in the mother or the child which enhance or decrease the possibility of transmission. Pregnancy itself can be a very stressful time for a woman. When the woman is also HIV positive, the extra burden of having to make decisions which may affect the health status of her future child can be unbelievable. Women need to be supported through the process to lessen any guilt or shame that they may feel later should their child turn out to be infected.

The HIV status of a baby born to a positive mother may not be clear for many months after the birth of the child. Often the test for the presence of HIV is an antibody test and it is not possible for such a test to differentiate between maternal or child HIV antibodies. Maternal antibodies may not disappear from a child's system until well after the first year of its life. Parents may have to live with the uncertainty of having an indeterminate diagnosis on their child for many months. More centres are now able to offer tests which detect the virus itself and are not dependent on the presence of antibodies (Chapter 2). Such tests should be able to give a clear diagnosis of the child's HIV status within the first few months of life and their wider availability needs to be encouraged as they will help reduce anxiety about the child and provide an earlier basis for future care planning.

The impact of giving a clear diagnosis, whether it is perceived as good or bad news, should never be underestimated. The relief of hearing that their child is not infected may well be tinged with new worries and regrets for the parent. Not being there to see their child grow up, worrying about who will look after the child should they fall sick or die, and having to disengage from paediatric staff who have supported the parent and family up until that time, are just some of the thoughts that have been expressed. In a few instances it has been recorded that the mother's health has seriously deteriorated after confirmation that her child has not been infected. A contributory factor to this deterioration could be that she no longer felt she needed to be strong in case her child fell sick.

Progression of HIV in children

Infected children show a wide range of medical and physical problems, many of them similar to the kinds of illnesses noted in positive adults; for example, illnesses such as PCP, CMV infection and lymphadenopathy all occur in children. Other opportunistic infections in children include candidiasis and recurrent ear infections. Infected children are also more likely to pick up ordinary childhood illnesses, and these can often last longer and have a more pronounced effect because of the child's reduced immune system functioning. There are also some notable differences from the presentation in adults; for example, the incidence of Kaposi's sarcoma is much rarer in children than in adults.

In children who have been infected vertically, HIV will have been present whilst bodily systems are developing and subsequent problems may arise because of the damage caused by these effects. Developmental delay and failure to thrive occur commonly in children with HIV infection, although it must always be remembered that such presentations could be due to a whole variety of other factors as well. The kinds of developmental problems seen most noticeably in infected children are either those which affect motor functions or those affecting expressive abilities. Motor problems can range from a slowness to acquire some of the early developmental milestones or a mild weakness or increased tone in some of the limbs, to the presence of severe spasticity preventing mobility. Expressive weaknesses include slow acquisition of speech, reduced communications and interactions or an inability in older children to sustain attention and effort. Other common problems noted in infected children are poor appetite and feeding difficulties which are sometimes, but not always, associated with poor growth. Early interventions such as establishing adequate nutritional intake and eating routines can help prevent or can delay the progress of some of these problems, and medications such as AZT have been found to help promote progress and enhance quality of life for some children.

Infected children will vary in the range and the time of onset of symptoms associated with HIV. The diagnosis of AIDS is used less frequently in the paediatric setting; instead terms such as asymptomatic, mild or severe symptoms of HIV infection are much more frequently used. Whilst individual children vary in the manner in which symptoms progress, there does appear to be at least two main ways of progression. In one group (known as fast or rapid progressors) severe physical symptoms of illness appear early in life and many such children have a major physical illness within the first months of life. For this group of children prognosis is poor, and they usually do not survive after the first few years, although new medications and better care and nutrition are prolonging or increasing the quality of the lives of these children.

The second group of children (known as slow or non-progressors) may appear symptom free or have only mild symptoms for several years. Indeed some children may be well into school before there are any obvious signs that anything is wrong. The needs of these children and of their families will be very different from the former group. The children themselves have greater awareness of what is going on and may have questions and concerns which need to be considered. Further the chances of illness of a parent or other family member or of changes within the structure of the family are greatly increased for this latter group. Support systems will need an awareness of the unpredictable nature of the progress of paediatric HIV infection, and must be able to take on board the changing needs of children as they grow older and become more aware of what is happening.

Testing and diagnosis

An initial diagnosis of HIV infection for a woman or a child is frequently made at a time when stress or vulnerability is already present, for example during pregnancy or at a time of illness. It can be the child who is the first member of the family to be identified as being HIV positive. Often when this happens the child is sick and has an illness which suggests that HIV may be a possible underlying cause. Most parents whose child is sick will agree to investigations which help to identify the cause of the illness. Where testing confirms a child to be HIV positive, the result obtained has implications about the status of the mother, and this needs to be considered when consent is being obtained for testing of the child. It also has implications for the pre-test counselling for the parent. In such situations, consideration of where, when and who tests the mother and/or the father and maybe other children in the family also needs to be made.

If the mother is well, she may not want to be tested immediately and may not be emotionally ready to take on board new information until she has had time both to understand the implications of her child's diagnosis and also to see him or her recover from the presenting illness. However other parents find that the anxiety and uncertainty of not knowing their own status, or that of other children in the family, is worse than the possible upset of taking on board new or upsetting information, and they will request testing straightaway. Testing at a time and pace which takes into account individual differences can help prevent any further trauma or distress which may hinder the later process of acceptance. The following case illustrates such a situation.

Jenny's 8-month-old son was admitted to the paediatric ward and found to have PCP. Jenny agreed that he be tested for HIV and he was found to be positive. She immediately wanted to be tested herself and requested that this be carried out on the paediatric ward. As this was not thought to be appropriate, arrangements were made for her to see the health advisor and adult physician in the genitourinary medicine clinic at the hospital. She was accompanied by a support worker from the paediatric department.

When she received her positive diagnosis she appeared quite calm but rather detached. In the new few days she was extremely tearful and restless, not able to concentrate on her sick child or herself. Later on when her son was better and both had returned home, she mentioned that if she could she would like to turn the clock back and wait to be tested; even though in her heart she knew she must be positive she was not really prepared to hear the words and have it confirmed. She thinks she was so preoccupied with what she had been told about her diagnosis that she could not focus on her baby when he really needed her.

Jenny's partner, the father of the baby, was also offered the test at this time. He did not want to be tested and up to the time of writing has not wanted to know his HIV status. He has distanced himself from Jenny and the baby since the diagnosis was made.

Jenny, like many parents faced with an HIV diagnosis for themselves or their child, did not inform any friends or family about the diagnosis and all the personal support systems which can usually be called upon when such devastating news has been given could not be accessed. In time many parents do identify someone in their family or community to share the diagnosis with, but at the early stages most choose to cope alone. The fear of rejection, stigma or shame which is still associated with HIV appears greater than the need for sharing and personal support. This can lead to an exaggerated need for secrecy and confidentiality. Isolation is further exacerbated in cases where there is a single mother who may be caring for several children by herself. These are key features when the emotional support of parents is being considered. Understandably an over-dependence on statutory support systems can and does occur in such situations.

Unfortunately there have been instances where parents have either not realised that an

HIV test was being carried out on their child, or have not been made aware of the consequences if the result should be positive. Where a positive result was obtained, this led not only to extreme distress, anger and often denial, but also to a lack of trust in the services at that hospital or clinic. In some circumstances the family have refused to engage further with the hospital and have sought care elsewhere. If a decision is taken to test for the presence of HIV, even if the child or parent is perceived to be of low risk, the consequences if a positive result is obtained must always be considered and planned for.

> Stephen was 10 years old and although he had been a rather sickly boy who was not growing well, the question of HIV had never been contemplated as the cause of his ill health. He was admitted to his local hospital with meningitis and underwent a whole battery of tests to investigate the cause of his illness. Although informed that the blood being taken would be tested for HIV, his parents were given the impression that this was just a routine. When the test showed a positive result, both parents and staff were devastated. The situation was not helped by the diagnosis being given on a busy ward with no preparation or privacy. It appeared that the infection had resulted from a blood transfusion in Stephen's early life, at a time before all blood products were tested for HIV. These parents refused to return Stephen for care to the hospital of diagnosis as it took them a long time to believe the diagnosis. They were obsessed with issues of confidentiality.

Living with HIV

Discordant parents

The reactions and needs of uninfected partners of HIV infected adults can be diverse and their needs may be marginalised in the care provision of those who are infected. In a family situation this can affect the relationship between the partners, but may also change roles within the family. In working with mothers who are HIV positive there will be some situations where her partner will be HIV negative. He may have to cope with the illness and possible death of his partner and/or child, and may also face becoming the main carer of other children in the family.

> Peter's wife and baby son both tested positive for HIV, while Peter and his older daughter tested negative. He remarked how initially he felt so guilty and helpless: 'Why couldn't it be me instead of them; I'd do anything to take the place of my son'. The relationship with his wife was strong and, although initially there were some difficulties dealing with how she had become infected, they were able to provide mutual support for each other through the illness and eventual death of their baby son. Following his son's death the father withdrew from the family for a while; he did not know who he could approach or who, if anyone, could really understand what it was like for him. All his contacts were at the hospital and centred around the health issues of his wife and son. His wife is now unwell and the father has returned to care for his daughter. This main parenting role is unfamiliar for men from his ethnic group.

Family and cultural factors

Diverse family configurations are found within the population of families living with HIV infection. There are many single parent families, usually a positive mother, where the parent is looking after one or more children, some of whom may also be HIV positive. Issues of isolation and support as well as present and future child care may be paramount for these families. There are also many families with a more complex set of relationships. There may, for instance, be a number of adults – e.g. grandparents, brothers, sisters, aunts, uncles, cousins, in-laws etc. – who have a primary role to play in all matters concerning the index family. Parents may have several children from different relationships. There may be several adults and/or children who are HIV infected within these families. Family members may have different levels of knowledge about HIV; they may also complicate the issue of confidentiality. Families are not static bodies but systems in which there are frequent changes, both in the persons present and in the intensity of the relationships that exist. Health related problems can confuse relationships where HIV is present.

In the London population, for example, there is a wide cultural mix of families living with HIV. A large percentage of the parents originate from sub-Saharan African countries, although many European and Asian countries are also represented. Some adults have lived, worked or studied in the UK for many years, but others may be recently arrived and seeking asylum. Whatever their country of origin or residence status, there will be compounding factors for such families who are living outside their community of origin. These include:

- Language barriers
- Isolation due to separation from wider family and support networks
- Different attitudes to illness and disclosure of information
- Different child rearing practices
- Different family roles and expectations of men, women and children
- A lack of familiarity with, or trust of, counselling and other psychological support which may necessitate different approaches to help engage with or support such clients.

Finally, for all parents and families where someone is identified as HIV positive, there may be financial and other practical or social difficulties to be resolved before aspects relating to health and emotional well-being can be dealt with; for example, providing ongoing support at a clinic or centre may be wasted if the parent has no money to travel there or if no facilities for young children exist at such clinics.

Support needs

Most people living with HIV infection face enormous emotional stress and concerns. These may be compounded in family situations where there is more than one infected person and where there are young affected and infected children. The following issues need to be considered with regard to children living in such families:

- Uncertainty and confusion
- Confidentiality and sharing of information
- Multiple change and loss
- Future care plans.

Uncertainty and confusion

Preparation and decision making can be difficult when outcomes and consequences are unclear. The kind and speed of progression of illness is very uncertain with HIV infection. Children who are infected themselves and know of their diagnosis may wonder how long they will be able to do all the things their friends can, and whether they will still be treated normally etc. Being seen as different can be a source of upset for many children and there is an ongoing need to maintain ordinary routines and activities. Others who do not know about the diagnosis, either of themselves or someone else, may be bewildered or confused by new events or changes in their lives and routines. There may be many new people visiting their home and talking quietly to the parent, more hospital visits, periods of separation, and maybe also new caregivers to get to know.

Whilst it may not be possible to help children cope with all the concerns about the progression of the illness, many of these other events can be explained and sometimes prepared for. There is much literature, both from the fields of other chronic childhood illnesses and from the study of children's emotional development, to show that if children are prepared and involved in what is happening to them, their adjustment is better, they are less anxious, and they worry less that what is happening is their fault or is out of control.

Confidentiality and sharing of information

Children can be the last people in a family to be told about the presence of HIV. Parents are often reluctant to disclose the diagnosis to their children because of fears about what the child might do with the information. There is a need to protect the child and themselves from any adverse consequences if the news were to spread. They fear the rejection and stigma that is still associated with HIV.

It can help if understanding is seen as a process, with disclosure being only one part of this process. Honest explanations about what is happening may be as important as giving a full diagnosis; for example, when asked questions such as: Why is mummy always tired? Why are they taking blood? etc. Working towards full disclosure by giving age appropriate explanations can help reduce adult anxieties and children's concerns that maybe they are to blame for any illness or upset. Deciding when, how, and who should give new information also has to be addressed. Ideally a parent telling their child about his/her HIV status probably promotes the best trust and comfort for the child. But this can be upsetting for parents and access to someone who can discuss ways of doing this, or provide some subsequent help for the children, may give greater confidence.

It also needs to be remembered that some families or cultures are less open about discussing personal subjects with their children than the professionals expect. If the pace of disclosure is uncomfortable to parents, they may disengage with the professionals which in turn will not benefit the children. The following example shows how a child was able to cope with the news of HIV as long as he was aware of who he could share it with.

Steve was eight years old and quite a chatterbox at school, never able to keep any secrets. His mother wanted to tell him that his father was HIV positive and sick, but she was worried that he would tell all his school friends and she feared that if they told their parents and teachers no one would want to play with him. Steve became more distressed and difficult at school; he worried about his dad and it seemed he was blaming himself because he knew something was wrong. His mother decided she needed to tell him what was happening and she identified a teacher at the school whom she felt comfortable with telling, so that Steve had someone to talk to. Steve was told about the HIV and was able to spend some special times with his dad before he died. He has never told his friends the name of the illness, but if they ask tells them his daddy had something wrong with his blood.

Multiple change and loss

Coping with the many and often complex losses which continually impinge on families is a common reason for referral for support. Losses include those to do with health and future expectations as well as death. For some children the changes that occur when they and/or another loved one show behavioural or neurological changes, resulting from the effect of the infection, can be particularly stressful. Children may have to face seeing their parents become frail or disturbed and perhaps unable to care for them. Others may be aware that they themselves or their brother or sister are not able to do something they were previously able to do. Separation can add to these changes, as the following example illustrates.

Johnnie, aged 6 years, and his mother, Rose, were both HIV positive. They had been diagnosed soon after their arrival in the UK (as refugees from Zaire). Johnnie and his mother were both ill and had simultaneous separate hospitalisations. Johnnie spoke no English and was confused and upset by being in unfamiliar surroundings. It was the added loss caused by their separation which hindered both Johnnie and his mother in recovering from their presenting illnesses. Plans were made to try to maintain contact and encourage visiting time when either had to be admitted.

Giving honest, age-appropriate explanations can help most children cope with very upsetting or adverse situations. Children often know much more about illness, loss and death than adults realise, and with preparation and support they will be able to share in the rituals around death and the funeral. They must also be allowed time to grieve. It is crucial not to assume that children cannot cope and seek to keep the truth from them out of a misguided wish to protect the child from an unpalatable reality.

Planning for future care

Planning for the long-term care of their child after their death is perhaps one of the most emotionally painful tasks a parent can undertake. It reflects a time when one of the most important of human relationships – the bond between parent and child – comes to an end. If plans can be made when the parent is well and feels in control of the process, there is the opportunity for careful consideration of the options available and time for children to be involved in the plans where appropriate.

It is important, wherever appropriate, to involve the child in the discussions and planning. For children who are faced with the death of a parent or loved one, and possibly with their own death, the question 'who will be there to care for me?' is a prime one. It is important that the child should be reassured that this has not been forgotten, and that the child's wishes should, as far as possible, be taken into account. Without this the chances of the child adapting successfully to whatever the future holds are likely to be much reduced.

In the UK at the moment the majority of infected children are still living with at least one natural parent. However, as time passes there will be an increasing number of children, especially the uninfected children of infected parents, who face a future with foster parents, adopting parents or with other carers. Some infected children will also outlive their parents and need care from others. Plans for this eventuality need to be made early where possible, and appropriate contact established between the child and those who will care for him or her when the parent becomes sick or dies. This avoids a situation of the child having to face at the same time the death or serious illness of a parent and being looked after by strangers.

Children feel more secure when regular routines are in place and when they can stay in familiar surroundings. These are important considerations in building up a care package. It is also important, wherever possible, to maintain links with the family of origin, even if it is not possible for that family to look after the child directly. Building up memories with the parent, assembling mementoes and providing appropriate cultural experiences are also important in helping the child to prepare for the death of a parent and for life afterwards.

A package of care needs to take into account short-term as well as longer-term considerations. Parent(s) and child may become sick unexpectedly and, in some cases, at the same time. A comprehensive plan needs to take into account planning for the hospital admission of the parent. Who will look after the child or children? There needs to be planning for respite care for the parent and, often, for child care support which can work alongside the parent to reduce the strain on them and support the family. Day care provision may be needed for the child either on a continuing basis or on an occasional basis while the parent attends hospital appointments or feels too unwell to cope.

This sort of planning cannot be done at the last moment in a panic. It is important to make forward plans as early as possible. It is better to plan properly, even where such planning may be distressing to the parent at the time, than to leave matters until an emergency occurs and the parent cannot cope with either planning or the child. Knowing that their child will be looked after properly if they die is usually a great comfort to parents, and the short-term upset of planning for such an eventuality is much less than the worries of uncertainty if plans are not made. If the plans turn out to be unnecessary, no-one is likely to be too unhappy about it.

Overview

Whilst paediatric HIV infection is still a relatively rare illness in the UK, there are increasing numbers of affected children who are living within families where there is someone who is HIV positive. The needs of these children may be marginalised or given little consideration within health and support systems, which tend to concentrate resources on the infected person. Consistency of care and access to normal routines and resources must be features in the lives of all these children, whether infected or affected.

There is increasing evidence that family clinics and family centred care are the preferred systems for providing ongoing care and support. However, within such a system some individuals will also need to be given the option of personal counselling or therapeutic support, and this should be available for the children as well as the adults. The quality of all these children's lives must be of continuing concern to us all.

Further reading

Ammann, A.J. (1994) Human immunodeficiency virus infection/AIDS in children: the next decade. *Paediatrics*, 93(6), 930–35.

Barnett, R. & Blaikie, P. (1992) *AIDS in Africa*. Belhaven Press, London.

Bor, R. & Elford, J. (eds) (1994) *The family and HIV*. Redwood Books, Wiltshire.

Cates, J.A., Graham, L.L., Boeglin, D. & Tielker, S. (1990) The Effects of AIDS on the Family. *Families in Society*, **ZI**, 95–201.

CDR (1990–1994) *Communicable Disease Report 4*. PHLS Communicable Disease Surveillance Centre, 61 Colindale Avenue, London NW9 5EQ.

Eiser, C. (1990) *Chronic Childhood Disease: An Introduction to Psychological Theory and Research*. Cambridge University Press, Cambridge.

Levine, C. & Stein, G.L. (1994) *Orphans of the HIV Epidemic*. The Orphan Project, 121 Avenue of the Americas, New York 10013.

Melvin, D. & Sherr, L. (1993) The child in the family – responding to AIDS and HIV. *AIDS Care*, 5(1), 35–42.

Tasker, M. (1992) *How Can I Tell You?* Association for the Care of Children's Health. Maryland, Bethesda.

Walker, G. (1990) *In the Midst of Winter*. W.W. Norton & Co, New York.

References

ECS (European Collaborative Study) (1992) Risk factors for mother-to-child transmission of HIV. *Lancet*, 339(8800) 1007–1012.

Pizzo, P. & Wilfert, C. (eds) (1994) *Paediatric AIDS: The Challenge of HIV Infection in Infants, Children and Adolescence*, 2nd edn. Williams and Wilkins, Baltimore.

Chapter 11

The Worried Well

John Green and John Kentish

The term 'worried well' has undergone a change in meaning. Originally it simply meant someone who was worried about HIV or AIDS but had not been tested and had no symptoms. Today it is used to refer to someone who is excessively worried about AIDS or HIV infection despite being known to be uninfected or being objectively at little or no risk. The huge amount of media coverage given to HIV and AIDS has resulted in many people becoming anxious and seeking testing. Each time there has been a publicity campaign on HIV and AIDS, genitourinary medicine clinics have seen a sharp rise in the number of patients seeking testing for HIV. Of these people some will be reassured by pre-test counselling or their negative test result, whereas the 'worried well' are not reassured and remain convinced that they have been infected.

To most clinics offering the test, the worried well individual is a familiar sight. Often highly anxious, they seem to have little to worry about in reality.

Mary was a 58-year-old woman who had been celibate for six years since her husband died. Following a mild bout of illness, probably influenza, she became worried that she had contracted HIV infection. She worked in a busy shop and felt sure that she had been in contact with someone who was infected. She thought that they had passed on the virus to her by giving her money with 'body fluids' on it; possibly someone had licked their fingers before giving her a bank-note. She worried about HIV for much of every day; it was seldom far from her thoughts and she interpreted every minor illness as the result of AIDS. At the time of coming for testing she had already put her affairs in order and was coming for final confirmation of what she already 'knew' to be a fact, that she was infected and would soon die.

Sometimes individuals who are worried well do have some very small theoretical risk of being infected.

Jim had travelled widely on business. He had, on two occasions over the past three years, had sex with a prostitute in New York in a hotel. On both occasions there had been some oral sex first but intercourse had been with a condom. Over the past year, with all the information about AIDS in the media, he had become convinced not only that he had become infected with HIV but also that he had infected his wife and children. At the time of presenting he was in a thoroughly wretched state of anxiety or depression.

Presenting symptoms

The worried well are a mixed group, but there are some common themes to their histories. Initially, something makes them believe that they have been at risk of infection. Sometimes there is no real risk but the patient is misinformed or uninformed about the transmission of HIV. Sometimes there has been some slight risk but at a level at which most people would not allow it to dominate their thoughts. Thoughts of being infected by HIV then become a consuming obsession on which they ruminate constantly. As a result they may develop the somatic symptoms of anxiety and these can be so dramatic that they begin to feel that they are physically ill and this tends to confirm their worst fears.

Miller *et al.* (1988), in a study of 19 worried well patients, found that the most common presenting symptoms included fatigue, sweating, skin rashes, muscle pains, intermittent diarrhoea, slightly swollen glands, sore throat, slight weight loss, minor mouth infections and dizziness. Superficially some of these symptoms appear to the patient to be those which can accompany HIV infection, but most of these symptoms can also occur as a result of anxiety.

Categories of the worried well

Careful examination of the cases of those who are worried well shows that they fall into several overlapping categories.

Misunderstanders

These are people who have misunderstood the way in which the virus is transmitted and consider that they have been at risk. Most people understand that certain activities are very risky (e.g. unprotected intercourse), whilst other activities are safe (e.g. shaking hands), but there are some activities such as kissing, about which there remains a degree of uncertainty in people's minds. This uncertainty is often based on rumours that circulate in any community about certain activities being more dangerous than was previously thought. Misinformation in the media can also counteract the effects of health education campaigns run by government and voluntary groups. Generally such individuals can overcome their fears by being provided with clear, precise information and they are much reassured by a discussion of the issues.

Hypochondriacs

In every age and in every place there are people who worry about their health to the extent that they believe they have whatever disease happens to be fashionable or attracting attention at that time. It is interesting to compare what is being written about in the newspapers or covered on television against what illnesses people feel they have at any given time. In the past few years there have been bursts of people with food allergies of various sorts, with post-viral syndrome, with legionnaire's disease, even with problems associated with strip-lighting following publicity on these problems. This is not to say that these problems are not real ones, nor that people do not suffer terribly from them. But undoubtedly many people present at hospitals utterly convinced that they have these problems when, in fact, they do not.

It is likely that many people in the population feel generally unwell for much of the time. They seek an explanation of this, initially from their doctor and later, when he or she cannot help, through their own reading and research. They are often extremely well informed about the illness which they feel they have. Sometimes if they are convinced that they do not have one illness they will switch to another.

Alan, a gay man, became convinced that he was infected with HIV despite repeated blood tests which were negative. After many sessions of counselling he was finally convinced that he was not infected. After the end of the treatment he contacted the hospital to say that he was sure he had contracted legionnaire's disease.

The guilty

A surprising number of people in the population suffer from chronic unresolved guilt; in particular guilt about past sexual behaviour is very common. Green and George (1988) found that in a sample of 30 worried well, 19 patients reported moderate or severe feelings of guilt about some past event in which they broke their own concept of moral behaviour. Very often this was an affair or a time at which they committed some sexual act of which they did not approve, or of which they felt those close to them would not have approved. Guilt is one of the most under-researched human emotions and yet it would appear that it may be a powerful factor in many people's inner lives. Few of these people seek any sort of counselling or advice about their feelings, but the appearance of AIDS has provided a focus for their anxiety and guilt and it may be that sometimes there is also a self-punitive element in their fears.

In 1981 Peter had had a brief affair with a woman at work at a time when his marriage was going through a bad patch. He felt her to be promiscuous at the time and had vaguely disapproved of her. He had terminated their relationship. He had always felt very guilty about this affair and had striven to be a model husband when it ended. The woman had subsequently moved to another firm. Recently quite by chance he heard that she had become seriously ill. He immediately thought of AIDS and gradually became more and more convinced that he had caught HIV from her and had passed this on to his wife, and probably to his children. The family dog had been unwell and he half-wondered whether he might not have passed the virus to the dog through some cut on his hands, even though he knew this to be ridiculous.

AIDS as an addition to psychiatric illness

A small proportion of the worried well are individuals suffering from psychiatric conditions with concerns about AIDS as a more or less incidental feature. Worries about AIDS occasionally appear as features of schizophrenic delusions or as part of a paranoid delusional state. Rarely they appear as a mono-symptomatic delusion. More commonly they appear either as features of depressive illnesses or as part of obsessional states, particularly those obsessions concerned with cleaning. The issues of both depression and obsessions are covered in more detail in Chapter 12.

It is worth separating those worried well in whom AIDS has become incorporated into a pre-existing psychiatric condition, from those frequent cases in which worried well patients have, as a result of their worries, become depressed, anxious or obsessional.

In a busy clinic dealing with individuals who are very ill with HIV-related conditions, it is easy to ignore the worried well and treat them as a nuisance. In fact a disturbingly high proportion of them turn out to be quite depressed or highly distressed. Worries about AIDS can often produce levels of depression and anxiety far higher than those seen in an individual with AIDS itself. Suicidal thoughts and suicide attempts are not uncommon, and some suicide attempts are successful.

Dealing with the worried well

Pre-test counselling

Pre-test counselling is likely to be much the same with the worried well as with those who are objectively at higher risk. The level of risk should be established early on in pre-test counselling. The time taken for pre-test counselling is likely to be less for the person with no risk, simply because some of the issues discussed will not be particularly relevant. The person will not, for instance, require a detailed discussion of some risk behaviours because they simply do not engage in them.

On the other hand it is important not to skimp on pre-test counselling for several reasons. First, good pre-test counselling is an educative process which will help the patient understand why he is not at risk. It is important to feed back to the patient a realistic assessment of their risk. Secondly, someone who is at low risk at the moment may, of course, start to engage in higher risk behaviour in the future and pre-test counselling provides an opportunity to educate. Thirdly, it will prepare them to understand the blood test results when they come back. Fourthly, because pre-test counselling in itself serves to reassure patients tht they are not at risk, it reduces the anxiety level of the patient while they wait for the results. Finally, it is worth bearing in mind that being worried about HIV does not in itself serve as a protection against getting it. Some people who appear highly anxious do, in fact, have some degree of risk. A few of them will actually be infected.

When explaining these issues to patients it is important to inform without attempting to offer reassurance (Saikovskis & Warwick 1986). Informing in this case means giving the facts to the patient and then helping them to draw their conclusions. Offering reassurance by saying, 'You have nothing to worry about, you are perfectly healthy', or, 'There is absolutely nothing wrong with you', will conflict with the patient's own beliefs and inner feelings that there is something wrong with them, and so the patient is likely to dismiss such reassurances.

Post-test counselling

At post-test counselling the counsellor is almost certain to be holding a negative test result for the worried well patient. It is important at this stage to discuss the patient's worries in detail and to try to convince them that the test result is accurate. This can only be done by relating the negative result to the fact that the patient has been at no risk or at minimal risk. With many worried well patients the test result in itself does not serve to reassure more than temporarily. In most countries with testing facilities there are numbers of worried well individuals who travel from test site to test site seeking repeated blood tests, simply because they do not believe the results they have been given. In a study by Green and George (1988) of 24 worried well who had had HIV tests, 12 had had more than one test, with one man having had as many as nine.

At post-test counselling it is also important to try to assess how likely it is that the patient is actually reassured. If they are not reassured it is important to assess whether they have actually understood the information they have been given.

For patients who still appear anxious about HIV after counselling, and even after they have understood the facts about AIDS, it is particularly important to try to discover the reason why they remain worried. The patient should be assessed for anxiety, depression and obsessions, and carefully questioned about past contact with psychiatric services in a way that does not imply that the counsellor feels that the patient is mentally ill.

It is also important to discuss with anyone whose result is negative any risk behaviours they may have and to seek to ensure that these are reduced. For their future health and peace of mind it is also important to ensure that those who are unnecessarily worried now understand the true facts about the virus.

Further referrals

Where the patient remains worried, there are two choices available to the counsellor. He or she can undertake either to try to help the patient himself/herself, or can refer the patient on for specialist help. The decision is likely to be based on the level of anxiety and depression, on the counsellor's confidence that he can deal with the problem, and on the amount of time available to the counsellor. Clearly, a patient who is very depressed or actively suicidal is in need of specialist help as a matter of urgency.

It is crucial for any counsellor to have good mental health facilities as a back-up. Referring on worried well patients in need of psychiatric support is a necessary skill for a counsellor. It is important to be frank with the patient and to stress that they appear anxious and depressed and that sometimes these feelings can make it difficult to accept the results of a blood test, but that if these feelings can be dealt with the patient will feel better and, hopefully, stop worrying about HIV.

Patients who have come thinking they have AIDS are sometimes rather unhappy about the suggestion that they should be referred for psychiatric help. It needs tact on the part of the counsellor and, if they do decide to be referred, it needs knowledge of HIV and tact on the part of the mental health worker who takes the referral. Sometimes the counsellor may feel it best to see a patient a few times himself until he feels that the patient has built up sufficient trust to agree to being referred. It also helps greatly if the referral can be made to a mental health professional whom the counsellor can vouch for and can discuss with the patient by name.

If the counsellor decides to try to help the patient himself he will be aiming to use the same sort of skills which are used in dealing with anxiety, depression and obsessional behaviours and thoughts in the HIV positive patient. The types of approaches which can be used are dealt with in detail in Chapter 12.

In addition to dealing with any anxiety or depression, discussing the patient's worries with them can be of considerable value. In particular, those who are guilty about some past sexual episode may want to talk over the issue with the counsellor or try to find some resolution in their own minds. This can be a valuable process but it is always important to keep an eye on the patient and to make sure that they are, in fact, becoming less worried or guilty. If they are just using the service as a prop but not making any progress, the counsellor is still going to need to pick up the issue and to think in terms of referral.

Individuals who are worried well can often be frustratingly difficult to deal with. However it is surprising just how successful simple interventions can be with those who are not suffering from major depressive symptoms or other major psychiatric conditions.

Anthony was a 36-year-old man who had no previous psychiatric history. Following the break-up of his marriage three years before, he had gone through a very bad period. He had stopped going out socially, his only social contact being at work. He lived alone and spent most of his leisure hours reading or watching the television. He had had one brief affair with a woman he met in a pub. It had been an unpleasant experience because they had split up under strained circumstances with her accusing him of being an 'inadequate person'. He had not liked her and had only had sex with her for the company. Later he had noticed her in the pub with several different men, and formed the view that she was 'promiscuous'. Shortly after breaking up with her he began to worry about AIDS and this anxiety built up until he was thinking about the issue most of the time.

On assessment Anthony was sleeping a normal amount, eating well and, though he felt life was 'pointless', he denied suicidal intentions. He did not enjoy much in his life but he did have a few things which brought him pleasure. He felt himself, accurately, to be mildly depressed and he was also anxious. When he thought about AIDS he sometimes felt rather dizzy and, while he did not have panic attacks during the day, he was troubled by vivid and unpleasant dreams and sometimes woke in the night sweating heavily.

He was somewhat reassured by the information he was given about AIDS. However, he still continued to worry that he might have it, despite realising rationally that this was not so. He benefited from discussion of his life with the counsellor. The counsellor also taught him relaxation skills which he found very helpful in reducing his physical anxiety symptoms. At the same time he was encouraged to increase the level of pleasurable activity in his life. The counsellor and patient drew up a list of activities which he enjoyed and could carry out, including visiting places he enjoyed. At the same time he began building up his social life, inviting people at work round for dinner, taking every opportunity to go out with them and looking up old friends he had lost contact with.

His level of anxiety began to reduce and he became more cheerful and less depressed. He also began to feel that he was coping much better with his life. After six sessions he reported that he only thought about AIDS occasionally and was enjoying life much more.

It was agreed that he would continue to work on his own but come back in three months for follow-up. In the intervening period he could come back if he felt that things were not going well. At follow-up he reported that he was continuing to feel better, that he thought about AIDS infrequently and that when he did think of AIDS it no longer worried him as much as it used to. He had begun to go out with a woman with whom he got on very well. He had high expectations of the relationship and these seemed to be justified from his account.

Suggestions

The case study above illustrates several useful techniques. The following suggestions from Green and Davey (1991) may be helpful.

(1)   The patient should be discouraged from taking a disproportionate interest in information in the media about HIV or AIDS.
(2)   They should be encouraged to find other ways of spending their time. This may involve taking up old interests or developing new activities.
(3)   They should be encouraged to reduce the time spent thinking about HIV. Patients should be encouraged to monitor their thoughts and as soon as they start thinking about HIV, to think about something else or to do something that distracts them.
(4)   The patient needs to try to resolve as far as possible the issue of guilt.
(5)   Where there are outstanding problems in the patient's life, particularly decisions which should have been taken, the patient needs to be encouraged to take action and restore control.
(6)   The patient may need direct help in reducing anxiety levels. Teaching relaxation techniques may help.

Overview

Sometimes it is difficult in the middle of the HIV/AIDS epidemic not to feel rather resentful about the time and energy the worried well can absorb. However they, like those who have HIV-related diseases, do have a real problem and like those with the disease itself have a right to be counselled to try to reduce distress and to promote well-being. Furthermore, without too much difficulty, it is possible to help most of these people.

References

Green, J. & Davey, T. (1991) The worried well. *AIDS Care* 3(3), 289–93.
Green, J. & George, H. (1989) *Treating the Worried Well.* Presented at the International Conference on AIDS, Stockholm, June 1989.
Miller, D., Acton, T. & Hedge, B. (1988) The Worried Well; their identification and management. *Journal of the Royal College of Physicians*, 22, 550–52.
Saikovskis, P. & Warwick H. (1986) Morbid preoccupations, healthy anxiety and reassurance: a cognitive-behavioural approach to hypochondriasis. *Behaviour Research and Therapy*, 24, 597–602.

Chapter 12

Dealing with Anxiety and Depression

John Green

Anxiety

Some degree of anxiety is virtually universal in individuals who have a positive antibody test result. Even for someone who has adjusted to being infected there are likely to be occasions when he becomes anxious, perhaps when a friend dies of AIDS, or when he reads something disturbing about AIDS in the newspaper, or when he feels that he is not well. However, anxiety can be long-lasting and intense and it can make people's lives unpleasant. Since anxiety can usually be reduced with the right intervention, it is important to assess for it and to intervene if anxiety is long-lasting or if there are frequent bouts of anxiety.

Anxiety has four different components:

- A somatic (physical) component
- A cognitive component (changes in thought patterns)
- An affective component (changes in feelings)
- A behavioural component.

One or more of these components may be missing, particularly in someone who is only mildly anxious. Moreover the actual pattern of anxiety differs quite a bit from person to person. People who are very anxious usually have elements of all four components.

Table 12.1 shows the symptoms of anxiety. It is important with all seropositives to check whether they have these symptoms and how frequent and intense they are. Looking at the physical symptoms of anxiety it is clear that many of them are, individually, seen in physical illnesses. For instance, individuals with pneumocystis also show shortness of breath. Those with meningitis have headaches. Those with opportunistic infections of the gut have diarrhoea. This overlap between the symptoms of physical disease and anxiety can cause people to worry that they are physically ill when in fact they are showing normal symptoms of anxiety. It is also the basis of some of the difficulties with dealing with the worried well.

In assessing for anxiety one is, as with all other assessments, looking for a pattern of symptoms. Where there is any doubt about whether physical symptoms are the result of anxiety or of disease they should always be thoroughly investigated to reassure the patient as well as to ensure that nothing is missed. However, frequently physical symptoms are obviously the result of anxiety because the pattern shown does not resemble physical illness

Table 12.1   Symptoms of anxiety.

Somatic symptoms	
Muscular	Tension headache
	Pains in muscles and joints
	Shaking
	Feelings of tension in the muscles
Cardiovascular symptoms	Increased heart rate
	Sensation of heart pounding
	Peripheral vasoconstriction causing cold hands and feet and whiteness in extremities
	Flushing
Breathing	A feeling of tightness in the chest
	Difficulty in breathing
	Excessive yawning
	Overbreathing (hyperventilation)
Sweating	Sweating on palms and soles of feet
	Excessive sweating in axillae
	Generalised sweating
Dizziness	
Blurred vision	
Loss of libido	Loss of desire
	Impotence
	Lack of arousal
	Lack of vaginal lubrication
	Failure to reach orgasm
Sleep disturbance	Delay in getting off to sleep
	Very light fitful sleep
	Frequent waking
	Disturbing, vivid dreams
Gastro-intestinal	Nausea
	Lack of appetite
	Diarrhoea
	Frequent bowel movement
Frequency of micturition	
Affective symptoms	
	Feelings of anxiety
	Feelings of panic
	Feelings of being 'out of control'
Cognitive symptoms	
	Difficulty in concentrating
	Preoccupation with problems
	Narrowing of attention
	Excessive worrying over minor issue
	Feeling that things are out of control
Behavioural symptoms	
	Avoidance of particular situations
	Rapid speech
	Jerky or sudden movements
	Increased levels of overall activity

and because the patient is able to identify the link between physical symptoms and cognitive, affective and behavioural symptoms.

Anxiety comes in two types: steady or fluctuating high background level of anxiety, or intense bursts of very high anxiety – panic attacks. Many people have a mixture of the two types. Sometimes people have one panic attack and then never have another. In some there may be very frequent panic attacks, sometimes only lasting a few minutes at a time but repeated over and over again.

There are several steps to take in dealing with anxiety.

Explaining to the patient what is happening

The symptoms of anxiety, the physical ones in particular, are very dramatic. Many patients think that they are physically ill when they have them; sometimes people in panic attacks even think that they are going to die or go mad. They need to be given a clear explanation of the meaning of the symptoms.

Table 12.1 shows that many of the symptoms of anxiety are those of general excitement. Indeed physiologically the changes seen in anxiety are much the same as those seen in someone violently in love or very angry. They are the result of a generalised physiological reaction which has been called the 'fight or flight' response, because it prepares the body for action. The exceptions are symptoms like tension headaches, which are the result of prolonged increased muscle tension, and sleep disturbances, which are the result of the carry-over of anxiety from the day. It is helpful to explain this to the patient, as with Paul:

PAUL: 'So, why do I get these physical sensations?'
COUNSELLOR: 'They are intended to prepare your body for rapid action, for fighting or
               for running away.'
PAUL: 'But I don't have anything to fight or run away from.'
COUNSELLOR: 'That's right, but your body doesn't know that; it has the same primitive
               response to all sorts of stresses. Somewhere part of your mind knows you
               are under threat, but it doesn't know quite what threat so it prepares you
               for any eventuality.'
PAUL: 'But why do I get these particular symptoms?'

The answer is actually very straightforward. Each of the symptoms of anxiety serves a purpose. In general they are aimed at making rapid vigorous muscular effort easier or more efficient.

There is a rise in heart rate and in cardiac output (pounding heart) to increase blood flow. When someone engages in violent physical activity they need increased blood flow to the muscles; in the fight or flight response this occurs in advance of the physical effort so that the person is prepared for when muscular activity starts. At the same time blood is shifted away from non-essential areas so that it can be concentrated on the muscles; the blood vessels of the hands, feet and skin contract so the person goes pale and their extremities go cold. Blood is diverted away from the stomach and this contributes to the feeling of 'butterflies in the stomach'.

There is increased sweating on hands and feet because wet skin is tougher than dry skin and slightly damp skin grips better. More general sweating is aimed at preparing for the sweating needed to dissipate heat generated by muscular effort.

Emptying the bowels and bladder has obvious advantages. Loss of appetite is partly the result of changes in blood-flow away from the stomach, and partly for survival reasons. If our ancestors were being chased by lions it paid not to stop to eat a banana. It also paid not to stop to have sex, hence the effects on libido. Basically all appetites and needs are reduced and concentration is shifted to the main aim, survival, the changes in concentration being particularly obvious in some anxious subjects.

There is an increase in muscle tension designed to prepare for vigorous rapid muscular action. If this is sustained over long periods it can lead to tension headaches and muscular pains. The breathing changes are interesting in themselves because they can often be quite crucial to the experience of anxiety. Most people when they are anxious overbreathe, some quite substantially. Overbreathing is aimed at increasing the oxygen content of the blood; it simply means breathing too much for the immediate needs of the body. Obviously it prepares for the increased oxygen requirements of active muscles. However if overbreathing is sustained for long periods it causes excessive loss of carbon dioxide. This, while a waste product, is crucial to blood chemistry and can lead to an interesting situation:

- When carbon dioxide loss becomes excessive the brain acts to shut down the breathing and bring blood chemistry back into balance. It does so in part by increasing muscle tension in the chest. The patient thus feels a 'tightness' in the chest.
- In part because of the disrupted blood chemistry the patient feels that he is not getting enough oxygen and tries to breathe more rapidly.
- The patient struggles to breathe while the brain struggles to cut down on breathing.

It is an interesting struggle which occasionally results in the patient fainting; this returns breathing to normal and the patient is fine. However, this is unusual. Generally overbreathing occurs on a much less dramatic scale, with the patient complaining of episodes of breathlessness and tightness in the chest. Episodes of dizziness and faintness can often be traced to overbreathing.

It is important to go through the reasons for the symptoms of anxiety with a patient. It can make a tremendous difference to the success of intervention in anxiety. It is also important to make it clear to the patient that anxiety can spread. Someone who is already anxious about one thing will be likely to react with greater anxiety to something else which would, in the normal course of events, elicit only a small amount of anxiety. This is particularly the case when there is a strong physiological component to the anxiety.

Teaching relaxation techniques

Relaxation techniques can be extremely helpful in dealing with anxiety. All patients who are anxious should be taught relaxation methods. The basis of this is covered in Chapter 19.

Talking over why someone is anxious

Often anxiety is the result of real worries in someone's life. This chapter is all about finding out what problems people have and trying to help them to deal with them. This in itself is likely to reduce their anxieties. Just talking over worries – ventilation – is often extremely effective in reducing anxiety. As people talk they are able to put their problems into perspective.

However, sometimes the cause of the anxiety cannot be eradicated, for instance the fact of being seropositive. Or the anxiety can actually get in the way of solving problems so that it needs to be reduced before the patient can take any action. Or it can take on a life of its own. Anxiety can feed on itself; just being anxious can make people more anxious, particularly if they are interpreting anxiety symptoms as the result of physical disease.

Looking for factors affecting anxiety

It often helps to try to find out under what circumstances anxiety is reduced or increased.

COUNSELLOR: 'Are there times when you are less anxious?'
PATIENT: 'Yes, when I'm with other people, talking to them, I forget myself and my symptoms disappear.'
COUNSELLOR: 'What about things which make you more anxious?'
PATIENT: 'Well, I get anxious when I am on my own in the house during the day. If I got out and do something I tend to feel better. It's when my mind is unoccupied that I feel most anxious.'

This sort of situation is common. Often anxiety is greatest when someone has nothing to do and therefore has time to worry. The patient can be helped to become more active. However different people get anxious under different circumstances and it is important to look for these.

In some cases giving up things actually makes anxiety about them worse. This tends to be the case when patients have panic attacks in particular situations, for instance when they are in company or going into busy social situations. Avoiding those situations leads to the patient finding it increasingly difficult to go into them, so may actually increase overall anxiety. Increasing the amount of time a person spends in these situations will, over time, reduce anxiety. They should be encouraged to make efforts to put themselves into such situations as frequently as possible. They should not leave an anxiety-provoking situation until their anxiety level drops. They should remind themselves what the symptoms really are, i.e. symptoms of anxiety, and that although unpleasant these will cause them no harm and they should, if possible, use relaxation techniques to reduce their anxiety.

To find out the factors which cause changes in anxiety it is often helpful to get people to keep a diary. Most people find it easy to make a rating of their anxiety level on a simple scale:

1 – No anxiety
2 – Slight anxiety
3 – Moderate anxiety
4 – Strong anxiety
5 – Overwhelming anxiety.

They can use the scale to make a diary recording what they were doing, how anxious they felt, what they did about the anxiety and what difference this made. A diary entry of this sort is shown in Fig. 12.1. They should also include the date and time of each recording (not

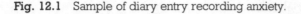

What doing	Rating	What did then	Effect
Reading newspaper article about AIDS	4	Got up, went out for walk	Anxiety dropped to 2 within ten minutes

Fig. 12.1 Sample of diary entry recording anxiety.

shown above). It is easy to make up sheets of paper divided into the headings shown and give them to the patient. It is important when giving someone a diary to explain the rationale, otherwise many patients will not compile the diary as it is rather time-consuming.

> COUNSELLOR: 'This diary will help us in two ways. First of all, we'll be able to see the sort of things which make you more anxious and those which help to reduce your anxiety. It's often not all that obvious what these are. But if we get a record over several days we can often pick out a pattern, even one you may not have noticed yourself. Secondly, we are going to try to work together to reduce your anxiety. We want to make sure that what we are doing really is having an effect. By keeping a diary we'll be able to see what impact we're making and, if we are not making an impact one way, we'll be able to change to attack the problem in another way. Does that make sense to you?'
>
> PATIENT: 'Yes, I understand that.'

You should also take an example of a time when the patient has been particularly anxious and fill in the diary with them, to make sure that they grasp what needs to be done from a worked example. The patient can then take the example with them as a guide to what they should be doing. An example is often worth a thousand words of explanation.

Diaries are also useful in trying to help a range of other sorts of problem. For instance, a similar diary can be used to monitor length of sleep and factors affecting the quality of sleep in someone with sleep problems. Or it can be used to record how many rows a couple have, what they row about, how intense these are and what ends the row and how they feel afterwards. Diaries not only help to elicit what affects particular psychological reactions, they are also vital in measuring whether possible solutions to particular problems are working.

Drugs

There are a number of drugs available which can reduce anxiety, but these all have problems. Some can induce drowsiness which may make driving or operating machinery hazardous, or may increase feelings of fatigue. However, there are three particular problems with them which severely restrict their usefulness. The first is that they are not a cure for whatever is causing the anxiety and so when they are stopped the anxiety tends to return. Secondly, many anxiolytics cause dependency in a large proportion of patients who take them. Thirdly, after a time they become less effective in relieving anxiety in many of those who use them.

These characteristics mean that the use of anxiolytics for more than a few weeks at most is undesirable. They can be helpful for very short-term control of high levels of anxiety until other interventions can be made to work. However they are not in any way a cure in themselves.

Referral

Because anxiety is often a highly treatable condition it is important to refer on to specialist mental health workers patients who either appear particularly anxious or who fail to respond to simple interventions such as those outlined above.

Depression

Everyone gets depressed from time to time. Certainly anyone faced with having HIV or AIDS is likely to have hours or days when they are depressed. Periods of depression may come and go, interspersed with periods when they do not feel depressed at all.

However, depression can be more than a passing mood. It becomes a matter of concern either when it lasts for more than a few days at a time or when bouts of depression are very frequent or very intense. This section addresses that sort of depression, rather than passing moods of mild depression, as it undermines people's ability to deal with the problems of everyday life, it makes life a misery for them and, ultimately, it can lead people to commit suicide, although even among people who are very severely depressed only a small proportion are actively suicidal.

When dealing with people with AIDS, seropositives, the worried well or partners and carers, it is important that the counsellor should assess for depression and should keep a careful eye on proceedings to make sure that the individual concerned does not become depressed.

It is a mistake to assume that prolonged or intense depression is 'natural'. Among people with AIDS we are seeing only a minority show depression at a level which requires specific intervention during the course of their illness. There is some evidence to suggest that professionals sometimes fail to intervene in cases of depression in those with life-threatening disease, simply because they regard the individual's depression as natural. People with AIDS are ordinary people, usually with no history of psychiatric problems, faced with the strains that having AIDS can bring. It would be a major surprise if they showed very high levels of severe depression.

Assessing depression

As with anxiety, the symptoms of depression can be split into four main headings:

- Somatic symptoms
- Affective symptoms
- Cognitive symptoms
- Behavioural symptoms

In assessing for depression it is important to look for a pattern. A single isolated symptom does not usually mean that someone is depressed. In general the greater the number of the symptoms (explained below), the more depressed an individual is. However, the intensity of the symptoms has also to be taken into account; someone with slight anorexia, a slightly depressed mood and slight gastrointestinal symptoms is hardly likely to be severely depressed.

It is also worth bearing in mind that many people who are depressed are also highly anxious and so it is common to find a mix of the symptoms of anxiety and depression. It is, thus, important to look for the symptoms of both.

Affective symptoms of depression

Depressed mood

The single most common feature in depression is people complaining that they feel depressed. People can often give you a good estimate of just how depressed they are by comparing their current mood with their mood at other times when they have been depressed in the past. However there is something of a snag in only using people's subjective estimates of whether they are depressed or not. Because people's thinking about themselves and the world changes when they become depressed, they may not see themselves as being depressed at all, or they may underestimate the extent of their depression. Instead they may see their situation as being hopeless and pointless, and may think this is being realistic, or they may see themselves as being worthless.

It is important to ask about mood not just currently but over the past few weeks.

Changes in enjoyment

A moment's thought about what it is like to be depressed (and most people have been at least a little depressed at one time or another) will show that one of the key elements in depressed mood is that life no longer seems pleasurable. Everyday events which normally give pleasure instead become a chore. People who are depressed may become extremely bored. Ultimately lack of enjoyment in life can lead to people simply stopping doing anything.

One of the most important questions to ask someone about depression is, 'What have you enjoyed doing over the last two weeks?'. This does not simply mean big events, but also small pleasures: watching television, drinking coffee, talking to friends, doing the garden. Someone who can think of nothing or very little that he has enjoyed, is likely to be depressed.

Loss of libido

Lack of interest in sex is common in depression. Sex itself may become unpleasurable. There may also be a lack of arousal; a man may find it difficult to get an erection or ejaculate, and a woman may not lubricate properly or may fail to reach orgasm. It is a change in these aspects which relates to depression; some people have long-lasting sexual problems which are quite unrelated to depression.

It is important to ask whether there have been any changes in the patient's interest in, or enjoyment of, sex recently.

Irritability and increased emotional lability

People who become depressed are often much more irritable; things which would not normally bother them may make them very angry. They change not just in terms of how easily they are angered but also, often, in terms of how easily they are upset or moved to tears.

It is important to ask whether the patient has become more irritable recently or whether they have found themselves more easily upset than usual.

Cognitive changes

When people are depressed their view of themselves and of their world changes in several ways.

Loss of self-esteem

People who are depressed often feel worthless and unlovable. They look at themselves in a negative way, seeing only their failures and shortcomings. Depression should always be suspected in a patient who seems to be taking an unrealistically harsh view of themselves.

These changes are sometimes combined with a change in perception of their own body. They feel not just personally but also physically unattractive. They may start as a result to neglect their appearance, or they may start to exaggerate some real blemish. They may, for instance, feel not only that a small Kaposi's sarcoma lesion on the face is glaringly obvious to everyone, but also that everyone knows what it is.

It is important to ask patients how they feel about themselves, whether this has changed recently and whether they feel less attractive than they used to.

Guilt

People who are depressed sometimes start to feel guilty about things they did in the past which were actually quite minor or were not their fault at all. Sometimes this can be quite severe.

> One patient had absent-mindedly driven away from a petrol station without paying several years before. Whenever he became depressed he was racked with guilt about this and made repeated attempts to give himself up to the police. They sought to reassure him – one policeman admitting that he had done the same himself – before driving the patient home. He even 'confessed' to the garage owner, who made him coffee and told him to forget it. None of this made him feel any less guilty.

However, guilt is often more subtle. Patients blame themselves for infecting others, or blame themselves for engaging in particular high-risk sexual activities and getting infected, although many could not have known that they were at risk or putting others at risk. They may, indeed, in some cases have behaved unwisely but their feelings of guilt are out of all proportion to what they have done.

Gay men sometimes blame themselves for being gay when they become depressed, and reject all aspects of being gay, including other gay men. It is important to ask patients whether they feel guilty about anything.

Feelings of failure

The person who is depressed often feels a failure. Looking back over a successful and happy life he may tend to see only the bad points, situations which went wrong for him and the things he failed to do. One patient, when asked about his career as a salesman, talked about an order he had lost and implied that he was likely to lose his job as a result. Further questioning showed that he was the most successful salesman the company had and that not only was the order in question small but the loss had not been his fault at all.

It is very difficult to come up with a single question or a few questions to elicit a person's view of his past. However the information usually comes out in discussion and in history-taking. The counsellor can compare the objective details of someone's life against the patient's assessment of that life. This often reveals the gap in the patient's perceptions.

Loss of hope

For people who are depressed the future looks bleak; there is nothing to look forward to. They anticipate that anything they do will end in failure because of their lack of ability to carry out the task. Depressed people often say things like, 'I'll try it, but I know that I won't be able to do it'. In fact there is very little loss of ability in people who are depressed; they just think that they will fail. The feeling of helplessness – that nothing they can do will make any difference and failure is inevitable – is common in depression.

It is important to ask patients what they are looking forward to in their lives. Unrealistic expectations of failure are usually very obvious when talking through plans for the future.

Feelings of changes in thinking

People who are depressed frequently report changes in how they are thinking. They report difficulty in concentrating on something for more than brief periods, and say that when they are thinking their minds are painfully slow. They also frequently report difficulties with their memory. Often they feel that something is wrong with their brain. The mental symptoms of depression are often misinterpreted by people with AIDS as early signs of encephalopathy, and cause intense anxiety. In fact, objective measurement of mental functioning usually shows no real change in cognitive efficiency.

It is important to ask patients whether they feel they are thinking less clearly than they used to. It is also important to reassure the patient about the nature of any changes they report.

Obsessional thought patterns

Obsessional thoughts and obsessional behaviours are sometimes seen in depression. Brooding on past behaviour or on negative and unpleasant thoughts is quite common. This is covered in more detail below.

Somatic symptoms

Sleep disturbances

Disturbances in sleep are common in those with depression. Particularly common in severe depression is waking up early and not being able to get back to sleep, often at four or five o'clock in the morning. Difficulties getting to sleep are also seen, particularly in those who are also anxious, which many depressed people are. The sleep problems are often combined with a feeling of great fatigue and tiredness during the day. There may also be nightmares.

Occasionally people who are depressed show a great increase in the amount that they sleep and they spend much of their time in bed.

In assessing sleep disturbances it is important to look for any changes in their sleep pattern. Some people are, and have always been, poor sleepers. Patients should be asked whether they have noticed any changes in their sleep pattern recently.

Anorexia

Anorexia is common in depression, although the opposite state, eating excessively, is also seen in some people, particularly those who have always used food as a comfort. The anorexia in depression is characterised by a loss of appetite, loss of interest in food and a loss of appreciation of food generally – it may not taste as it used to. Eating is often an effort.

Again, it is the change in eating and attitude to food which matters; some people have never had much interest in food. They may also be anorexic because they have pain on eating because of some physical condition, and this possibility should be eliminated.

Patients should be asked whether there has been any change in their appetite or enjoyment of food recently.

Gastro-intestinal symptoms

Changes in bowel motility can occur. Constipation is fairly common, sometimes linked to changes in eating. However, in the individual who is very anxious diarrhoea is sometimes seen.

Patients should be asked whether they have been constipated or have had diarrhoea recently.

Multiple physical complaints

People who are depressed sometimes report multiple physical complaints: headaches, joint pains, palpitations, stomach problems and so on. These are often, when examined closely, symptoms of anxiety. People who are depressed often interpret such symptoms as signs of physical disease.

Patients should be asked about any physical symptoms they may have. Naturally physical complaints are seen also in physical conditions so any possible organic illness should be eliminated.

Behavioural symptoms

Lack of energy

People who are depressed feel that they lack energy, that everything is too much effort and too much trouble. They may be unable to 'get going' in the mornings or even to get out of bed. They may 'put off things until tomorrow'.

Patients should be asked whether they have noticed that they are any less energetic recently.

Reduction in overall levels of activity

People who are depressed tend to do less then they used to. They go out less, they find they do less at work, and they find that they do less at home, often simply sitting in a chair or in bed.

Patients should be asked whether they are doing less then they used to.

In extreme cases retardation is seen. The depressed person shows a slowing in movement and/or speech which is obvious to the observer. In rare cases this may become so extreme that the patient simply sits mute in a chair or lies in bed doing nothing at all unless prompted.

Suicidal thoughts and actions

Many people who become depressed contemplate suicide at some time. There is a spectrum of thoughts about suicide, from the person who feels that 'it's not worth going on' but has never actually thought of killing themselves, through the person who has daydreamed about it, through the person who has made plans but has no intention of carrying them out, to the person who expresses an intention of killing themselves or makes an attempt. It is a dangerous myth that people who intend to kill themselves do not tell anyone else but just go ahead and do it; the majority of successful suicides have told someone else that they were thinking of suicide in the days leading up to the attempt.

It is also a myth that suicides can be divided into 'real' attempts and 'cries for attention'. People who actually attempt suicide tend to take a calculated chance, with different people balancing that calculation in different ways. Some people take very little risk that they will die; they may take pills in front of others for instance. Others take a greater risk: they take tablets knowing that it is likely (but not certain) that their partner will return before they die and find them. Others stack the chances firmly in favour of death. A man who shoots himself with a shotgun is certain he is going to die.

People who have made suicide attempts in the past are more likely to do so in the future. Past attempts may have been weighted heavily towards being found and saved. Future attempts may be weighted more towards dying.

It is important always to ask the depressed patient about suicide. Counsellors are often reluctant and embarrassed to ask about this issue but they should not be; it can be a matter of life and death.

COUNSELLOR: 'When people get depressed they often think about killing themselves. Have you thought about that?'

PATIENT: 'Yes I have. I've even thought that if I was to do it, I'd take tablets.'

COUNSELLOR: 'Have you thought like that recently?'

PATIENT: 'I thought about it quite a lot over the weekend.'

COUNSELLOR: 'How likely do you think it is that you will actually do it.'

PATIENT: 'I won't kill myself, but sometimes it comforts me to think about it as a way out if I get very sick.'

If someone is actively planning suicide and intends to carry out the plan they will, very often, tell you so if you are sympathetic. Often it is a great relief to them to tell you. An active suicidal intent is a psychiatric emergency and arrangements should always be made to bring in advice from specialist mental health workers.

Where someone is contemplating suicide but has no active intent, a careful eye should be kept on them to monitor changes in their mood. If they become more depressed there is a danger that they may become more active in planning to kill themselves.

Interpreting symptoms

The list of symptoms above suggests the sort of questions that need to be asked. It is, of course, the pattern of symptoms which is being looked for. It is also helpful to ask patients:

● When did the symptoms start and how long have they lasted?

- Are they constant or does the level of depression fluctuate?
- How intense are the symptoms?
- Have you been depressed at any time in the past?
- Have you ever had treatment for depression? If so, what was it and how successful was it?
- Are you currently receiving treatment for depression?

Using standardised measures of depression

There are a number of questionnaires which can be filled in by the patient, and a number of observer-rating forms to assess depression. These can be helpful because they usually make it possible to assess how depressed a patient is in comparison with others. They give a numeric value for the level of depression. They do not, however, remove the necessity to ask patients about depressive symptoms.

Introducing standardised methods as a routine part of assessing patients can be helpful. There are many different scales, each with their advantages and disadvantages. In order to select the right scales it is helpful to discuss them with mental health professionals who will be aware of what is available, will probably have or be able to obtain suitable ones, and can usually advise on their use and interpretation.

Taking action

The first decision is whether the counsellor should attempt to deal with the depression himself or whether he should pass the patient on for advice from specialist mental health services. Anyone who is severely depressed or actively suicidal should always be the subject of urgent referral to specialist services.

There is a range of antidepressant medication available which can often be very effective in relieving depression. This does not provide a complete answer but it can 'lift' very depressed patients sufficiently to make it possible to help them deal with their problems. In some cases psychiatric admission may be required.

For individuals who are mildly depressed and who are not actively suicidal there are steps which the counsellor can take to help. It is worth reviewing these.

Putting things in perspective

As with anxiety it helps just to tell patients that they are depressed and to explain to them that the symptoms they are experiencing are those of depression. It is also important to tell them that, however they feel at the moment, they will feel better in the future. The symptoms given above provide a framework to talk about the sort of experiences which go with being depressed.

It is also a fact that, at least in cases where people are reacting to some life event, they will eventually almost certainly feel better even if no intervention is undertaken. Depression does eventually tend to lift either of its own accord or because events in the person's life change so that the factors causing or supporting the depression disappear or become less important. This is why the brief depressions we all get usually tend to pass off after hours or days and not to become fixed features.

It is important to reassure patients that they will not always feel like this; it is a passing phenomenon and in the future they will feel better.

Sorting out problems

The chapters of this book look at various ways of helping people to solve their problems. Where depression is the result of specific problems, dealing with those problems can in itself often relieve depression.

Increasing activity

Our mood is maintained at least in part by the pleasures of life; pleasant things tend to keep us on an even keel. People who get depressed tend to get less pleasure from what they do. As a result they stop participating with the result that they have even less pleasure in their lives and get more depressed. It is a vicious circle and can lead to people going further into depression.

It is helpful to get people to increase their overall level of activity. At first the activities may not be pleasurable, but they should be told that they will have to do more first and then they will start to find things more pleasurable later. There are several steps:

- Go through activities that the patient enjoyed in the past.
- Make a list of these.
- Make up a simple diary sheet for the week with a slot for each hour, or use a commercial diary.
- Go through with the patient and fill in something they can do each hour. This need not be a particularly complicated or elaborate item; some examples might be: ringing up an old friend and asking how he is; eating some specially liked food for lunch; going to an exhibition; going out and buying a book; going to the cinema; going for a walk in a favourite park. Whatever is agreed needs to be realistic.
- Get the patient to tick off the items in the diary as they are done and to give them ratings on a five-point scale from unenjoyable (1) to very enjoyable (5). It is also helpful to get the patient to rate how well they feel they carried out each task (regardless of the enjoyment) on a scale from 1 (not carried out well) to 5 (very well). These ratings help both the patient and the counsellor to keep an eye on progress.
- After the first week the patient should be encouraged to fill in their own diary, either at the beginning of the week or each evening for the following day.

It is surprising what a difference such an apparently simple intervention can make. People's mood often improves dramatically over a few weeks. The most difficult part of the process tends to be getting people started. Because they are depressed they tend not to want to start. It is important to encourage them as much as possible. Once they get going it usually gathers its own momentum because patients start to feel better.

Identifying inaccurate thoughts

The cognitive symptoms list earlier in this chapter shows that people who are depressed tend to have an inaccurate view of themselves. For instance, they may feel that they are unattractive when they are not, or that they have behaved badly when they have not. When this sort of thought is identified in a patient it is useful to challenge it, to explain that it is inaccurate and to look for ways of dealing with it. The challenging of inaccurate thoughts is one of the elements of cognitive approaches which are the subject of books in themselves. There are other elements from these approaches which can be easily used, as described in the following sections.

Testing out

Quite often patients hold views which are not in accordance with reality but which they can test out to see if they are true.

> One patient expressed the view, 'Now I have AIDS I don't even bother seeing my friends any more; they wouldn't want to see me anyway.' He agreed that this was testable and that, while he was sure he was right, there was no harm in trying out his view to see if it was true. He was encouraged to select several friends he had been close to in the past and to invite them round for a meal (which a friend would help him cook). He rang around and, to his surprise, many people asked him why he hadn't been in touch before and said they would be pleased to come.

When getting patients to test things out it is, of course, important to ensure that they succeed. It was agreed in the case above that the patient would plan well in advance so that people were less likely to be already committed. The fact that not everyone he rang would be able to come for a meal on a given day was also discussed. Getting a friend to help him cook also ensured that the occasion would not fail because he was unable to make the meal.

Writing down thoughts and talking them through

It can be helpful to get someone to make a list of the negative thoughts they have about themselves, and for the counsellor and the patient to go through and look at each of these in turn to examine how realistic they are.

> A successful businessman became depressed. He had had a career with many successes and few failures. However, he concentrated on the failures and ignored the successes. The counsellor and the businessman compiled a list of failures and the way that he had dealt with these, and also of successes. The successes markedly outweighed the failures but also it was clear tht he had usually managed either to learn from failures or to turn them to his advantage.

Rewarding and encouraging

For the depressed patient the world is a rather unrewarding place. However, few patients who are moderately depressed find it totally unrewarding, just more so than before. The counsellor needs to provide clear encouragement to the patient to solve his problems and to increase his activity levels or whatever else is agreed.

It is important that the counsellor should look out for achievements and give clear praise to the patient. A partial failure is also a partial success and it is important to get the patient to look at the success element. Praise from the counsellor is also rewarding in itself. To hear someone say, 'You've done very well' is a boost to almost anyone's confidence and mood, and while it appears a simple point it is surprising how many counsellors concentrate on what has gone wrong, and fail to give praise for success.

If the patient's depression does not lessen

It is unreasonable to expect someone to move from being depressed to being happy or in a normal mood in a few days or even a few weeks. However, some progress should be seen over the first few weeks of intervention. If there is no progress, it is time to refer the patient on. If they start to get markedly worse, they should also be referred on.

Obsessions

Obsessions come in two overlapping types: obsessional behaviours and obsessional thoughts.

Obsessional behaviours

Nothing appears more odd initially than obsessional behaviours.

> Edward began to worry that he had left a plug in the electric sockets in his house when he went to bed at night and that this might cause a fire. He spent up to three hours per night checking and rechecking the electrics.

> At a party Mary had sex with a man she said was 'very dirty'. She began to worry that he had infected her with some disease and spent several hours a day checking her vagina with the aid of a mirror, trying to work out whether it looked normal or whether she had any sort of rash.

> After David became seropositive he began to examine his skin in minute detail, looking for signs of Kaposi's sarcoma. He stared at the soles of his feet and worked upwards, always in the same order of checking. If he was interrupted or lost his place he would have to start again from the beginning. Sometimes he would finish and then feel he had not done it properly, so he would start again. This took up large parts of his morning.

These sorts of behaviour have their counterparts in everyday life: the child stepping over cracks in the pavement or counting up to particular numbers, or the person who is going on holiday driving to the end of the street and then coming back to check that he has turned off the gas.

A key feature of obsessional behaviours is that people who engage in them know that they are unreasonable but still feel compelled to carry them out. The most common types of obsessional behaviour are:

- **Checking.** Checking gas, electricity or locks, or checking for disease of one sort or another.
- **Cleaning.** Repeatedly and excessively cleaning, either objects or surfaces or one's own body; for instance the hand–washer who washes his hands for hours at a time.

No-one knows what causes obsessions. However, it is known that some cases of obsession are linked to depression and if the depression is treated the obsessions will disappear.

Despite the cause being unknown there are ways of dealing with obsessions. They tend to feed on themselves; the more they are continued the more people feel the urge to do them. The answer is to encourage the patient not to do them. This seems fairly obvious but it sometimes works rather well; it is even given a name in textbooks – response prevention. The key elements are:

- To discuss with the patient in a non-accusatory way the essential pointlessness and unreasonableness of the obsessional behaviours.
- To explain to the patient that the obsessions are self-sustaining and to provide a rationale for resisting them.
- To tell the patient that avoiding doing the rituals can get rid of them and that this will inevitably involve some discomfort but will be worthwhile in the end.
- To encourage the patient to notice those events which tend to set off an obsessional chain of behaviour and, as far as possible, to avoid such events or situations. Keeping a diary as explained for anxiety can help to pinpoint areas to avoid.
- To encourage the patient to use distraction to avoid the obsessional behaviours. For instance, if a patient has an urge to wash the kitchen floor, he might be encouraged to go out for a walk. This takes him out of the situation and makes the behaviour less likely to occur.
- If the patient cannot avoid the situation he should resist it for as long as possible. The urge to carry out the ritual will, eventually, weaken (though it may return later). To deal with the urge some alternative activity is essential; carrying out relaxation exercises is often helpful.
- Obsessional rituals take a considerable amount of time. It is important to find alternative activities to fill the time, otherwise they will creep back into the free space.

If these simple interventions fail, it is important to seek specialist help for the patient.

In the case of David above, his checking of his body for Kaposi's sarcoma was reduced by a simple programme:

- He rarely checked at any time other than in the mornings when he went to the bathroom to wash. He was encouraged to get up, get dressed and go straight out without washing. This was a good deal less of a problem to him than getting stuck in the bathroom for hours.
- He had rigged up an elaborate system of mirrors so that he could see inaccessible bits of his anatomy. He was encouraged to remove all the mirrors in his flat.
- When he felt the urge to check he was encouraged to put it off as long as possible by using relaxation techniques or by doing something else active and incompatible with checking, such as cleaning the floor (which was not one of his obsessions), going out or ringing a friend.
- When the urge to check was overwhelming he was taught to put it off by engaging in self-talk along the lines of, 'I'll wait five minutes before I check'. If he succeeded for five minutes he was encouraged to try to postpone it another five minutes.
- He booked occasional appointments with the doctor who gave him a full examination, 'so that he wouldn't have to check himself'.

This simple programme, over a period of a few weeks, more or less eliminated his checking.

Obsessional thoughts

Obsessional thoughts are sometimes called ruminations. They differ from everyday worries, with which they overlap, because of their rather stereotyped nature. They often involve a sort of 'mental checking'.

Richard developed ruminations that he might have run someone over in his car on the way back from work, even though he knew this was ridiculous. He would sit in the evenings and go through his journey in minute detail over and over again, trying to work out if he had injured anyone. These thoughts distressed him greatly.

Barbara, an antibody positive woman, developed a fear that she might in some way have infected someone else in her everyday life. She reviewed her day minutely to make sure that she had not cut herself or had a nosebleed and exposed someone to risk. She even thought over the possibility that she might have had sex with someone without remembering it. She knew these ideas were ridiculous but she felt obliged to go through the ritual of thinking about them.

Obsessional thoughts can be the result of depression; indeed they are very common in that form. Sometimes in people with AIDS, obsessional thoughts are seen in the form of stereotyped worries about AIDS, or obsessional attempts to remember anyone they might have infected in the past.

Distraction is the first remedy to try in dealing with obsessional thoughts. Patients should be encouraged to monitor their thoughts and, when they begin to start ruminating, they should interrupt their train of thought and occupy their minds with something else active: talking to someone, singing, adding up their bank balance, anything which distracts them.

Trains of obsessional thoughts are often easy to interrupt, although they tend to come back again. Some psychiatrists and psychologists have advocated that the patient should actually shout out loud 'Stop!', or they should pinch themselves or do something else dramatic to divert their attention as soon as they detect obsessional thoughts starting (this is called thought-stopping). Then they should distract themselves with alternative activities.

The following are suggested steps in dealing with obsessional thoughts:

- The patient and the counsellor should discuss the obsessional thoughts and try to sort out any underlying realistic worries the patient may have
- If the patient is depressed they should be treated for this
- If the patient is not depressed or the depression improves but the obsessional thoughts do not remit, distraction should be tried with or without thought-stopping
- If the patient is anxious and anxiety increases their tendency to have obsessional thoughts, relaxation training should be tried
- The patient should be encouraged to keep their mind occupied as much as possible since obsessional thoughts tend to be most common when people's minds are unoccupied.

Obsessional thoughts are notoriously difficult to treat. Quite often they disappear on their own but they can persist for months or years and make life a misery for the patient. New treatment approaches are being developed to try to solve the problem, and if the patient fails to respond to simple interventions they should be referred on for specialist advice.

Chapter 13

Problem Solving

John Green

The problem-solving approach

People in the real world, unlike those reported in many textbooks, tend to have more than one problem and these problems tend to be mixed together. The result is that the counsellor is faced with a tangled web of problems which have to be sorted out before they can be tackled. For the patient the tangle of problems makes life particularly difficult; because everything is mixed together the patient feels there is no way in which they will ever find a sensible solution to their difficulties.

The problem-solving approach to helping people is simply a set of ways of breaking down a series of problems so that they become easier to deal with. Breaking down the problems into discrete blocks is a valuable process for the patient because it allows them to get their difficulties into perspective and these no longer seem so insoluble.

The whole process of problem solving is carried out jointly with the patient. The counsellor does not decide on the problems and the solutions; the counsellor and patient work together. There are several good reasons for this:

- It is important to check that what is being written down is correct. This is an opportunity to re-check that the counsellor has grasped the problems.
- As problem solving proceeds it will, in itself, generate questions which need to be considered. A history is seldom perfect; some matters will have been missed and others will need clarifying.
- It is useful to go through the approach with the patient because it is a helpful way of looking at problems which the patient can use for himself in the future.
- It engages the patient in the task of solving their own problems, which is vital. An individual is far more likely to implement solutions they have thought of themselves.
- The process itself helps to sort out the problems in the patient's own mind.

There are several steps to taking a problem-solving approach.

Taking a good history

The first step is to gather as much information as possible about the patient's difficulties.

The sort of information-gathering covered in Chapters 3, 4 and 5 should provide a good basis on which to start.

In taking a history it is always helpful to take notes, if the patient does not mind. Naturally the patient will wish to be reassured that such notes are confidential.

At this stage a fairly good overall picture of what is happening should be available.

Making a list of problems

The next step is simply to make a list of the problems the patient has. This list needs to be constructed with the patient, of course. At this stage it does not matter if the same problem appears on the list twice in different forms. Nor is it necessary to try to sort out the links between different problems or to look for solutions. That comes later.

Making a good list of problems is more difficult than it appears at first sight; in fact, it is probably the single most difficult thing to do. Consider these statements about patients which are typical of those that appear in notes or in discussions about patients:

- 'He is worried about AIDS.' [Worried about what aspects of AIDS? Is he afraid that he has it? Is he afraid that he will get it?]
- 'She is unable to cope because of her social problems.' [What sort of social problems? Unable to cope with what?]
- 'He is rather socially inadequate.' [What does socially inadequate mean?]
- 'She has sexual problems.' [Does she not want to have sex? Or does she get pain in intercourse? What exactly is the problem?]
- 'He doesn't have any friends.' [Does he want friends? Does he lack opportunity to make friends? Does he find it difficult to make friends although he has plenty of contacts?]
- 'He has sleep difficulties.' [Sleeps too little? Too much? Can't get off to sleep? Wakes early? Wakes up often?]

All the above statements may be correct. However they are unhelpful because they do not give a clear enough description of the problem. Clear descriptions make it much easier to come up with solutions. Better problem descriptions might be:

- 'He is worried that he will get AIDS because he engages in casual unprotected anal intercourse.'
- 'She is unable to keep herself warm because she does not have the money to heat her flat and this makes her miserable.'
- 'He finds that in company he cannot say what he wants because he is anxious that he has nothing interesting to say.'
- 'She has pain at the entrance to the vagina on penetration.'
- 'He does not meet people with whom he could make friends.'
- 'He is unable to get off to sleep at nights because he worries about HIV, but he sleeps well once asleep.'

These problem descriptions, while far from perfect, do at least suggest further questions to ask and the lines along which possible solutions might be sought.

The following example shows what might be done. The list of problems is shorter than it might be in reality since it is an illustration only.

David, aged 35, has symptomatic HIV disease. He is anxious about his future and finds that he constantly worries about the possibility of getting AIDS. It occupies his thoughts for most of the time. He checks himself every day in the mirror, looking for signs of Kaposi's sarcoma (KS).

Previously self-employed, he gave up his job, which involved a lot of travelling, because he did not feel well enough to carry on. Since then he has spent most of his time at home reading the paper and watching the television. He finds himself frequently bored. He used to have an active social life around the clubs but now finds he tires easily and does not want to go.

He lives with Ted and has been doing so for five years. They get on well but recently he has been unable to have any form of sexual activity with Ted because as soon as they start safer sex he starts to think about AIDS and becomes more and more anxious. He now finds he is unable even to cuddle Ted because he fears it might lead to sex. He suffers from spells of dizziness and sweating. These can occur at any time, but are more frequent when he is thinking about AIDS.

The problem list developed with the patient in this case was:

(1) He constantly worries about AIDS, particularly when he has nothing else to occupy his mind
(2) He spends half an hour first thing every morning checking his body for Kaposi's sarcoma and this makes him very anxious
(3) He stays at home most of the time and finds that he is very bored and unhappy because there is little interesting to do
(4) He enjoys seeing people but, since he stopped going to clubs, he does not see many people
(5) As soon as Ted touches him when they are in bed he thinks they are going to have sex and he begins to think of AIDS and cannot get aroused
(6) He cannot cuddle Ted or be cuddled because he fears this might lead to sex
(7) He gets spells of dizziness and sweating; these are more frequent when he is thinking about AIDS.

These have been entered on the problem chart (Table 13.1) in an abbreviated form for reasons of space. On the full chart they would be entered in full. In the explanations below they have also been abbreviated; however the counsellor would normally use the full description of problems.

Looking for links and hypotheses

The next step is for the counsellor and patient jointly to try to form hypotheses about the ways in which different problems are linked together and about possible causes of particular problems.

In the case of problem 1 – his constant worries about AIDS – it may be that:

- Because he has so much time on his hands which he is not able to use pleasurably and in which his mind is unoccupied, he has time to worry excessively.

Table 13.1 Problem chart.

Problem	Links/hypotheses	Possible solutions	Evaluation
(1) Worries constantly about AIDS	Linked to (3) and (4) because mind frequently not occupied. Linked to overall high level of anxiety. Linked to (2)? Obsessional thoughts?	Occupy time more effectively. Treat for anxiety. Try treatments for obsessional thoughts.	See text for explanation.
(2) Checks for KS	May be an obsessional behaviour either contributing to or resulting from (1).	Treat for anxiety. Treat as obsessional behaviour.	
(3) Stays at home and gets bored	Contributes to (1) and (2)?	Go out more. Draw up list of enjoyed things which can be done at home and carry out.	
(4) Doesn't see many people since stopped going to clubs	Failed to develop alternative social outlets.	Start going to clubs again. Invite people round more.	
(5) Can't get aroused because of thoughts of AIDS	Linked to (1)? Result of high anxiety.	Embark on programme of sex therapy. Treat for anxiety and see if arousal returns.	
(6) Cannot cuddle Ted or be cuddled	Linked to (5). May not feel in control of sexual relationship.	As for (5). Develop rule with Ted that cuddles outside bed don't lead to sex. Help him to be more assertive in relationship.	
(7) Spells of dizziness and sweating.	Result of high anxiety. Physical problem exacerbated by anxiety?	Treat for anxiety. Get medical done.	

- The problem is linked to high overall anxiety levels, both resulting from high anxiety and contributing to its maintenance.
- Checking for KS may be contributing to maintaining thoughts of AIDS uppermost in his mind.
- The thoughts may be obsessional in nature. This needs further investigation (see Chapter 12).

In the case of problem 6 – he does not feel able to cuddle Ted or be cuddled – it may be that:

- This is linked to problem 5 – difficulties in getting aroused in sex
- He may not feel in control in their sexual relationship, so he does not feel that he can call a halt if things are going too far for his liking.

These links need to be developed by the counsellor with the patient so that any which do not fit the facts can be eliminated.

Generating possible solutions

The next step is for the counsellor and the patient to look for possible solutions to each problem. At this stage it is often helpful to generate a large number of possible solutions and not to worry too much about how practical each is. Later, unsuccessful solutions may form the basis for more successful solutions. Because of this, some workers advocate coming up with any solutions, however ridiculous, even solutions of the 'perhaps I could get a spaceship and go to Mars' type. However, I have not felt that going this far is very helpful and it tends simply to produce more totally unworkable solutions, rather than ideas which can be turned to practical use.

On the problem chart it is possible to see some of the possible solutions generated for this case. In the case of problem 3, staying at home and getting bored and unhappy, possible solutions might be:

- Going out more.
- Drawing up a list of enjoyed activities which can be done at home and then planning a diary of these. They might include past enjoyed activities but also some new ones. The patient might, for instance, want to take up painting.

In the case of problem 5 – not getting aroused for sex – possible solutions might be:

- Embarking on a psychosexual therapy programme or finding a therapist to carry it out if the counsellor is not expert in that area
- Treating general overall anxiety about AIDS and seeing whether the problem disappears.

Evaluating solutions

The next step is for the counsellor and the patient to look at each possible solution in turn and try to evaluate it. In making an evaluation there are several important points to think about. Using the solutions generated for problem 3:

- What assets does the patient have to carry out a solution? For instance, if they have many activities which they like doing and which can be done at home, it should be relatively easy for them to make time at home more pleasurable.
- What difficulties are there with the solution? Going out more may not be possible for a man who is in ill-health, cannot drive, is not near public transport and cannot afford a taxi. The counsellor and the patient should look for practical solutions. Perhaps a friend could take him out in his car?
- Are there intermediate steps which need to be taken before a solution can be implemented? For instance, going out more may require an intermediate step of drawing up a list of places to go, or it may involve looking up old friends and telephoning them to arrange to meet.
- How practical is the solution? This should be the final decision when the above questions have been answered.

In Table 13.1 the evaluation section has not been filled in for reasons of space. However, against each possible solution it is helpful to jot down an indication of what was decided. With luck several different solutions may be possible for some problems. The decision then is which solution to try first, or whether to try a combination of different solutions.

Drawing up an action list

The final step is to draw up an action list from the problem-solving chart, with the patient. This needs to specify:

- What actions are needed to resolve the various problems.
- The order in which various actions will be tried. Some may be done first because they lead on naturally to the implementation of other solutions. At other times the most promising solution, or the quickest to implement, may be tried first and if that is not successful another solution tried.
- What steps are needed to solve a particular problem.

From the problem chart it might, for instance, be decided that the steps to take are as follows.

Stage one
Tackle the high level of overall anxiety and monitor the effects of this on the amount of checking for KS, frequency of spells of dizziness and sweating and ability to get aroused in sex. Steps would be:

- Developing a relaxation strategy and a relaxation tape with the patient (Chapter 19)
- Going through the procedures for reducing anxiety (Chapter 12)
- Keeping a diary to monitor levels of anxiety
- Keeping diaries of frequency and duration of checking for KS, spells of dizziness and sweating and of level of sexual arousal during times he and Ted attempt sex.

Develop a range of pleasurable activities which can improve the quality of time spent at home. Steps might be:

- Drawing up a list of activities which can be done at home and which have been enjoyed in the past or which the patient would like to do
- Drawing up a schedule for a week of such activities
- Monitoring enjoyment and satisfaction of each of these.

Arrange medical to ensure that there is no organic basis for sweating and dizziness spells.

Stage two
The next stage will depend in part on the results of stage one. The counsellor should always be prepared to try different approaches to solving a problem.

Try to extend the number of people seen at home. Steps might be:

- Get out old address books and ring up old friends. Invite some friends round for a drink one evening.
- Arrange a dinner party and invite people round.

Go out more socially. Steps might be:

- Draw up a list of places to go which are within the physical capacities of the patient; for instance, going to a cinema or the theatre might be enjoyed and might be less wearing than going to clubs
- Planning over the next two weeks when these activities will take place
- Making necessary arrangements: booking tickets, arranging transport and so on.

The reader might like to look through the other possible solutions in the problem sheet and draw up similar plans for the next stages.

Overview

The problem-solving approach suggested above is, of course, only one way of tackling problem solving. However, whichever way the counsellor approaches problem solving, it is helpful to work systematically through potential problems and try to develop systematic solutions. Writing down problems and possible solutions is often helpful for both the counsellor and the client. Problems which appear at first sight an unresolvable mass can resolve themselves into a series of manageable parts which can be dealt with effectively.

Chapter 14

Dying, Bereavement and Loss

Lorraine Sherr and John Green

Loss and bereavement

The literature on loss and bereavement relates largely to death itself, but this is not the only potential loss faced by those with AIDS and sometimes it is not the most important. However, lessons learnt from research into death and dying can be applied to the wider context of loss.

Theory of loss

There is no prescriptive theory of loss, that is no theory which says how people should feel about loss or how they should deal with it. There are only descriptive theories – theories which seek to categorise and describe features that people have seen when they have looked at people experiencing loss.

The best known theory is that of Kubler-Ross (1970), who has set out a series of stages that have been observed in people facing loss. Such approaches can be helpful in thinking about the issues surrounding death and bereavement. However, particularly in the field of death and dying, workers have sometimes sought to use such descriptive theories as prescriptive theories. They have come to feel that unless people experience certain feelings or deal with those feelings in certain ways they will suffer psychological or even physical harm.

Trying to force what happens to real people into rigid prescriptive theoretical models is at best unhelpful, and at worst it prevents counsellors from seeing what is really happening and makes them see only what they expect to see. Although descriptive models, such as that of Kubler-Ross, are helpful in thinking through the issues, our own clinical experience suggests they must be used with caution, since:

- One cannot assume that all individuals experience or ought to experience a similar set of reactions. Many individuals may experience some of the reactions; some may experience them all.
- Some may go through the stages in a different order, or entirely miss out a stage. There is no 'normal' grieving process and individuals show a wide variation in expression.

- Patients do not necessarily travel from the first stage to the last; they may move backwards and forwards between stages at different times.
- It is not clear that some 'stages' are in fact 'stages' as opposed to reactions.
- Terms which are used specifically by particular writers are sometimes used in a broader, looser sense by workers in the field.

Theory is thus limited but can still allow for a framework which may be helpful in anticipating, guiding, helping and understanding, and within these constraints it may be a useful tool for counsellors.

Shock

Kubler-Ross felt that many patients showed an initial shock reaction to news of a loss. The shock made it difficult to take in information and difficult to think or plan rationally. This reaction of shock was often, though not always, followed by a stage of denial.

Denial

The concept of denial is often used by other writers on loss too. In general use it has sometimes become a vague catch-all term which is used to describe a whole range of different reactions. Stripped to its barest bones it is often used to mean the patient or relative not viewing the situation as negatively as others think they should. This is, of course, in contrast to the more precise usage of Kubler-Ross.

At its most extreme, it may appear that the patient simply refuses to believe the diagnosis. We have not seen this extreme form of denial as a lasting response in our own patients, although it possibly appears as a fleeting immediate response to being told they have AIDS: 'It can't be, I feel so well.' On the other hand there are sufficient cases in the literature to show that it does exist as an emotional response. However, at least some cases of 'denial of diagnosis' have rather simpler explanations:

A patient referred from a distant hospital was sent because he was believed to be 'suffering' from 'denial' in that he kept asking whether he had AIDS. On being questioned he said he was sure that he did have AIDS but that no-one had said so in so many words. On contacting several doctors in the three hospitals he had previously been in touch with, each doctor ridiculed the view that he had not been told, each one saying that he had been 'told repeatedly'. Yet none of these doctors had given the patient the information themselves! When the diagnosis was confirmed with the patient he said he was relieved to know and no longer showed any signs of 'denial'.

Less extreme forms of this sort of problem are probably not that uncommon. Cartwright *et al.* (1973) showed the discrepancies between the desire for information expressed by terminally ill patients, and the provision offered by doctors. Such difficulties often referred to diagnosis and telling patients about the nature and prognosis of their condition.

While it cannot account for all cases of denial of diagnosis, there are probably occasions where apparent denial is simply the result of poor explanation. It is easy for a well-education professional to believe that he has adequately explained a condition to the patient, when he has in fact completely failed to get the message across in an under-standable form.

Probably a more common form of denial in people with AIDS is denial of the seriousness of a condition. In the early 1980s, when few patients with a history of pneumocystis could be expected to live longer than twelve months, many patients, despite asking about this and being told the answer, took the view that they were 'going to beat this thing'. This is an example of the fact that denial can be a healthy reaction; patients took the view that they might die, and made plans in case they did, but lived as though they were going to beat AIDS. There were no obvious adverse psychological sequelae to this stance; indeed such patients often appeared happier and more energetic in dealing with their condition. It is hard to believe that what was objectively an irrational view could be anything but beneficial for them.

Cognitive coping is a concept that may well contribute to the adjustment of any serious condition, especially HIV infection and AIDS. Such coping requires an appraisal of a threat, prior to an integration of the meaning of the threat for an individual. Some workers have shown that denial as a copying strategy has been adopted by many individuals. It is inter-esting to note that it sometimes seems to be the professionals who find denial more dis-tressing than the patient. Perhaps it disturbs their framework of belief about the world.

Anger

Kubler-Ross suggested that, after shock and denial, many patients exhibit an anger reaction. Outbursts of anger will be familiar to anyone who has worked with the dying, and they can take many forms. People may be angry at themselves, at others or at medical staff. Indeed Parkes (1972) reported that 25% of relatives of terminally ill patients exhibited anger towards staff. If irrational anger is shown towards them, staff must take care not to interpret it personally and patients should not face recriminations for angry outbursts by their relatives. Staff may pre-empt many such occurrences by open and honest two-way communications at all times.

However, anger is not always irrational; there may often be cause for it. It is easy to attribute anger to the internal emotional state of the patient or relative when, in fact, they have good reason to be angry. Studies on multiple bereavement (Sherr 1992) showed that those affected had significantly higher anger reactions than the singly bereaved. It may be anger at a partner who died before them, anger at the medical profession which can provide no cure, or anger at themselves for contracting HIV in the first place.

Bargaining

The next stage for many patients, in Kubler-Ross's formulation, is that of bargaining. The patient tries to strike a bargain, often with God but occasionally with their doctor, for more time along the lines of, 'Please, if I am good, give me more time.' This, in our experience, tends to be a rather fleeting reaction when it occurs and only occasionally takes on major significance. However, some individuals make arbitrary bargains with themselves; for example, that if they avoid certain behaviours they will survive longer. This can become very difficult when the behaviour is no longer avoidable or when circumstances change. One patient, for example, vowed never to have sex again if he survived for a long period. After some years with HIV, however, he met a new partner and wanted to initiate a new relationship. This meant severing his bargain.

Depression

Kubler-Ross suggested that patients then tend to pass into a stage of depression. Depression is a common feature in those experiencing loss. Times of brief transitory depression are almost inevitable in someone faced with death or other major losses. However, when such depression is profound and prolonged it should not be dismissed simply as a normal part of mourning. In many cases those suffering prolonged severe depression as a result of loss can benefit from counselling and support. Ultimately, where there is severe and persistent depression which is not relieved by counselling, it may be necessary to consider anti-depressant medication (Chapter 12).

Acceptance

For Kubler-Ross the final stage was acceptance, a coming to terms with the inevitability of death and an acceptance of it. However, acceptance is not unitary. Some patients accept comfortably, while they are still relatively well, that they will die, and use this as the basis for living their lives from that point onwards. For other patients acceptance of death is reached fully only when they have become very sick. Indeed for many patients who are in pain or tired of repeated infections, death is no longer something to be feared – it is something almost to be welcomed. Even here, however, it is a mistake to assume that things are straightforward.

> Martin had had repeated infections over a period of three months. Always rather difficult and unpredictable to deal with, he also had considerable charm. He developed a respiratory infection and appeared to be certain to die. He himself was sure that he would die. He appeared to reach a comfortable acceptance of his impending death. He asked several people he had had difficult relationships with to come and see him and had a series of reconciliations with them. Shortly afterwards the treatment unexpectedly started to make an impact and within a few days he was well again. He then became exactly as 'difficult' as he had been before, including falling out with one of the people he had been reconciled with. He continued to be determined to fight his disease.

It could be argued that this is not 'true' acceptance because he moved away from it, but this would logically suggest that acceptance can only be judged when someone is dead and cannot change his mind – which would make it a rather pointless concept.

How people cope

People are immensely complex in their reactions to death, as in their reactions to life. They find many different ways to cope. Some individuals may rapidly find a way to cope and others may experience prolonged adverse reactions. There may be oscillations, gradual changes and abrupt changes. How people are coping may vary according to how well other aspects of their lives are going, or according to other external factors. Anniversaries and special occasions can provide reminders which may bring on fresh mourning or cause changes in mood.

There is some evidence to suggest that multiple loss is more difficult to bear than single loss. If someone is faced with a sequence of losses they may find that their capacity to cope is further impaired and they need extra support.

Ultimately descriptions such as that by Kubler-Ross of the reactions of those faced with death or other losses can be very valuable in providing the counsellor with signposts in unfamiliar territory. However, to date all models are merely partial descriptions of very complex events, with many unsatisfactory features. It is important for counsellors to use such models to help them to see more clearly what is happening to a person, not as blinkers to blind them to things happening which are not in the model.

Spectrum of loss

People with HIV can experience a wide range of losses other than simply those associated with the imminence of death. The following is a partial list of some of the losses which people faced with AIDS or HIV infection may suffer.

Loss of certainty

We all have a (spurious) certainty about what will happen to us next week or next month. Although people are mortal and life is uncertain, they tend to live as though life is certain and they are immortal, at least while they are young. Even filling in a diary for next month is an expression of faith. Someone with a potentially fatal illness is brought face-to-face with the fact that this sort of view is, to some extent, a self-deception.

Future hopes

Most people have a range of hopes for the future – promotion, that small house in the country, having a family, going to places. These hopes can be lost.

Relationships

People can be rejected by their family or partners or friends either because they have HIV or AIDS or because their sexuality or use of drugs is revealed for the first time. Under the strain of diagnosis relationships may break down. However, there may be more subtle changes in the meaning of relationships as the other people involved change their behaviour and attitudes to the person who may be dying. A relationship based on equality may be unbalanced when the other person has to look after the person with AIDS (PWA). The avenues to forge new relationships, which might replace old relationships, may also appear closed.

Health

People tend to take their health for granted, at least some who are younger do. The automatic assumption of good health is lost in someone faced by HIV or AIDS. Loss of health also means for some people a restriction on the range of activities which they can undertake. When a patient becomes easily tired or short of breath he may be unable to do the things he used to.

Control

People generally have an assumption (sometimes exaggerated) that they are in control of their lives. For the PWA or the individual with HIV there can be a considerable loss of control. In extreme cases they feel that they are the helpless victims of an attack by the virus. However, there are also other control losses. They may lose control over their use of time because they find themselves forced to attend the hospital or clinic at particular times. If the issue of control is not understood by the hospital, patients may find themselves losing control over even their own bodies as others take decisions about their care. It is for this reason that decisions about care should always be taken jointly between the clinician and the patient.

Sexual losses

The range of sexual expression is restricted for someone infected with the virus. The patient may miss the intimacy that penetrative sex represents for some people. If he is unable to function sexually because of organically caused impotence or inability to ejaculate, as occasionally happens, he may find that his sex life is virtually ended.

Lifestyle

Changes in lifestyle are common, particularly in PWAs. Losses in this area may include:

● Loss of standard of living through loss of earnings in those who become unemployed, or those whose earning ability is restricted
● Loss of housing
● Loss of ability to obtain mortgages and insurance
● Loss of freedom to travel and settle in some countries.

Loss of body image

Particularly where this involves weight loss or extensive KS, people may feel that they are no longer physically attractive, not just sexually but also in everyday interaction with others. Often this feeling is unrealistic, but sometimes it is realistic. There are steps which can be taken to help people make the most of their appearance. Sometimes treatment is called for on cosmetic grounds where on strict clinical grounds it is unnecessary, for instance in the treatment of facial KS. The use of cosmetics to mask KS and other skin conditions, and even the purchase of new, well-fitting clothes to disguise weight loss, can sometimes help.

Loss of lovers

Those with AIDS or HIV sometimes experience the loss of lovers from AIDS too.

Loss of status

What someone does for a living is not just a source of income, it is also often a part of social status. A bank manager who suddenly becomes unemployed loses not just the income but also part of his place in society.

Loss of dignity and privacy

Particularly where extensive tests and clinical interventions are carried out, there can be a perceived loss of dignity. Patients may find themselves festooned with pipes and tubes and with clinicians poking in every orifice with medical instruments. They may even be unable to go to the lavatory on their own and instead must call for a bed-pan.

Dignity and personal privacy are very important. Our dignity and privacy are a major part of our feelings about ourselves, and a major personal right. We have seen patients refuse treatment for particular conditions because, in spite of the best efforts of those working with them to minimise this loss, they can no longer tolerate the invasion of their privacy and the loss of dignity involved in treatment. If privacy and dignity are not respected by everyone dealing with the patient, such refusals are likely to be even more common.

Loss of hopes for children

For the HIV seropositive man or woman there may be a loss of the hope of having a family. Those who already have children may face the loss of seeing their children grow up, achieve and flourish. Their children may also be HIV positive and the loss of hope for the child may take on a different form. The natural history of AIDS in children is more dramatic than in adults and the parents may watch illness and death in their child. HIV in families is not uncommon and there may be a complex where there is the loss of hope for new children, loss of hopes for a current child who is ill, and even loss of hopes for other children who may be HIV negative but face a future alone.

Loss of security

Where there is prejudice against people with AIDS there is often a loss of the feeling of personal security. There is the fear that others will find out and that persecution will result.

Multiple losses

One of the problems with AIDS and HIV infection is the multiple nature of losses. An individual may face multiple occasions of loss, but within relationships, families and communities there is multiple loss of partners, friends and children. Such multiple losses can strain a situation and create a disaster type reaction. It also means that an individual may be in a state of bereavement when they themselves have to face new losses, and they are therefore unable to utilise all their coping resources.

Many people with HIV infection and AIDS are involved in self help and support groups. They are then often exposed to multiple bereavement in the course of their work whilst simultaneously facing their own mortality. This may lead to severe stress and even burnout or exhaustion. It is essential that these groups are fully resourced in order to ensure adequate support and respite.

Counselling those facing death

The single most important thing to remember about people who are dying is that they are living people. They are just as alive as the person talking to them. There is a danger of treating the patient as a 'dying person' rather than as just a person. For the person who is faced with death most of his problems are the problems of living, not those of dying. However, there are some specific issues.

Discussing death

In discussing death with PWAs there are two different approaches, which will be appropriate in two different situations. The first is the possibility for anyone who has AIDS that they may die in the near future. For most PWAs at most times it is simply not possible to answer the question 'Will I die?' with any certainty. New treatments are being developed which may turn a probable 'yes' into a 'no' in the future. The patient may be a long-term survivor. However, both the counsellor and the patient know that most people with AIDS do die from the disease sooner or later. In discussing death with the patient it is important to acknowledge this and to answer any questions honestly and straightforwardly on the balance of probabilities.

PATIENT: 'Will I die from AIDS?'
COUNSELLOR: 'I don't know, no-one knows. It is quite likely that in the future you may die from AIDS. On the other hand you may not, because...'

An assessment of probabilities will take into account not just currently available treatments or those the counsellor knows may come into use in the future and the possibility of being a long-term survivor, but also the current clinical state of the patient. Clearly a man with a history of repeated opportunistic infections who has gradually responded less and less well to treatment for them has a worse outlook than a man who is well except for some KS.

The second situation is that of the person visibly close to death because they are not responding to treatment, or are so weak that they are clearly dying, or they have some untreatable tumour. If the patient asks, 'Am I dying?' the answer can only be, 'I think you are'. If the patient does not ask, there is no need to make the fact that they are close to death verbally explicit. However, it is important not to treat such a patient as though they will live forever. They will know that they are very ill, they will know that they may well die, and they need to be encouraged to take those steps which they would like to take concerning their death (these issues are covered in more detail below).

When to discuss death

Death will naturally be discussed at certain times – at the time of diagnosis and, sometimes, when the patient becomes very ill. However, counsellors often worry about whether they should bring up the issue at other times, particularly in cases where the patient does not bring it up. In part this stems from a reaction to anxiety. Counsellors are often anxious about discussing death; they do not wish to evade the issue because of their own anxieties, so they react by going to the other extreme and seeking every opportunity to talk about death. Sometimes this can have interesting results.

> One of us visited a PWA at home late one evening to see how he was getting on. He did not seem terribly keen on discussing anything very profound so the conversation turned to sport. After a few minutes the PWA suddenly said, 'Thank God you've come round; you're the first person that's come to see me today that hasn't wanted to go on and on about death and AIDS. Can't they talk about anything else? It's so incredibly boring.'
>
> He spoke with considerable good humour. He had had a number of visitors that day from various statutory and voluntary agencies, each one determined not to 'evade the issues', each one unaware of what the others were doing.

The counsellor should aim to take his lead from the patient. If the patient wants to talk about death, the counsellor should be willing to do so. If the issue of death comes up naturally as part of something the counsellor is saying, he should not go out of his way to avoid the issue. On the other hand there is no point in forcing a patient to talk about death simply because the counsellor thinks either he or the patient ought to talk about it.

Planning for death

Anyone faced by a possibly life-threatening illness should 'put their affairs in order'. If they do not eventually die they will not have lost anything. Aspects which they might cover include:

- Making a will.
- They may need to take steps to secure their partner's financial future, particularly with gay couples where the partner does not have the legal status of next-of-kin, as a wife or husband would have.
- Stating any special request or making special arrangements for the funeral. Sometimes people want special music or a special oration. Sometimes people go even further; several PWAs we have seen have made all their own funeral arrangements as far as possible, down to choosing the sort of coffin they want.
- Any religious requirements they may have either at the time of death, or as death approaches, or after death.
- Deciding where they want to die. Some people have a clear wish to die at home if at all possible.
- Anyone they would want to be with them when they are dying.
- Who should be informed when they are dying.
- Putting personal papers together and leaving any special instructions about their affairs.

Once these matters have been arranged they can be forgotten and the person can get on with their life. Tackling this sort of issue should be presented as insurance, something which it is wise to do, not as a sign that death is imminent (unless it is).

Clearing up loose ends

For some people there are loose ends in their lives which they want to tie up before they die. These can be of many types: people they have fallen out with whom they would like to be reconciled to, things they have not done that they feel it important to do, or people they have not seen for a long time whom they want to see again.

Spiritual matters

Some people have deeply held spiritual beliefs, some find such beliefs when they are faced with death, while others have none at all. It is helpful for the counsellor to find out about these and to make any necessary arrangements for the person to see a chaplain or rabbi or priest, or whoever else can deal with these issues with the patient.

Doing things they have always wanted to do

Some people have things they have always wanted to do but have put off. The point where they are facing death is often the point where they want to do these things. Within the limits of the patients' physical abilities it is important to help them as far as possible to achieve what they want to. Sometimes this creates a conflict with clinical issues. Patients may want to travel and there may be a question of whether they will become ill abroad and find themselves in difficulties. As far as is possible, though, they should be helped to travel even at some small risk that things may go wrong.

Treatment or not

Patients may have strong views about the extent to which they want treatment if they are dying, or whether they want to be resuscitated. These views should be respected and followed.

What happens when you die?

A number of patients want to know about what happens physically to the body when they die. What does the hospital actually do, for instance? In these cases, a full and sensitive explanation should be given.

Reassuring patients

For many patients fear of death is less important than the fear of dying alone or in pain. They should always be reassured that this will not be allowed to happen. Someone will be there with them when they die and adequate medication will always be given to suppress pain.

Sometimes patients ask a similar but distinct question, 'Is it painful to die?' The answer is that it is not. We know this because some people have died and been resuscitated and they do not report it as an unpleasant experience. Experiences of seeing other people die peacefully can also be discussed.

Carers

The person facing death is often not the only one who wants to talk through the issues above. It should be remembered that carers and lovers may also need to go through these issues with the counsellor and they should be given every opportunity to voice anxieties and have them addressed.

Living wills

For many people with AIDS, decision making is not straightforward. There are no clear answers and much is unknown; there are many fears and uncertainties. Some people wish to be involved with the decision making about their future. The process of living wills may be helpful in providing an opportunity for dialogue between a patient and carers. It may also provide an opportunity for someone to express their desires and have these recorded. Case management becomes much easier if the clear views of the individual are recorded. Obviously the optimum time for this is prior to an emergency situation. Although the level of cognitive impairment with HIV infection and AIDS is relatively low, the fears of dementia or decline are widespread. It is reassuring for such people to have their wishes and desires explored in case they are not capable of doing so later. However, the process is often not simple. People change their minds, relatives may hold different views and it may be difficult to carry out all wishes.

The death of a child

There is a growing level of paediatric HIV infection and deaths in children of all ages. The death of a child is seen as an untimely death and requires much specialised input. Initially there is the need for disclosure of the terminal issues with the family and the child. Children are often excluded from information about their own condition despite the fact that they may have a clear idea that something is wrong. The aura of secrecy and social stigma which surrounds HIV infection and AIDS makes this more difficult.

Children who are themselves dying, or whose parents or siblings are dying, need full explanations, careful handling and someone who can answer their questions openly and honestly at a level commensurate with their cognitive ability. For many children this is not a one-off process, but requires regular opportunities to explore questions. This is often difficult if the parent(s) are also facing HIV illnesses (Chapter 10).

Unrecognised deaths

Hidden deaths can cause extreme bereavement reactions which are unnoticed. Many of these are associated with AIDS, for example, termination of pregnancy in the presence of HIV, or the ending of relationships.

End of life decisions

No discussion of dying, bereavement and loss in the context of AIDS can ignore some of the important end of life decisions. As HIV usually strikes those in younger age groups, death has not necessarily been pondered. As there is no cure for AIDS there are many decisions associated with the end of life when individuals examine both the quality and quantity of life. These range from individual decisions to end their own life, to decisions about the manner of death, the place of death and the surroundings of death. There may also be decisions by carers either to withhold treatments or to administer treatments which may directly or indirectly influence end of life.

Those left behind: death and the carer

In this context 'carer' means exactly what it says: lovers, wives, husbands, friends, family and anyone else emotionally affected by the death or possible death of the patient. Carers often need as much support and help as the patient, and sometimes considerably more. There is a particular problem with carers because they are often reluctant to say that they are having problems. There are several reasons for this:

- They feel that they have to be 'strong' so as to be able to help the patient
- They feel that it is the patient who should be getting all the staff time, not them
- They feel that their problems are trivial in comparison with those of the patient.

Because carers are so often reluctant to come forward for help they need to be given every possible opportunity to express any difficulties they may be having. The counsellor will have the opportunity to talk to the carer when the patient has come into hospital or is being visited at home. It is helpful to set aside some time to talk to carers and to find out how they are getting on. It is surprising how many will say they have difficulties if asked.

Every effort should be made not to downgrade the importance of the carer. It is easy for carers to think that their usefulness is limited compared with the 'real experts' of the hospital. As far as possible they need the chance to talk to staff, and it needs to be emphasised how valuable their contribution is to the care of the patient, being careful not to corner them into a situation where they cannot admit it if they are not coping.

Sometimes a carer needs to be 'given permission' to withdraw. They simply cannot cope any more and the hospital must say, 'You have done everything it is possible for one person to do; we will take over the physical burden now but you still have an important role in being there'.

When a person is approaching death, as much as possible should be done to prepare the carer for what is going to happen: if they are going to be there, what the death will be like and what will be done after the death.

Tying up loose ends

Carers themselves may have loose ends to tie up with the patient: things they have never said, things that have been difficult between the two of them for years, things they need to discuss for their peace of mind. The carer too has needs and rights. He or she should be encouraged to sort out anything before the patient dies. Leaving matters settled makes dealing with death easier.

A PWA's mother had been taught from her earliest years onwards not to show emotion. She had never been able to tell her son that she loved him. She had shown her disapproval of his being gay and had never been willing for him to bring his lover to her house. When she saw that he was dying she began to regret this. She at last found the strength to tell her son she loved him. She saw how upset the lover was and found she understood that he too loved her son. They talked and got on well, much to the patient's delight. After the death they were able to support each other and became friends, indeed the lover became something of a son himself.

The carer as patient

It is important to remember that carers are often themselves infected with HIV or have AIDS. In this case they will need just as much counselling as the patient, or even more, since they may be facing a double stress.

Bereavement

The time of a death is a busy one for everyone concerned. It is important that carers should not get 'lost' in the process. They will continue to have their needs and require support and help, often through an extended period.

For people suffering a bereavement the first few days after the death are often a terrible shock. There are often sympathetic people around who will share the burden of loss and who are willing to talk over the death with the carer. After a short while, however, carers are expected by the world to 'pull themselves together'. It is considered that they are grieving too long, or 'being morbid'. The friends who flocked around at the time of the death now begin to get on with their own lives again. The amount of support that the carer gets drops off, even though they may feel worse than they did immediately after the death.

There is no 'natural' length of mourning. A person can mourn for days, or weeks or months. Even over many years they may still get pangs of mourning, particularly on anniversaries or when some favourite piece of music that they both shared is played. There is a difference between mourning and depression, although normal mourning may have days of depression in it, and the counsellor should be careful to pick up the carer who becomes depressed after the death (Chapter 12).

There are several things the counsellor can do which will help the carer cope with bereavement.

Reassuring the carer

Some bereaved carers feel they are in some way failing by not coming to terms with the bereavement quickly enough, a message all too often echoed by their friends. They need to be reassured that it is all right to mourn, it is natural. It is also all right to cry sometimes and all right to be depressed from time to time. Above all, they must be reassured that the counsellor has time for them.

Not all carers mourn after a death. They may feel a sense of relief, particularly if the patient had been very ill before the death or had been suffering from severe dementia. They can feel that they are abnormal in this respect and should be reassured that they are not. There is no evidence for the commonly held view that someone who fails to mourn will come to great psychological harm. What is harmful is the carer who is mourning but is not able to express that mourning, usually because of the behaviour of others.

Discussing the dead person with the carer

Many people who are bereaved want desperately to discuss the dead person with someone. They want to talk about them partly to put things into perspective and partly because talking about them eases the pain. They find sometimes that friends are reluctant to discuss the dead person in case the carer becomes 'upset'. In fact discussion, if the carer wants it, is the best thing. Talking things over with the carer and listening are the two best ways that the counsellor can help.

Dealing with guilt

Few people who are bereaved escape without at least some guilt. They look back over their lives with their loved ones and see only events that they regret: arguments, things they feel they prevented the other person from doing, things they failed to do. They need time to talk these through, but they also need gently to be brought round to thinking of all the good times the two of them had together. They need to be helped to put the good and bad into perspective. It is also helpful to reassure them that feelings of guilt are natural.

Accepting the good and bad parts of the deceased

'Speak no ill of the dead' is an old adage, but not a very sensible one. Few people are saints and carers will have to come to terms with the good and bad aspects of the deceased. At first they may well tend to idealise them; however, as time goes on they will come to take a more realistic and integrated view. The counsellor should stress that the deceased was a real flesh-and-blood person with a real person's faults and qualities. If they had not been, would the carer have loved them in the first place?

Dealing with avoidance

Sometimes carers are reluctant to go to particular places which they visited with the deceased, usually places where they have been happy together. They may be reluctant to visit the deceased's grave, not because they do not want to go – which can be a perfectly natural reaction ('there's no point in going, he's not there anyway') – but because they are afraid to go. They should be gently encouraged to go; they may feel bad at first, but many people find great comfort from going to places where they have been with the deceased, once they get over the initial anxiety. It helps them to feel close to the loved one.

Duration of grief

There is no clear view on how long people grieve. Studies have shown severe depression still apparent a year after a loss. Some theories suggest a permanent attachment which allows someone always to have a sense of grieving for the individual who has died, but to balance this with the continuation of life. When the passage of time does not see any form of reconstruction or resumption of normal life, it is described as a syndrome variously labelled as pathological, atypical, morbid, abnormal or extended grief. Intervention in the form of a dialogue is often helpful for such people. It allows them to air some of their deeply felt emotions and to move forward with their grieving.

'The shrine'

It occasionally happens that, after a death, the carer makes the joint home, or part of it, into a sort of shrine, keeping it exactly as the deceased left it and resisting all attempts to change it. This is rarely helpful; the deceased does not live on in material objects, but in the memories of those left behind. In this context it is often helpful gently and gradually to encourage the carer to make necessary changes, a little at a time.

Memories

The process of bereavement and grieving is not one of forgetting, denial or disassociation. Rather it is one where an individual finds a place for uncomfortable emotions. This involves the active creation of memories rather than the denial of them. Help comes in the form of allowing an individual to feel and experience their emotions rather than denying or blocking them or pretending. If their social surroundings do not allow space for the creation of memories, other alternatives can be found. Such exercises as memorial services, donations in an individual's name, remembrance quilts and dedications all serve this vital function.

Talking to the dead

Where there are issues which the carer and the deceased have not resolved, it sometimes helps to get the carer to actually talk to the deceased. Whether this is in the form of going to the graveside and talking to the deceased, or setting up an empty chair and talking to that, or simply talking, it can help immensely. The carer can say all those things they did not say when the deceased was alive. A technique we have sometimes used is to get the carer to write a letter to the deceased and then burn it (a sort of way of 'sending' it).

No belief in after-life is needed in the carer to make these things helpful. They are symbolic rather than magical or religious acts. They work because so many bereaved people feel the closeness of someone who is dead.

Odd experiences

Odd experiences after death are very common. The carer may 'see' the deceased, perhaps fleetingly in the street but sometimes in the house. A feeling that the dead person is close, or actually in the room, is very common. These experiences often distress people greatly. They may think they are going mad, or they may think they have seen a ghost.

It is only when the subject is touched on by the counsellor that carers will sometimes admit that they have had these experiences. They should be reassured that they are quite natural, normal experiences. If a carer feels that they are spiritual experiences no attempt should be made to argue by a sceptical counsellor. On the other hand it is possible to explain the experiences in terms of normal products of the mind which is mourning, a part of the process of coming to terms with grief and mourning, a benign and helpful process.

Letting go

After a time the image of the deceased often becomes weaker in the mind of the carer. They may find that they can no longer clearly picture the face or imagine the voice of the deceased. This can cause great distress if, for the carer, the deceased seems to live on only in memories. The carer can be reassured about this. The image will often return in the future and can, in any case, be strengthened again through photographs of the deceased.

Thinking what the deceased would want

One great ally which the counsellor has is the deceased person. In general, if the deceased had loved the carer, they would want the carer to have a happy life. Talking through what the deceased would want, with the carer, and trying to come to some conclusions is often a liberating and pleasing experience.

References

Cartwright, T.A., Hockey, L. & Anderson, J.K. (1973) *Life Before Death*. Routledge and Kegan Paul, London.

Kubler-Ross, E. (1970) *On Death and Dying*. Tavistock, London.

Parkes, C.M. (1972) *Bereavement. Studies of Grief in Adult Life*. Tavistock, London.

Sherr, L. (1992) Unique Patterns of Bereavement in AIDS and HIV Infection. *J. GU Medicine*, Nov.

Chapter 15

Changing Sexual Behaviour

John Green

For the counsellor in sexual health, helping people to reduce their risks of HIV infection is a key task. The benefits for an individual of safer sexual behaviour are not limited to HIV. While the pattern of transmission of different sexually transmitted diseases differs somewhat, it is broadly true to say that the same changes which protect an individual against HIV also protect them against other sexually transmitted diseases.

Background

The lifetime incidence of known sexually transmitted diseases is high (Laumann *et al.* 1994; Wellings *et al.* 1994), and many individuals in the population are not aware that they have sexually transmitted diseases. Individuals with gonorrhoea, chlamydia, herpes, warts and HIV are often asymptomatic or have such mild symptoms that they overlook them. Sexually transmitted agents other than HIV not only cause immense physical and psychological suffering but also they can have severe and sometimes even fatal consequences; pelvic inflammatory disease and cervical cancer are examples.

In most countries the coming of HIV has been accompanied by an unprecedented amount of information about the disease, its risks and the sorts of changes which can protect against it. However, many people continue to put themselves at sexual risk, particularly heterosexuals. In part this probably reflects the fact that, for many people, safer sex is less desirable in itself than 'unsafe sex'. Many people dislike condoms; they find them uncomfortable, find that they reduce sensation and interrupt the 'natural flow' of sex, and they feel that they reduce intimacy. The widespread success of condom programmes with prostitutes ironically illustrates this issue. For the prostitute, reducing intimacy with the client is a bonus, while for most couples engaging in unpaid sex it is a disadvantage. Many prostitutes will use a condom with clients, if they can, but will not do so with their regular partner.

For heterosexuals in particular, non-penetrative sex is often seen as a poor second-best to vaginal or anal intercourse. Oral sex or mutual manual stimulation is 'foreplay' rather than the sex itself. This is not to say that people will not move towards safer sex. However, if it was easy and just as much fun to move to safer sex, most people would have done so already – but they have not. Putting safer sex into practice involves taking important decisions and taking trouble to ensure that safer sex is built into a pattern of sexual behaviour.

The counsellor is, in theory, particularly well-placed to offer help to people wanting to change their sexual behaviour. General health education through leaflets, education programmes and the media are important, but such approaches have certain limitations. They are important in creating a climate where people appreciate the risks and what they might do to reduce them. They undoubtedly allow some individuals to make necessary changes. However, while they tell people what they can do, they do not necessarily tell them how to do it. They tend to offer general advice not necessarily applicable to particular cases.

Mary was a 34-year-old unmarried woman who had lived with the same man for four years. They had one child. During that time she had twice contracted chlamydial infections from her partner. She was aware of the fact that he, from time to time, had unprotected sex with other women. She would have liked him to either give up having sex with other women or to wear a condom when they had sex together. When she raised this with him he always assured her that the incidents when he had had sex with other women were isolated ones and 'he would never do it again'. If she asked him to use a condom he would become angry and accuse her of not trusting him. He argued that if she did not trust him, there was not much point in their continuing the relationship. She felt that if he left her she would not find anyone else, her child would be left without a good father and she would find it very difficult to cope.

This is clearly a case where Mary knew what steps would protect her, but did not know how to implement them. Providing her with more information, demonstrating how to put on a condom or urging her to consider the risk of sexually transmitted diseases including HIV, were unlikely to help her change her behaviour. What she needed to do was to try to solve some of the practical problems preventing her from implementing safer sex strategies.

The case also reflects a common problem for women: the difficulty they can have in getting their partners to implement safer sex. There is very often a power imbalance between man and woman which puts the woman at a disadvantage when it comes to implementing safer sex. Interventions which are successful in changing sexual behaviour in men often fail to change sexual behaviour in women (Cohen 1992a,b). Indeed the woman's view of her partner's attitude to, say condoms, may be more important in whether she changes her risk behaviours than her own attitude (McCusker *et al.* 1993). Knowing that one should change does not imply that one is able to change.

Such situations are common. Background health education is vital, because otherwise individuals are not aware that they have to act at all, but they may need individual help in generating strategies for change and in this the counsellor can help, in ways which information alone cannot.

Features of sexual behaviour

Motivated behaviour

In order to help people to implement safer sex it is important to consider certain features of sexual behaviour. Most people conduct their sex lives the way they do for a reason. It is necessary to understand those reasons in order to help them to change.

Most sexual behaviour is motivated behaviour. In other words an individual's sex life is the way it is for a reason. There are many reasons why people conduct their sex lives the way they do, but these can be summarised as two basic reasons: because they like it that way, or because they do not feel that they have any alternative.

Roger was gay and conducted most of his sexual contacts in 'cottages' (public lavatories). While most contact was oral sex or masturbation he occasionally had anal sex either in the cottage or, more usually, in his car or at his, or his contact's, residence. His concern was that he had experienced a number of condom breakages from men who were performing insertive sex on him, and that he was putting himself at risk of HIV infection. He felt that it was difficult to ensure greater safety with men whom he hardly knew and with whom there was little conversation. He had a number of concerns about cottaging generally; he felt that he sometimes put himself at risk of physical violence (although he had never been attacked) and he was concerned that he might be arrested. However he particularly enjoying cottaging since he liked the variety, the anonymity and the fact that sex was usually quick and commitment-free.

Roger's sexual behaviour is motivated behaviour. He does it that way because he likes it, even though he finds safer sex in that particular context very difficult and even though he feels he runs other risks. On interview he saw no likelihood that he would give up cottaging or that he would cease to have occasional anal intercourse with people he met in cottages. To do either of these would make his sex life unacceptably less interesting and enjoyable. The question then became how he could manage the situation to reduce the risk of condom breakage and to minimise the possibility of other adverse consequences.

Cottaging is an interesting example of positively motivated sexual behaviour because many people who have never done it, both heterosexual and gay, cannot imagine that it is enjoyable. It has been frequently suggested that there must be a compulsive element in cottaging. How else could one explain that someone should choose to have anonymous sex in a cold uncomfortable public toilet with the risk of arrest? However, when we researched the issue (Church *et al.* 1993) we found that cottagers did it because they liked it. Few regarded it as compulsive and few wished to stop. Just because a behaviour is not what the counsellor would choose, does not mean it is not fun to others.

Not all sexual behaviour is positively motivated. Some sexual behaviour is motivated not by specific enjoyment but by a lack of perceived alternatives, not just alternative sexual partners but alternative ways of behaving. The case of Mary above illustrates this, but many cases in clinical practice show the same problem.

Jane was an attractive 26-year-old heterosexual woman who had had 40 partners in the past 18 months. She had very low self-esteem and felt herself to be dull and unattractive. Her sexual behaviour also made her feel bad; she felt dirty and 'used'. She had a particular pattern of sexual behaviour. She would be invited out by a man (which was a common occurrence) to dinner or to a club. Since she was lonely and had a low opinion of herself she would be flattered by this and would accept whether she liked the man or not. Typically, half way through dinner she would run out of conversation and would feel that she was boring her companion. The more she became concerned about this the more anxious she became, and the more anxious she became the less she could think of to say. Eventually she would take him home to bed with her out of sheer desperation. She did not enjoy sex and the following morning would feel humiliated and upset with herself and would reject the man and never see him again.

Jane had clear problems in her perception of herself and of the behaviour and expectations of others. She could only believe that a man would want to take her out in order to have sex with her. If she did not have sex with him, he would not want to know her and her feelings of self-worth would be reduced even further. Such negatively motivated patterns of sexual behaviour are not uncommon in both men and women. Fear of displeasing or losing a partner should perhaps be put into this category. It is covered in more detail below.

Social behaviour

Sex fulfils many functions other than the physical, including social and emotional functions. In concentrating on the mechanics of safer sex and the gadgetry of condoms, dental dams, lubricants etc., it is easy to forget that sex is not just about orgasms and physical contacts.

> Alan was a 33-year-old man in late stage AIDS. He became very depressed for reasons which seemed unconnected to his physical state but which he would not expand upon. Finally he told the counsellor, 'Look at me, I'm dying and for what? I've had sex with many men and I did anything they wanted. I never enjoyed sex with any of them, I only did it because I was lonely.'

Sex can be a social event, a way of getting close to people and, in some cases, of meeting people. Changing one's sexual behaviour often means changing social behaviour generally.

Emotional relationships

Sex can also be a statement about the emotional relationship between two people. One of the apparent oddities of HIV is the number of partnerships in which one individual has HIV and the other does not, and in which they seem to 'take a risk' with infection.

> Colin and Angela were married. She had contracted HIV during a period of IV drug use in Holland in the early 1980s. She was becoming unwell although she did not have an AIDS diagnosis. It transpired that they were having unprotected sex regularly and had been for some years even though he was seronegative. When this was discussed with them she expressed anxiety about this. However Colin said that he wanted to be close to her, particularly now that she was becoming ill and might not be around for long. He saw sex with her as an affirmation of his love for her and was willing to take the risk of infection. He said 'If it happens, it happens; we've shared our lives together and I'm willing to take the risk.' He said that he was anxious about being infected but would rather run the risk than 'treat her like a leper'.

Several attempts had been made by well-meaning and exasperated health workers to make Colin see 'the error of his ways'. In fact he could see the risks in front of him every day in the shape of his own sickly wife. These attempts had achieved nothing except to make both of them more anxious, without changing their behaviour. Getting some change was impossible without recognising the need which having unsafe sex fulfilled in both of them. It was an affirmation of their closeness and of their willingness to deal with any problem together. It might not have made rational sense to the dispassionate observer, but it was how they felt and where they started from.

Chain of behaviours

Sexual behaviour is a chain of behaviours with each leading to the next. The importance of this can be seen by looking at a common problem for health educators: how to persuade people to wear condoms with new partners. To look at this it is helpful to draw up a typical pattern of heterosexual behaviour, in this case a first sexual encounter with a new partner:

- Jane and Peter meet at a party in the kitchen while they are both getting a drink.
- They chat generally and then he asks her to dance.
- They dance together closer and closer. She kisses him.
- They move through to a quieter room where they talk more and kiss more. He has his arm around her.
- The party is coming to an end. Neither has a car with them. They agree to share a taxi.
- When they arrive at her flat she asks if he would like to come in for coffee. He agrees.
- While she puts on the coffee, he puts on a record and they sit together on the settee.
- They kiss and begin 'heavy petting'.
- Clothing removal begins.
- They are both sexually excited and they go through to the bedroom and have sex.

This pattern is played out with variations by many people starting their sex life with a new partner, whether that relationship lasts a day or a lifetime. The pattern raises a number of interesting questions. People are usually advised to insist that their partner uses a condom or to negotiate condom usage. Sometimes they are advised to find out as much as possible about their partner before going to bed with them. However at what point in this chain of behaviour will they do these things? Inspection of the chain suggests that there is a strong possibility that the answer is 'never'.

The couple are carrying out a complex dance of interaction in which the initiative flows backwards and forwards over time and each is keen to find out, subtly, how far the other is prepared to go, while avoiding as far as possible the chance of getting a rejection.

Another interesting point is that they may very well never discuss the fact that they are going to have sex, until they are actually doing it (and very probably not even then). The process is one of tacit agreement at every stage, of people 'feeling their way', sometimes literally so. It may be tacit because for either to admit what they were hoping for would invite rejection and they might have misunderstood the signals right up until the end. However, if they do not actually acknowledge that they are going to have sex it is difficult to see how they are going to negotiate the use of condoms. The reader might like to think about where they would discuss condom usage. In the kitchen over the peanuts? While dancing? In the taxi? On the settee? Or when they are already in bed and otherwise engaged? In the same way it is clear that advice to find out about their partner (code for finding out about their past sexual behaviour) before going to bed with them is unlikely to work in a chain like the one above.

However, the chain does suggest one way for the parties involved to implement safer sex successfully. If they do not discuss having sex and they do not discuss condoms, neither party is likely to refuse to use a condom. It would therefore seem most sensible if she puts a condom on him and does not discuss it at all. Similarly he can put on a condom without discussing it. This puts the onus on the partner to object, which they are probably unlikely to do. If they do object it is easy for the woman to say 'I'm not on the pill' or 'I like to be safe' or 'it's the responsible thing to do'. The man can use similar responses. At the point of penetration negotiation is unlikely to be protracted, and if it is, the objective of finding an opportunity to negotiate safer sex has been achieved.

Sex is a chain of behaviours with each leading on almost imperceptibly to the next. It is necessary to look at the overall pattern of what happens. Simply putting the condom on, or on one's partner, is not the usual advice on what to do in these circumstances. However, while overt condom negotiation is a viable strategy for some people, for many people discussing sex – let alone negotiating about it – is very difficult, and the situation makes it much more difficult. Under these circumstances, putting the condom on is likely to be a more reliable strategy for many people than trying to discuss it.

The example above is a useful way of drawing generalised conclusions about the sort of strategy that might be effective. However, when it comes to the sex life of the individual, it is important to find out in detail how he or she conducts his or her sex life, and why that individual conducts it in that way. Only then is it possible to work with them to find out how they can change it. This means looking at examples of how they have behaved in the past, looking for the chains of behaviour. As the old adage says, 'the devil is in the detail'. It is almost impossible to help someone implement safer sex by dealing in generalities.

Interaction between at least two people

One of the difficulties of helping people to change their sexual behaviour is that there are usually (at least) two people involved. The behaviour of each person affects the behaviour of the other. It is important to see sex as an interaction and to consider the position of each individual in the relationship in order to see what scope they have for change. For an individual who does not have a settled partner, it is important to understand what sort of partner they have.

> Justin was a 29-year-old gay man. He tended to form relationships with older men whom he perceived as stable and financially settled. He earned a reasonable but intermittent income as a freelance artist and led a chaotic lifestyle punctuated by bouts of heavy drinking and failure to pay bills and deal with everyday life issues. When he had a partner he tended to hand over responsibility for everyday life to his partner, including responsibility for deciding what sort of sex they should have. His relationships tended to be short-term since once he had handed over responsibility for his life to someone else he quickly began to find their involvement restricting and even suffocating. He saw his sex life in a very negative light, feeling that he exchanged his youth and physical attractiveness for someone to look after him, and he felt that this was not an 'adult' way to behave. He also often found himself involved in sexual activities he did not like. He usually left decisions about safer sex to his partners, despite great anxiety about HIV.

Justin felt that he needed to try to find sexual partners whom he was not likely to put into a 'parental' role. In order to get control over his sex life he needed to think about the sort of partner he set out to find.

The relationship between partners is also an issue in longer term relationships which can influence the scope people have for changing their sexual behaviour. If a partner cannot accept particular changes, either the individual will find change difficult or the relationship may break down.

> Tanya was a 28-year-old prostitute with a young daughter. She had a boyfriend with whom she lived and who was ambivalent about her prostitution. He had a steady and modestly-paid job. She would have liked to give up her trade but he was a heavy gambler and drinker who usually brought almost none of his income home. Consequently she supported her daughter, their home and often him, financially. She was stuck with being a prostitute. She was afraid that if she lost him no-one else would want her, given her occupation and history.

The power balance is an issue in many relationships which restricts the scope for change.

> Graham was a 38-year-old man who was conducting an affair with a 29-year-old married woman. He had just contracted herpes from her. She had an ambivalent relationship with her husband, who was seeing other women. Graham wanted her to leave her husband and move in with him. Some weeks she would say that she would and they would make plans together; the next week she would change her mind and nothing would happen. He felt unable to address the issue of the herpes with her because she became upset whenever they tried to discuss it, so he was unable to put safer sex into place, unable to get her to change her behaviour and unable to bring himself to end the relationship.

Sometimes a specific sexual behaviour takes place because it is what a partner wants. Many people engage in sex, or in particular types of sex, because that is what their partner wants or because of social pressure. A fair proportion of women in the US have their first sexual experience under such circumstances (Michael *et al.* 1994). However, examples of such circumstances are common even in established relationships.

> Jane was a woman in her mid-thirties. She was married to a man who liked to watch her have sex with other men. A number of their friends had similar interests. They went to parties at which he would encourage her to drink and then have sex with another man while he watched. She enjoyed this at the time but needed to be drunk to do it and, on balance, would have preferred not to do it.

This is a rather obvious example. Less obvious cases are probably common.

In order to understand someone's sexual behaviour it is important to understand their relationship with their current partner and their relationships with past partners, the balance of power within relationships, and the meaning of these relationships to the individual.

People are concerned with specific risks not general risks

There have been numerous attempts to model the sexual behaviour of individuals, to try to find out what makes them fail to adopt safer sexual practices. They have mostly been built around ideas about general risks – the extent to which an individual feels globally at risk of contracting HIV or other sexual health problems. Unfortunately such models have proved very poor predictors of how people behave in the real world. People's ratings of their global risk of catching HIV does not relate very strongly to their behaviour. Our own research (Green, Taylor and Fulop, in preparation) and that of others suggests that we should be using a specific risks model. People's behaviour is determined not by their estimates of their own risks of catching HIV but by their subjective estimates of the likelihood of a particular partner being a risk to them. In short, people will take precautions to protect themselves (all other things being equal) if they believe that their partner may present a risk to them, but if they feel that their partner could not be infected they will be much less likely to take precautions. This is one of the reasons why people are less likely to adopt safer sexual practices with those they are madly in love with; they often cannot believe that the love of their life could have an STD. The counsellor needs to discuss this issue with the patient very explicitly. It is not, in real life, usually possible for the average person embarking on a relationship to reliably determine who is and is not a risk to them. The criteria people use to assess the riskiness of others make matters worse since they tend to be based on appearance and personality, neither, of course, any guide to risk. Helping the patient to overcome the very human approach of trying to weigh up the other person, and to move towards more global self-protection, is probably central to helping people to change their sexual behaviour.

Helping people to change

In helping people to change their behaviour it is important to note several points at the outset. It is not possible to force people to change their behaviour against their will, even if the counsellor feels that this is desirable. It is characteristic of sexually transmitted diseases that the infected person can put others at risk, possibly of their lives but certainly of their health. However, few societies find it acceptable to lock people up just because they have a disease and might infect others. In any case the history of control of sexually transmitted diseases shows many attempts to use legal means – including confinement to prevent the spread of infections – all of which were failures. The counsellor can only seek to help the individual to change; what they do once they are out of sight is not subject to observation. This does not mean that the counsellor should not take all possible steps to encourage change in someone who is putting themselves, or others, at risk. But this can only realistically be done by working with the patient. Trying to force people to do what they are unwilling to do (even for their own good) usually results in them not coming back, rather than in them changing their behaviour.

Helping people to change means trying to find out as much as possible about the context and nature of their sex life, and then working jointly with the patient to generate solutions which fit their particular situation. Potential solutions to problems seldom come ready-made. If it was easy for most individuals to change their behaviour in order to reduce risk or distress, they would already have done so. This does not mean that the counsellor should not have a range of possible tactics or approaches available, or that they should not draw on their experience of how others have dealt with particular problems. However, these need to be seen as elements which can be suggested as part solutions. The answers to problems come from a full understanding of the problems themselves. It is my impression, from training counsellors in the field, that many people in sexual health are unwilling to pursue the details of people's sex lives because they are afraid that they will come up with problems for which they do not have an answer. In fact it is surprising just how often solutions readily suggest themselves once a full picture of the problem is obtained.

There are several steps involved in helping people to change their sexual behaviour.

Understanding and negotiating what they want to change

Most health professionals and volunteers have their own opinions of how they believe others should lead their sex lives. Whether these are good or bad ideas is usually less relevant than the fact that this can colour their perception of what an individual actually wants to achieve. The following extract from a transcript shows the problem.

PATIENT: 'I'm embarrassed to tell you this but, well, what's worrying me is, you see – I go to prostitutes a lot and, you know, I like them to tell me off and things – sometimes spank me. Then we have sex; we always use a condom but I've been very worried lately, if I might have caught something.'

COUNSELLOR: 'So you want to give up using prostitutes?'

To which the patient might reasonably have responded that the counsellor was not listening to what he was saying. However, patients are usually much too polite to point out the obvious. The first step is to try to help the patient to articulate what they concerns are and what they would like to change.

PATIENT: 'I've slept with a lot of men over the last ten years and it just hasn't worked out for me.'

COUNSELLOR: 'Why's that?'

PATIENT: 'They've stayed for a while and then they've gone. I just don't seem to have been able to find someone to share my life with and I'm not getting any younger.'

COUNSELLOR: 'You'd like to find a long term relationship?'

PATIENT: 'Yes, that's right.'

It is important not to leap in at this stage with a series of questions about condom usage or exactly how many men they have slept with. There is time to get to these points later.

Sometimes patients will come up with unrealistic solutions rather than aspects they want to change. It is important to recognise the difference and to pick up the problem rather than the solutions.

PATIENT: 'I want treatment to make me heterosexual. I don't want to be gay any more.'

COUNSELLOR: 'Why is that?'

PATIENT: 'I hate the gay scene and with AIDS it's just too risky.'

Here the patient's concerns turned out to revolve around fear of infection and a dislike of the behaviour of the gay men he was meeting. He met potential partners exclusively in clubs and gay bars. He has presented an unrealistic 'answer' however – not being gay any more – rather than the problem. Starting at this point is hopeless; it is important to go back to the problem and start from there, thinking about all the possible ways of dealing with that problem.

The counsellor need not be passive in dealing with patient problems. It is sometimes desirable to try to influence a patient's thinking about what needs to be done, but this needs to be approached tactfully.

PATIENT: 'I was pretty unlucky catching gonorrhoea. I would never have gone with her if I hadn't been drunk. I'll just have to be more careful about the women I pick in the future.'

COUNSELLOR: 'When you were in the waiting room there were quite a few women waiting with you. What did you think of them?'
PATIENT: 'Well, I'm not sure ... there were some pretty attractive women there.'
COUNSELLOR: 'Could you tell which of them had gonorrhoea?'
PATIENT: 'Well, no, I don't suppose I could. Did some of them?'
COUNSELLOR: 'Very likely. Do you think you can always tell whether a woman has a sexually transmitted disease just by looking at her?'
PATIENT: 'Not really. It doesn't make sense does it?'
COUNSELLOR: 'Maybe we can think of some other ways you can protect yourself?'

Sorting out realistic objectives is often a process of working together with the patient. It should never be a matter of telling the patient off and instructing them as to their future conduct. Aggression seldom gets anyone anywhere.

COUNSELLOR: 'Look, this is the third time in two years you've been in here with something. You've had gonorrhoea, non-gonococcal urethritis and once you thought you had herpes. You can't go on like this, can you? What are you going to do to make sure we don't get you back in here next month?'

To which the probable answer is, 'go to another clinic'. Again, it is worth considering that if the patient had found it easy to change they would probably have done so already.

Finding out about the patient's sexual life

The next stage is to find out about the patient's sex life, which usually means taking a sexual history. The purpose of taking a history is to get as much detail as possible about the three Ws:

- What they do
- Who they do it with
- Why they do it.

The order of getting the information is a matter of taste but it is usually best to start at the present and work back.

Peter was a 32-year-old gay man who came regularly to the sexually transmitted disease clinic for screening. He was seronegative and concerned that he was putting himself at risk of HIV infection. He was inconsistent in using condoms when having anal sex, both insertive and receptive. Discussion of his objectives suggested that he was keen to use condoms consistently but that he found this difficult. Otherwise he was happy about his sex life.

COUNSELLOR: 'Do you have a sexual partner currently?'
PATIENT: 'Not at the moment. I split up with my last partner about six months ago.'
COUNSELLOR: 'Had you been together long?'
PATIENT: 'About six years.'
COUNSELLOR: 'Why did you split up?'

PATIENT: 'It was mutual. We sort of drifted apart and eventually I called a halt. We'd more or less given up having sex together a couple of years before that. We both had quite a few other partners in the time we were together. Eventually there didn't seem any point in going on; it was over. So he moved out and got his own place. We still see each other sometimes but I don't think we'll get back together.'

COUNSELLOR: 'Have you had any sexual partners since?'

PATIENT: 'Yes, twice. I wanted a bit of a rest from things for a while but over the last month I've had sex with two men.'

COUNSELLOR: 'Tell me about the last one. How did you meet, what happened?'

This is important. Getting a clear account of particular episodes of sexual behaviour gives a much better idea of what might be done than getting the patient to relate a series of unhelpful generalisations.

PATIENT: 'I met him in a club. I sort of knew him, he was a friend of Terry's – my ex. I'd always quite fancied him and he was on his own and we got talking and then we went back to his place.'

COUNSELLOR: 'You knew you were going to have sex with him when you left the club?'

PATIENT: 'Yeah.'

COUNSELLOR: 'What happened when you got back to his place?'

PATIENT: 'We had a few drinks, and then he put on a video.'

COUNSELLOR: 'Porn?'

PATIENT: 'Yeah. Pretty tame stuff about a building site; made no sense and nothing much happened, but he obviously liked that sort of thing.'

COUNSELLOR: 'Did you talk about the fact that you were going to have sex or did you just do it?

PATIENT: 'I told him I was negative and asked him whether he was. He said he was, as far as he knew.'

COUNSELLOR: 'Did you discuss safer sex?'

It is my impression from taking many sexual histories that gay men are more likely to discuss safer sex than heterosexuals; however, it is far from universal even among gay men.

PATIENT: 'No, not really, we just left it at that. Then he went down on me.'

COUNSELLOR: 'He sucked your penis? Did you use a condom?'

PATIENT: 'No, I didn't have one. Maybe he did, but we didn't discuss it.'

COUNSELLOR: 'Did you come?'

PATIENT: 'Not while he was sucking me. I've usually got good control. A few times when I've been sucked I've come without meaning to, but not this time.'

COUNSELLOR: 'OK, so you didn't come although sometimes you do. What happened then?'

It is helpful to feed back to the patient one's understanding of what they are saying as a way of checking that you have understood the story correctly. But do not do it to the extent that it interrupts the patient's flow of conversation.

PATIENT:	'He asked me to fuck him.'
COUNSELLOR:	'Anal sex?'
PATIENT:	'That's right. He produced some lubricant but he didn't mention condoms and I didn't ask.'
COUNSELLOR:	'So did you do it?'
PATIENT:	'No, I didn't feel like it so I messed around for a while and then I brought him off with my hand.'
COUNSELLOR:	'What made you do that rather than have anal sex with him?'
PATIENT:	'I was tired by that time and I wanted to get it over with. I'd lost interest a bit. Also, I guess I was a bit nervous about not using a condom.'
COUNSELLOR:	'What did you say?'
PATIENT:	'I didn't. I took hold of him and just did it. I talked about what I'd like to do to him and what he needed and he seemed to quite like that. He came off pretty quickly. Then he sucked me some more and I came over his chest.'
COUNSELLOR:	'You pulled out or he took his mouth away?'
PATIENT:	'I pulled out. I was a bit anxious about coming in his mouth.'
COUNSELLOR:	'Were you worried that you might have an infection you'd pass on?'
PATIENT:	'I was pretty clear that I didn't have anything but, well, in the current climate you can't be too careful.'
COUNSELLOR:	'Does worrying about sexually transmitted diseases interfere with your enjoyment of sex sometimes?'
PATIENT:	'Quite often, more recently. Several of my friends have died of AIDS or become sick with it in the last year.'

Further discussion of this episode showed that the interaction had been a one-off occurrence. The patient had found his contact rather dull and after having a lunchtime drink the following day had gone off without any further sexual activity. Listening to the story immediately raised a number of questions and interesting points:

* The patient had been motivated to avoid putting his partner at risk of a sexually transmitted disease. Concerns about the risk had interfered with his enjoyment of sex.
* The patient had not had a condom or lubricant with him, even though he knew he was going to go back for sex. In fact he had gone to the club with the intention of meeting someone. Condoms were available in the club but he had not taken any. He said that if he had had a condom he might have had anal sex as requested.
* They had discussed their serostatus but not safer sex or condom use. Serostatus is a poor guide, of course, because they could have become infected since their last tests or immediately prior to the last test. In any case they may have had other sexually transmitted diseases.
* The patient was very much in control of what happened.

Discussion then moved to the previous time he had had sex. Again, the contact was someone he knew vaguely whom he had met in a club. They had gone back to his flat and had had oral and anal sex. He had penetrated his partner, with a condom, and then had fellated his partner to orgasm without a condom. The following morning they had had mutual masturbation. He had found his partner only moderately attractive and although he had promised to ring him he did not do so.

COUNSELLOR: 'We've looked at a couple of times you've had sex recently. How typical were those?'

PATIENT: 'Pretty typical of the way things have been over the past couple of years.'

COUNSELLOR: 'You met both partners in clubs. Is that where you usually meet partners?'

PATIENT: 'Yes, almost always. Once or twice I've chatted up people in the street if I've fancied them enough and they've given me some encouragement, but I don't usually.'

COUNSELLOR: 'Do you feel that you put yourself at any risk of HIV or anything else on either of these occasions you've described?'

PATIENT: 'Well, on the last one I was pretty safe, I think, at least from the point of view of HIV. The time before that I sucked the guy off without a condom. I reckon the risks of HIV are pretty low from that, but maybe not nil. I just hate the taste of condoms so I don't think that that's an option for me for oral. I know you can get flavoured ones but who wants to suck a black-berry-and-rubber-flavoured penis?'

COUNSELLOR: 'But sometimes you feel you run a greater risk?'

PATIENT: 'Yes, sometimes I take a big chance.'

COUNSELLOR: 'Tell me about the last time you felt you put yourself at risk?'

PATIENT: 'It was last year. I met this guy at a party at my next-door neighbours . . .'

The key question now is: in what way did the times he behaved unsafely differ from the times when he behaved more safely. He recounted that he had met a man at a party and they had gone back to his flat. He had had receptive anal sex with a man without using a condom. He had had condoms in his flat but had not used them, even though he knew he should be using one while they were having sex.

COUNSELLOR: 'So you had unprotected receptive sex with this man even though you felt at the time that you should be using a condom?'

PATIENT: 'That's right.'

COUNSELLOR: 'But at other times you've wanted to use a condom and you have done. What was different this time?'

PATIENT: 'I was very attracted to him. I think I find it more difficult when I'm very attracted to someone. I just don't feel that I can ask them to use something; I hope that they'll just offer.'

COUNSELLOR: 'And he didn't.'

PATIENT: 'No. I guess it was me that was at risk, not him.'

COUNSELLOR: 'Did you discuss safer sex at all, or anything about risks?'

PATIENT: 'No, I just left it to him to take the lead.'

COUNSELLOR: 'You felt less in control with someone who was very attractive?'

PATIENT: 'I think that's it. I'm OK with people I don't really fancy, but when I really go for them I have a problem.'

COUNSELLOR: 'Are you afraid that if you don't give them what they want they'll reject you?'

PATIENT: 'Yes, I think I am. I know they won't really. Once it gets to that stage they'll go on anyhow and they're usually protecting themselves as well as me by keeping to safe stuff.'

COUNSELLOR: 'Any other reasons why you didn't use a condom?'

PATIENT: "No, not that I can think of.'

COUNSELLOR: 'You were at a party – had you had anything to drink, or taken any drugs?'

PATIENT: 'I'd had a few drinks, but nothing I couldn't handle. I don't think it makes much difference whether I drink as to whether I have safer sex or not.'

COUNSELLOR: 'How typical was that of times when you have felt you ought to be safe, but have been unsafe?'

PATIENT: 'Pretty typical.'

At this point it is worth obtaining some more examples. It is possible that these might yield other reasons why condoms are not always used. The patient was asked about other occasions. He mentioned an occasion when he had met someone in a bar, gone back to their flat and had engaged in bondage and then unprotected anal receptive sex. He particularly focused on the bondage.

PATIENT: 'I didn't like being tied up like that. It's OK with someone you know but it's not good with a stranger.'

COUNSELLOR: 'Why's that?'

PATIENT: 'Once they've got you tied up they can do what they like to you. There were those guys recently who got murdered by someone who tied them up. It makes me nervous not being able to do anything if things get out of hand.'

COUNSELLOR: 'Why didn't you refuse to let him tie you up?'

PATIENT: 'One thing led to another. It was quite exciting being out of control, but then once he got me tied up I began to panic, even though I knew I could get out ... he hadn't tied me up that tight.'

COUNSELLOR: 'And what about the anal sex?'

PATIENT: 'I guess I was so relieved nothing bad had happened that unprotected sex didn't seem a problem at all. It was only afterwards that I began to think.'

COUNSELLOR: 'Were you particularly attracted to him?'

PATIENT: 'Yes, I wouldn't have let him go so far if I hadn't fancied him so much.'

Clearly only snippets of the picture have been outlined above. The patient had much else to say about his sex life. In particular he went over the three long relationships he had had. Safer sex was a part of the last two of these, the first being prior to HIV. All three had tailed off sexually within a year or two of starting and he had had other partners during the course of them. Novelty was an important part of his sexual functioning. He foresaw himself continuing to have multiple partners in the future but wanted to keep it safe.

It is not necessary, or usually possible, to go over every sexual encounter or every partner. The objective of the process is to build up a picture of typical chains of behaviour and it is necessary to get sufficient accounts for both the counsellor and the patient to feel that they have built up a good picture of the patient's sexual behaviour, their partners and their motivations.

COUNSELLOR: 'Why do you think that your sex life with steady partners tailed off each time?'

PATIENT: 'I think I just became bored. Maybe we both did. There were particular reasons why each one came to an end. John, one of them, was into some things that I didn't like very much.'

COUNSELLOR: 'OK, so there were some specific reasons each time and some things you don't like doing sexually. That's important – let's come back to that – but let me ask you about getting bored.'

The counsellor is indicating to the patient that they have been heard, and while selecting one path is indicating that they will come back to the other points. The problem for the counsellor is making sure that they keep a track of a host of different issues and making sure that they go back over them at some point. Keeping rough notes helps but some people find it difficult to listen, ask questions and take notes at the same time, in which case it helps at the end of the session, or at some convenient point, to write down the main points of what has been discussed.

Reviewing the material

Once the counsellor has gathered what appear to be the main issues, it is important to try to pull everything together and build up an overview of the situation. This can then be discussed with the patient so that some overall formulation can be arrived at jointly. It is worth taking a few moments to consider what the patient has said.

COUNSELLOR: 'Let me just think about this for a moment. We've discussed quite a lot in this session and I just want to try to get the issues straight in my mind, then we can talk them through.'

Reviewing the material also shows where there are gaps in what has been discussed, and these can be gone over in a straightforward fashion.

COUNSELLOR: 'I forgot to ask you. You said that you keep condoms at home. Do you also keep lubricant?'

Once some sort of pattern has been discerned, it is helpful to discuss this with the patient.

COUNSELLOR: 'Let me go through what I understand you have told me. I want to make sure that I've got this right, so you tell me if what I think I've heard is OK. You see yourself continuing to have a number of partners and you think that you are likely to have anal sex with at least some of those.'

PATIENT: 'That's right. I think that's realistic.'

COUNSELLOR: 'You'd like to try to make this as safe as possible even though condoms are not 100% safe?'

PATIENT: 'Yes.'

COUNSELLOR: 'Most times when you have sex you feel in control, but sometimes you just give up that control to the other person.'

PATIENT: 'That's right, when I'm really attracted to someone I get sort of tongue-tied, at least as far as talking goes.'

COUNSELLOR: 'And then you sometimes end up doing things that you don't want to do.'
PATIENT: 'That's right.'
COUNSELLOR: 'You always have condoms and lubricant in your flat but when you go out you don't always take them with you, even when you think you might be going to try to have sex with someone.'
PATIENT: 'Even then.'
COUNSELLOR: 'You don't like using condoms for oral sex but you don't like people coming in your mouth or coming in their mouths.'
PATIENT: 'I don't feel it's safe and that puts me off.'
COUNSELLOR: 'But you have good control; you know when you're going to ejaculate, at least most times.'
PATIENT: 'I can always control it if I set out with a clear idea of what I want to do in the first place.'
COUNSELLOR: 'You mean if you've decided that you're going to pull out before you come, you can always manage that?'
PATIENT: 'Yes.'
COUNSELLOR: 'Does that go for other sexual activities? If you decide before you go back with someone what you are going to do, do you usually stick to that?'
PATIENT: 'Usually. If I know what I'm willing to do before I go back with them, I don't usually go any further than I want to.'

This shows one of the interesting aspects about discussing formulations with patients. The formulation tends to generate ideas in both counsellor and patient about what may be going on. It furthers discussion and serves to crystallise issues. In this case the discussion forms the basis for further links to be made.

COUNSELLOR: 'Does how attractive you find someone affect whether you decide in advance what you are going to do?'
PATIENT: 'Yes, it does. With very attractive men I'm more concerned with getting back with them. With someone I can take or leave, I've usually decided what I want to do or am willing to do before we get back home, because that's the only reason I'm taking them home.'
COUNSELLOR: 'So it's deciding what you want to do in advance that governs whether you'll stay in control? Or is it fear that attractive men are more likely to reject you?'
PATIENT: 'A bit of both, but mainly I think it's making my mind up in advance. That way I feel in control whether they're attractive or not.'

This puts matters in a different light. The first hypothesis about how attractiveness and lack of control are linked looks less important than it seemed, and a new link has been found. It is always worth keeping an open mind about whether formulations or strategies are right until they have been tested.

Generating possible solutions

COUNSELLOR: 'Let's see if we can review where we want to get to. As I see it you want to make sure that you always wear a condom and that your partner always

	wears a condom for anal sex. You don't want to come in other people's mouths or to have them come in yours, and you want to have more control over what you do sexually, because then you'll be able to say no to bondage or whatever.'
PATIENT:	'That's it.'
COUNSELLOR:	'And deciding what you are willing to do and what you don't want to do is important in keeping you in control.'
PATIENT:	'I've never really thought about it that way, but yes, I do think that's right.'
COUNSELLOR:	'How could you put that into practice?'
PATIENT:	'Well, I could decide before I took someone back what I was willing to do. In fact I know what I will and won't do, at least as far as possible. I could even write it down.'
COUNSELLOR:	'Maybe you should?'
PATIENT:	'Writing it down is going a bit too far, but yes, I could make up my mind what I wanted to do.'
COUNSELLOR:	'Would taking a clear decision about what you are and are not willing to do make a difference?'
PATIENT:	'I think it would. I know really when I'm going out whether I'm in the mood for sex. I could go over what I planned before I set out.'
COUNSELLOR:	'It's no good planning to use condoms if you don't have any.'
PATIENT:	'That's not a problem. I could put some in my pocket before I go out.'
COUNSELLOR:	'Would you be likely to do that?'
PATIENT:	'I can't see why not.'
COUNSELLOR:	'You haven't in the past.'
PATIENT:	'I do sometimes, but if I change my jacket I sometimes forget to swap the condoms over.'
COUNSELLOR:	'How could you solve that?'
PATIENT:	'I could keep them in my wallet; I usually have that with me.'
COUNSELLOR:	'Or put some in each of your jackets.'
PATIENT:	'Why not?'

It is important to try to get patients to generate their own solutions because these are often best adapted to what the patient can achieve. However there is no reason at all why the counsellor cannot make suggestions. The important point is to engage the patient in the process and not let it degenerate into a lecture by the counsellor about how the patient should behave. It is also important for the counsellor to act as devil's advocate and test out how realistic various solutions are, both those generated by the patient and those generated by the counsellor. It is easy to get carried away into a fantasy world of what is achievable. A degree of mild cynicism about human nature comes in handy.

COUNSELLOR:	'OK, you have your condoms, you've decided what you will do, you meet a man, you're off to his place full of good intentions. Do you stick to your good intentions?'
PATIENT:	'Probably.'
COUNSELLOR:	'Probably. What might go wrong?'

PATIENT: 'I might get carried away once we get started. Once I've got his penis in my mouth I might not stop.'

COUNSELLOR: 'What if he objects to what you want? What if he wants to do things you don't want to do?'

PATIENT: 'That could be a problem.'

COUNSELLOR: 'How could you handle that? It can be a bit of a slippery slope, can't it? Once you've got so far you might as well go the "extra mile".'

PATIENT: 'Yes, but maybe I need to tell them what I will and won't do.'

COUNSELLOR: 'How would that help?'

PATIENT: 'It would help me because they'd know what I'd do and what I wouldn't do. It would stiffen my nerve and if they don't want to stick to the rules I wouldn't go back with them, or anywhere for that matter.'

COUNSELLOR: 'What would you say?'

PATIENT: 'I'd say, "I only do safer sex".'

COUNSELLOR: 'When will you say it – in the club, or when you get back to their place?'

PATIENT: 'There's no reason why I can't say it before I go back with them, before we even leave where we are. The other thing is, maybe it would be better if I always took them back to my flat. I'd feel more in control there.'

It is important to 'enact' solutions both in order to test how realistic they are and in order to improve the chances that they will be adopted. So it is important to get the patient to think through the details of how they are going to implement particular strategies, down to the finest detail possible. Once solutions have been generated the next step is for the patient to try them out. The patient then needs to meet with the counsellor to review how they have gone. Feedback from trying out strategies allows new solutions to be found and new approaches to be adopted. It is important for anyone trying to make changes in their lives to feel that they have support and are not tackling the problem by themselves. Regular appointments are essential until the patient feels comfortable with a new approach.

Dealing with more than one patient

The case outlined above is that of a single individual. His sexual behaviour is complex – but so is everyone else's. Given that sex is usually a two-player game, it often seems a good idea to try to see someone's partner. There is some evidence that dealing with both members of a couple can make the implementation of safer sex more likely (Allen *et al.* 1992). Many counsellors find this a particularly attractive course of action.

Marie was a 36-year-old woman living with a man who had had a number of affairs. She was aware of this fact although he lied to her about it. She knew he had had a child by at least one of his other girlfriends in the time they had been married. She was still very much in love with him but despite her pleadings he still carried on with other women, although he had become a bit craftier at hiding his affairs. Matters came to a head when he contracted pubic lice and passed them on to her. They argued about this and it came out that he had not used a condom with the woman (although this would not have protected him against the lice anyway). Marie was disgusted and arrived at the clinic in great distress. Her complaint was simple: 'If he must do it he might at least protect me.' It was hard not to be sympathetic to this view.

It is very tempting to get the partner in and try to sort things out between them. However there are various problems. First, there is the danger that he will start out as the villain of the piece, even if he is prepared to come at all. This may be justified (although he is likely to have his own story) but it is hardly likely to put him in a receptive frame of mind. Secondly, it is easy to ignore the fact that Marie is in fact someone capable of action in her own right. It is sometimes all too easy to side with one partner and go into battle on his or her behalf and therefore fail to consider what he or she might do to improve the situation. It is best generally to deal with the person in front of you. Where two members of a couple are to be seen it is important to see each separately, and where resources allow, it can be helpful to ensure each member of a couple is seen by a different counsellor.

The most difficult way of dealing with matters is usually getting both parties together in one room and trying to mediate. It is worth considering that international peace conferences usually fail, and where they succeed most of the hard work has been done by the mediators with the two parties in advance outside the meeting. The lesson is to work with each party individually before getting them together. Even this is not guaranteed success, as one of my own early cases of marital disharmony shows. Having carefully worked on both parties beforehand, I had been assured by both of them individually how much they loved their partner and wanted to make the marriage work. I then decided, unwisely, to stage a reconciliation scene. The scene was a short one:

ME:	'Now I've spoken to you both and you've both told me what this marriage means to you.'
HER:	'I love him very much and I'd like to make it work.'
ME (to the man):	'And how about you?'
HIM:	'Er, well, it's like this, er, if it wasn't for the kids I'd leave her.'

I am still not quite sure why he said this, but I am sure that I had not sorted out the issues in the way I thought I had. Instead, I had managed to create a scene destined to end the relationship. It is very easy to do.

Overview

Helping people to change their sexual behaviour is difficult. Most of the published research on the use of standardised interventions has been very disappointing. Evaluating the available research can be difficult because so few authors provide enough information about their approach to show exactly what it consisted of, let alone to enable it to be replicated. When one reads of a study on 'counselling and testing' one is often left unsure whether the counselling was five minutes of exhortation to adopt safer sex, or something more flexible and complex.

Under the circumstances it is not surprising that it is often not clear whether pre-test and post-test counselling, or being tested at all for that matter, have any impact on sexual behaviour (Higgins *et al.* 1991). Even in studies where there appears to be an effect, it is often rather modest. High rates of new sexually transmitted infections in both seropositives and seronegatives have been reported (Zenilman *et al.* 1992). In many studies it is difficult to separate the impact of being tested from the impact of being counselled.

Few studies of attempts to change sexual behaviour have produced large changes in behaviour, even where the change was sufficient to be statistically significant, and many of these have used individuals at relatively modest risk (Kotloff *et al.* 1991; Wenger *et al.* 1991; Cohen *et al.* 1992a,b; Mansfield *et al.* 1993; Turner *et al.* 1993). It is noticeable that most studies which have found an effect have actively involved the patient in the change process, through role-play or discussion (Winter & Goldy 1993). Few studies relying on the counsellor simply telling patients 'the facts' have made any impact on behaviour at all.

Many testing centres provide much worse counselling for seronegatives than for seropositives, seeing the latter as their priority. There is little doubt that this is a grave error. Most clinics have far more negatives than positives at high risk and there is worrying evidence that individuals who get a negative test result may actually increase their level of risk in the period after the test (Otten *et al.* 1993). Certainly, many will fail to reduce their risk (Dawson *et al.* 1991).

Undoubtedly much counselling aimed at changing sexual behaviour is doomed from the start. It sets out with a particular reason why people cannot implement safer sex: perhaps they are ignorant of the facts, or they do not know how to use a condom, or they need to understand how to eroticise safer sex, or they do not have the skills to negotiate condom usage, or they have a belief in their own invulnerability. Any or all of these might be true in a particular case, but a hundred patients might come up with a hundred different reasons why they are not able to implement safer sex. Starting out with a narrow, formulaic package of change is only likely to help some people. Those whose needs are not met by that package are unlikely to change. It is for that reason that this chapter puts forward a model which is based on first finding out why a particular individual is not adopting safer sex, and then trying to build up individual solutions aimed at that particular person.

We are all seized from time to time by strange enthusiasms, whether it be some new method of eroticising safer sex, or training people in safer sex negotiating skills or of looking at interactions. These are important. They give ideas about solutions in particular cases and they add to the armamentarium of the counsellor. However, it is rare for one of these stock solutions to provide a complete answer in any particular case, and most are applicable to a minority of cases. Slick off-the-shelf solutions can serve to distract from the steady careful work needed to help an individual to change. If counsellors know how they are going to deal with a particular case before they have heard what the patient's problems are, then they are probably going wrong somewhere.

Finally, it is worth reiterating the crucial point. It is usually difficult for people to change their sexual behaviour. They are hardly likely to seek the help of a counsellor to achieve something which they can easily achieve on their own.

References

Allen, S., Serufilira, A., Bogaerts, J., Van de Perre, P., Nsengumuremyi, F., Lindan, C., Carael, M., Wolf, W., Coates, T. & Hulley, S. (1992) Confidential HIV testing and condom promotion in Africa, impact on HIV and gonorrhoea rates. *Journal of American Medical Association*, **268**, 3338–43.

Church, J., Green, J., Vearnals, S. & Keogh, P. (1993) Investigation of motivational and behavioural factors influencing men who have sex with other men in public toilets (cottaging). *AIDS Care*, 68, 347–8.

Cohen, D.A., Dent, C., MacKinnon, D. & Hahn, G. (1992a) Condoms for men, not women. Results of brief promotion programs. *Sexually Transmitted Diseases*, 19, 245–51.

Cohen, D.A., MacKinnon, D.P., Dent, C., Mason, H.R. & Sullivan, E. (1992b) Group counselling at STD clinics to promote use of condoms. *Public Health Reports*, 107, 727–31.

Dawson, J., Fitzpatrick, R., McLean, J., Hart, G. & Boulton, M. (1991) The HIV test and sexual behaviour in a sample of homosexually active men. *Social Science and Medicine*, 32, 683–8.

Higgins, D.L., Galovotti, C., O'Reilly, K.R., Schnell, D.J., Moore, M. & Rugg, D.J. (1991) Evidence for the effects of HIV antibody counselling and testing on risk behaviours. *Journal of the American Medical Association*, 266, 2419–24.

Kotloff, K.L., Tacket, C.O., Wasserman, S.S., Bridwell, M.W., Cowan, J.E., Clemens, J.D., Brothers, T.A., O'Donnell, S.A. & Quinn, T.C. (1991) A voluntary serosurvey and behavioral risk assessment for human immunodeficiency virus infection among college students. *Sexually Transmitted Diseases*, 18, 223–7.

Laumann, E.O., Gagnon, J.H., Michael, R.T. & Michaels, S. (1994) *The Social Organisation of Sexuality*. University of Chicago Press, Chicago.

Mansfield, C.J., Conroy, M.E., Emans, S.J. & Woods, E.R. (1993) A pilot study of AIDS education and counselling of high-risk adolescents in an office setting. *Journal of Adolescent Health*, 14, 115–9.

McCusker, J., Stoddard, A.M., Zapka, J.G. & Zorn, M. (1993) Use of condoms by heterosexually active drug abusers before and after AIDS education. *Sexually Transmitted Diseases*, 20, 81–8.

Otten, M.W. Jr, Zaidi, A.A., Wroten, J.E., Witte, J.J. & Peterman, T.A. (1993) Changes in sexually transmitted disease rates after HIV testing and post-test counselling, Miami, 1988–1989. *American Journal of Public Health*, 83, 529–33.

Turner, J.C., Korpita, E., Mohn, L.A. & Hill, W.B. (1993) Reduction in sexual risk behaviours among college students following a comprehensive health education intervention. *Journal of American College Health*, 41, 187–93.

Turner, J.C., Garrison, C.Z., Korpita, E., Waller, J., Addy, C., Hill, W.R. & Mohn, L.A. (1994) Promoting responsible sexual behaviour through a college freshman seminar. *AIDS Education and Prevention*, 6, 266–77.

Wellings, K., Field, J., Johnson, A. & Wadsworth, J. (1994) *Sexual Behaviour in Britain*. Penguin Books, Harmondsworth.

Wenger, N.S., Linn, L.S., Epstein, M. & Shapiro, M.F. (1991) Reduction of high-risk sexual behaviour among heterosexuals undergoing HIV antibody testing: a randomised clinical trial. *American Journal of Public Health*, 81, 1580–5.

Winter, L. & Goldy, A.S. (1993) Effects of prebehavioural cognitive work on adolescents' acceptance of condoms. *Health Psychology*, 12, 308–12.

Zenilman, J.M., Erickson, B., Fox, R., Reichart, C.A. & Hook, E.W. (1992) Effect of HIV post-test counselling on STD incidence. *Journal of the American Medical Association*, 267, 843–5.

Chapter 16

The Role of General Practitioners in HIV and AIDS

Christine Ford and Elizabeth Murray

Introduction

General practitioners can play a central part in the care and management of people with HIV infection. Indeed, GPs have a role at all stages: prevention, testing, early diagnosis, management of asymptomatic and symptomatic patients, and finally, in terminal care and bereavement counselling. The GP will often also be looking after the relatives and carers of a person with HIV infection, and can help them to come to terms with their feelings through counselling.

GPs have extensive experience in the management of chronic relapsing conditions (Pereira Gray 1994). HIV infection, although relatively new, shares many of the features of other chronic illnesses, and therefore GPs are well placed to look after HIV-positive patients. Moreover, education about prevention of HIV infection can be integrated into more general health education and health promotion.

Prevention

General practice has changed over the past few years, having acquired an increased role in health promotion and disease prevention. The main areas where preventative work can be done with patients are:

(1) Opportunistic intervention
(2) Consultations about contraception
(3) New patient health checks
(4) Travel advice
(5) Drug users.

Opportunistic Intervention

Every day most GPs see between 30 and 50 people. The rest of the primary health care team can easily see double this number. Every one of these contacts can be used as a vehicle for health education, with sexual health promotion and HIV prevention high on the list of issues discussed.

Consultations about contraception

Discussion about sexual health including prevention of HIV and other sexually transmitted diseases can be part of the contraceptive consultation. Every woman who is seeking post-coital contraception has by definition put herself at risk and this needs to be explored. The number of heterosexual women contracting HIV infection in industrialised countries is increasing (Lepri *et al.* 1994).

> Jane, aged 24 years, presented as a new patient complaining of severe recurrent thrush. She was in a stable two year relationship and did not see herself at risk of HIV infection. After counselling around the issues of HIV infection by the GP, she decided to have an HIV test, which came back positive. After the first consultation she had discussed the problem with her partner and discovered that he had used IV drugs several years before they had met. She had sought advice and contraception before starting this relationship but had decided on the pill.

New patient health checks

Under the 1991 GP contract (DoH 1989), GPs are obliged to offer all new patients a health check. HIV prevention can be approached at these checks with all patients, men and women, gay and straight.

Travel advice

Patients travelling abroad who attend for vaccinations are an important group to target for advice and counselling around HIV infection. Condoms may need to be part of the travel package.

> Mohammed aged 42 years lived in London but had business interests in India which took him there about four times a year. He was happily married with two children but tended to use prostitutes when on his trips to India. He was reluctant to see himself at risk and failed to use condoms on several occasions. He presented to the practice with AIDS related tuberculosis, unaware of his HIV status.

Drug users

More drug-users are being managed in general practice. This can be successful with the right training and support (Cohen *et al.* 1992). Safer drug use should be explored with all drug users, regular and occasional. Sources of clean needles and syringes require discussion. Directions to the local needle exchange can be given and information about pharmacy schemes needs to be available. GPs can provide clean needles and syringes if they feel comfortable about this or if there are no local schemes available (HMSO 1991). Many regular drug users have taken on board the message about not sharing but can only act on this if the equipment is available (Ronald *et al.* 1992). The tendency to share appears common among people who would not define themselves as drug users, e.g. users of drugs at weekends or parties.

> Chris aged 21, had recently arrived in London from Dublin to further his studies. When he had an HIV test before starting a new relationship he was shattered to find he was positive. He had only experimented with drugs and did not see himself as a drug-user.

To test or not to test

Patients will come to their GP to discuss the possibility of having an HIV test. If the doctor knows the patient quite well, and has some prior knowledge of the patient's background, they can ensure that the pre-test counselling is targeted to the patient. Areas that need to be covered in pre-test counselling include: Why does the patient want a test? Why now? What risks has the patient taken and what will they do in future to avoid further risk? Does the person understand what an HIV-antibody test is (not an AIDS test), and about the window period (time between infection and production of the antibodies detected in the test, usually about three months)? Where do they want to be tested (in general practice, at a genito-urinary medicine (GUM) clinic, or other)? How and when will they obtain their result, and will the result be filed in their notes or not? GPs often have to fill in health insurance or personal health forms which ask about risk factors for HIV. Who will the patient tell about having the test? Is there anyone they want the doctor to inform, e.g. hospital consultant? How will they cope if the result is positive? Do they want to bring a friend with them when they come for their results? (Chapter 3.)

Some GPs will feel that these areas are better dealt with by a specialist HIV counsellor working in general practice or by the local genito-urinary medicine clinic, while others will want to do the counselling themselves. However, any consultation in general practice about HIV testing is an opportunity to discuss risk-taking behaviour and its future modification.

After the test

A negative test result is an opportunity for the patient to take stock of their life, and decide how they are going to remain seronegative. This is often a watershed time in people's lives, and sympathetic counselling when giving a negative result can help patients make major lifestyle changes. The GP must also be prepared for a negative result to cause strong emotional feelings; the relief can often make patients break down and cry.

Patients who have received a positive result are often shocked despite knowing that they had put themselves at risk or despite preparation for a possible positive test result at pre-test counselling. Receiving a positive result follows the course of any other bereavement reaction. Patients go through the stages of shock, denial, grief and acceptance described by Elizabeth Kubler-Ross (1970). Understanding the grieving process enables the GP to realise when the normal grieving process develops into a clinical depression. Patients may well become clinically depressed after a positive HIV test, and this depression needs active treatment (RCGP 1995) (Chapter 12 and Chapter 22).

Peter, aged 58, was made redundant at the same time as learning he was HIV-positive. He had been infected by his boyfriend, who was diagnosed at the same time. His boyfriend ended the relationship at this point and became extremely angry. Part of his anger was expressed with violence towards Peter, which Peter found extremely shocking. Peter had a severe reactive depression which responded to treatment and counselling by his GP.

Early diagnosis

Patients may present to their GP with a seroconversion illness. This is seldom diagnosed partly because it is non-specific and partly because it may not be considered in a differential diagnosis of a flu-like illness. As GPs become more familiar with the condition, more patients may be diagnosed at this stage of the illness. The seroconversion illness can take the form of a glandular fever like illness with fever, malaise, myalgia, arthralgia, sore throat, erythematous rash and lymphadenopathy. It may occur up to six weeks after contact with an infected person and the HIV antibody test can remain negative for up to 12 weeks after this illness.

Monitoring the seropositive patient

As the number of positive patients increases, the specialised clinics may find it harder to provide the total care that they do now. GPs may find themselves providing more of the routine care of HIV-positive patients. Routine care of an asymptomatic HIV-positive patient is no harder than the routine care of a stable diabetic. Initially, GPs need support and education to enable them to develop confidence and competence in caring for HIV-positive patients, but we believe they will eventually be the major providers of medical care for people with asymptomatic and early symptomatic HIV disease. A routine check should include screening questions as to the patient's physical and psychological wellbeing, followed by an examination of the mouth, skin, and lymphatic system. Weight should be recorded regularly, along with CD4+ and full blood counts. Other investigations can be done as required.

This regular monitoring of the patient allows a therapeutic relationship to develop which in turn enables the doctor to counsel the patient sympathetically when problems arise. Patients will often discuss with their GP whether to accept prophylactic therapy or new treatments.

The GP as a point of first contact

Any intercurrent illness can be alarming for an HIV-positive patient (and often for the doctor too!). The GP needs to be readily accessible to the patient, since the GP may be easier to contact than the specialist clinic. Moreover, the GP will usually be able to distinguish between trivial, self-limiting conditions, those that can be managed at home, and those that need a specialist opinion.

Everyone is frightened of missing PCP, but patients with a dry cough may be brought back for review with the local HIV team.

John, aged 23 and gay, was diagnosed HIV-positive in 1991. He developed a high temperature with a sore throat and became unwell. His GP discussed treatment options with
him and decided to treat him at home with penicillin. A throat swab confirmed strepto-
coccal sore throat and after 48 hours he was much better. Unfortunately he developed an
allergic rash which needed anti-histamines and a change of antibiotics. This entire episode
was dealt with in general practice and John was glad he had avoided a hospital admission.

HIV-positive drug users (especially if they are already seeing their GP about their drug
problem) often prefer to see their GP than attend a hospital if they become unwell.
Sometimes their presentations can be further complicated by withdrawal symptoms.

David, aged 29 and an IVDU, had been HIV-positive since 1982. He developed a dry
cough, associated with fever and night sweats. He had not had an AIDS diagnosis, smoked
20 plus a day and drank heavily. He was on maintenance methadone and injected heroin
twice a week. His GP thought he had pneumonia and treated him with antibiotics. He did
not respond but did not want to go to hospital. Then Jill, his girlfriend, discovered that the
'friend' who had been collecting his methadone had been taking part of it himself. As soon
as Jill collected the methadone herself and gave it all to David he rapidly improved.

Continuity of care

Inevitably hospital clinics are largely staffed by junior doctors, who may move on to other
jobs. This can interrupt continuity of care, particularly as HIV-positive patients need care
over many years. The GP is in a good position to develop a long-term therapeutic relationship with patients. The GP can help patients by giving information about different
treatments and allowing them to talk through the options available. This includes discussions
of alternative treatments and even, on occasion, the option of no treatment. It can be harder
to do this in hospital practice with its emphasis on high-tech, curative medicine and the need
to enrol patients into the various research trials in progress.

Robert, aged 32, had an AIDS diagnosis in 1992. He felt pressured to continue on the trial
of a new drug he had started and even more so when he developed oesophageal candidiasis. However he was keen to try homoeopathic treatment and to take back responsibility
for his illness. Following counselling by his GP he decided to leave the trial and begin a
complementary treatment. Fortunately he improved and recovered from this episode of
illness.

Other support

GPs can be an important source of practical information about sickness benefits and other
allowances. GPs often have good links with the local social services and the voluntary sector.
They can also provide support with applications for disability allowances and provide
medical evidence to assist with re-housing.

Ann was a 30-year-old single parent with asymptomatic HIV disease; her two children were aged 7 and 9. The GP directed her to the local social services who provided a foster family to take the children when Ann was ill. She also got support from two local voluntary agencies who provided a buddy for her and a woman who took the children on outings. These trips were enjoyed by the children and allowed Ann some time for herself.

Care of patients with advanced disease

If the GP has formed a good relationship with the patient over the years, the GP is in a good position to provide counselling when a new illness or problem arises. The GP can encourage a patient to use various prophylactic treatments (e.g. thrice weekly cotrimoxazole to prevent PCP). Most parameters can be monitored in general practice, and arrangements made for repeat prescriptions. If it becomes necessary the GP can arrange admission to an acute ward or respite or hospice care. This is a stressful time for partners, friends and family of the patient, and sympathetic counselling from the GP can be extremely helpful. The GP's knowledge of the situation can also illuminate consultations which might otherwise be perplexing.

Terminal care

Most GPs have a wealth of experience in terminal care (Seamark *et al.* 1995), and the principles of caring for someone dying with AIDS are the same as for patients dying of any other condition. These include symptom control, teamwork and respect for patient auton-omy: patients should be offered a choice as to where to die (home, hospice, hospital); choices made may well change as the illness progresses. The decision when to change from active treatment to palliative care can be quite difficult. Good control of symptoms is vital at this time and must always be done with the total involvement of the patient.

Respite care can be arranged if desired by the patient and the carers. There are often many people involved with the patient at this point, e.g. partner, family, home support team, and buddies, so everyone involved must be clear as to their roles and responsibilities. It is important that the patient and carers understand the out-of-hours cover arrangements for the GP. GPs who use a co-op or deputising service may wish to be called personally for named patients. Getting this terminal care period right is vital for all concerned and the result can be very rewarding, not only for the patient, their family and loved ones but also for the doctor.

Matthew, aged 24 and a Ugandan refugee, was dying at home from late stage HIV disease. He had wasting and diarrhoea although he was not in pain. He was very clear through his last weeks that he wanted to die at home and wanted no further active management. This became increasingly difficult for his family and friends, and the GP became a source of support for them all.

Bereavement counselling – life after death

There are numerous practical issues to be dealt with after death and these can be bewildering for the bereaved carers. It is helpful if someone has sat down with the carers prior to death and discussed these issues. Written material can be left with the household, such as the leaflet *What to do after a death* (DSS 1990). Often patients will have strong views about the type of funeral they wish to have, but people are sometimes shy about discussing it. The GP may be able to help overcome these barriers, which can often be a great relief for patient and carers alike. It is also comforting for the carers to know after the death that they are fulfilling the wishes of the patient.

Once the patient has died a doctor needs to certify that life is extinct and then issue a death certificate. Doing this promptly and efficiently helps those left behind. Some undertakers are wary of handling an HIV infected body so it can be useful to identify a sympathetic firm in advance.

Partners, family and friends are often devastated by the death and are often so bewildered and busy in the immediate aftermath that practical support is often more helpful than counselling. The true grieving process may not start until later, when the GP will be able to monitor and counsel as necessary. Extra bereavement counselling should be available if necessary. It is important to note that the bereavement process may be complicated for those who are themselves HIV positive.

Factors precluding GP involvement

So far we have explained the many possibilities for GP involvement in HIV care. However, the reality does not match the ideal (Grun & Murray 1995). In the next section we look at the barriers to GP involvement and suggest some strategies for overcoming them. These can be divided into three areas:

(1)   Patient factors;
(2)   Hospital factors;
(3)   GP factors.

Patient factors

Gay men, like many young men, may often not be registered or are low users of general practice, but high users of other services such as GUM clinic. Until recently these men have continued to use the service they know and feel happy with. Many are now keen to be cared for in general practice and strategies need to be set up to facilitate this.

One problem is a perceived lack of confidentiality. This can be overcome by surgeries introducing a written policy on confidentiality, including a 'confidentiality statement' in the practice leaflet, and providing specific training for *all* the staff in primary care. During our staff training on confidentiality we found the weakest link to be the doctors, not the usually blamed reception staff!

Hospital factors

When HIV infection first emerged it was seen as new, different and difficult to manage. Specialist clinics saw large numbers of patients and hence were quick to develop expertise in management of clinical problems. Specialist services are also able to monitor the patient and offer instant access to investigative procedures. They can also offer access to new treatments via drug trials.

However, the steepest part of the learning curve is now over, and the management of many of the common problems that arise in HIV are now well documented. It may be argued that just as the management of hypertension or non-insulin-dependent diabetes has largely moved from hospital out-patient departments to GP surgeries, much of the routine care of HIV could be handled in general practice.

GP factors

Many GPs lack confidence in caring for HIV-positive patients. This is partly because it is a fairly new illness and many GPs feel that it requires specialist hospital attention, and partly due to the GPs' real fear of missing a life-threatening complication such as PCP. These fears are gradually being overcome as GPs gain experience in caring for HIV-positive patients. Specific training in HIV for GPs has gone a long way in persuading them that they have the necessary skills and knowledge to manage many of the problems that arise in patients with HIV.

Some GPs are reluctant to care for drug-using patients, seeing them as unreliable, demanding and responsible for their own problems. This stereotype is far from the truth for the majority of drug-users. A trusting, open relationship between doctor and patient can be developed with time. A wide range of treatment options can be offered, from a swiftly reducing dose of methadone to help someone with a short term heroin habit, to offering stabilisation on an opiate substitute. Although it is preferable to stabilise someone on an oral drug, the patient must be allowed to make the choice. Stabilisation on injectables with clean needles can be infinitely better than a reducing dose of oral drug supplemented by dirty street drugs with possible sharing of equipment.

As we move into the 'second wave' of the epidemic, more women and children will be affected. Women traditionally use their GPs more than men. Women who are HIV positive may wish to continue to see their GP if given the choice.

> Marian, aged 29, had recently arrived from Uganda. She presented at the surgery feeling unwell, with a temperature and rigors. Bloods confirmed malaria from which she recovered well. The issue of HIV was brought up by the GP after her recovery. Following counselling Marian had an HIV test which proved positive. Since then her illness has been managed by the local hospital and her GP.

The future

Fortunately many of these barriers to care in the community are being tackled and perceptions are changing.

Training schemes and educational literature have enabled GPs to become more informed and competent. Some surgeries are employing HIV counsellors on a sessional basis; they can see anyone from the 'worried well' to the terminally ill. Closer links with the local community drug team and the GP are improving care of drug-using patients in private practice. HIV clinics are realising that GPs are central to the patient's care and are beginning to improve communication and actively encourage the patients to become registered with a GP. Some formal shared care schemes are being tested. These work by good prompt communication between the hospital and the GP. However, shared care can also work in a less structured format via personal contacts or simple telephone communication.

HIV positive patients are also changing and many are developing closer relationships with their GPs. This is especially true of women and their children.

Ann, 26 years old, had been HIV-positive for two years. She had one child who was three years old and HIV-negative. Ann had moved into the area 18 months before and had used the surgery frequently, developing a close relationship with the GP over time. Ann presented requesting a pregnancy test, which was positive. The GP was able to counsel Ann around the issues of the pregnancy, its effects if any on her health, her feeling about the pregnancy and any doubts she may have had about continuing with the pregnancy. Ann decided to continue with the pregnancy and her ante-natal care was managed in general practice with good support from the obstetric team and the infectious disease team at the hospital. Following the birth the baby continues to be monitored at the baby clinic in the general practice, with support when necessary from the paediatricians.

Overview

As in any other chronic illness, the role of the GP is central to the care of the patient. The GP needs to be actively involved in prevention work with all patients, and alert to the possibility of HIV infection, achieving early diagnosis wherever possible. The GP can provide medical care and supportive counselling for the patients and their carers, lovers, family and friends.

References

Cohen, J., Schamroth, A. & Nazareth, I. (1992) Problem drug use in a Central London General Practice. *British Medical Journal*, **304**, 1158–60.

DoH (1989) *General Practice in the National Health Service: A New Contract*. HMSO, London.

DSS (1990) *What to do after a death*. Leaflet D49. Department of Social Security.

Grun, L. & Murray, E. (1995) Acceptability of shared care for asymptomatic HIV-positive patients. *Family Practice*, **12**, 299–302.

HMSO (1991) *Drug Misuse and Dependence: Guidelines on Clinical Management*. Report of the Medical Working Group on Drug Misuse. HMSO, London.

Kubler-Ross, E. (1970) *On Death and Dying*. Tavistock, London.

Lepri, A.C., Pezzotti, P., Dorrucci, M., Phillips, A.N. & Rezza, G. and the Italian Seroconversion Study (1994). HIV disease progression in 854 women and men infected through injecting drug use and heterosexual sex and followed up for up to nine years from seroconversion. *British Medical Journal*, **309**, 1537–42.

Lloyd, M. (1994) Disease prevention and health promotion in practice. *The Trainee's Companion to General Practice* (eds J. Rosenthal, J. Naish, M. Lloyd). Churchill Livingstone, Edinburgh.

Pereira Gray, D. (1994) *Shared Care for Diabetes: A Systematic Review*. Editor's preface. Occasional Paper 67. Royal College of General Practitioners.

RCGP (1995) *Defeat Depression: Depression from Recognition to Management*. Royal College of General Practitioners and Royal College of Psychiatrists, London.

Ronald, P.J.M., Robertson, J.R. & Roberts, J.J.K. (1992). Risk taking behaviour on the decline in intravenous drug users. *British Medical Journal*, 87, 115–6.

Seamark, D.A., Thorne, C.P., Lawrence, C. & Gray, D.J. (1995) Appropriate place of death for cancer patients: views of general practitioners and hospital doctors. *British Journal of General Practice*, 45, 359–63.

Chapter 17

Legal Aspects

Diana Kloss

There is very little legislation about medical problems in the UK; it is the common law as enunciated by the judiciary which determines the legality of most forms of medical intervention. This has long term advantages since it means that the law can be developed in the context of changing social mores, but it makes it very difficult in the short term for a lawyer to advise a medical practitioner exactly where the boundaries are set. However the reader should be aware of two important trends in the courts.

The first is the judicial awareness of the dangers of defensive medicine as practised in the USA, and a clear resolve that our law shall be steered away from the worst aspects of the system. English judges are clearly determined that health care professionals should be liable in the courts only for failures of care which members of their own profession would also condemn. The standard is that of the reasonable member of the relevant profession, as explained by an expert in that speciality.

The second trend is an underlying realisation that advances in medical science have created a new world which demands that the common law develops realistic responses to the new state of affairs, as in the prosecution of a man accused of murder whose main defence was that it was not he who had killed the victim, but rather the doctor who had switched off the life-support machine on which the victim had been placed after the attack (*R.* v. *Malcherek*). The court rejected the defence, holding that the victim had 'died' before the machine was switched off.

It is necessary to make these preliminary points, because the spread of HIV has given rise to many legal problems about which there has been no time for the courts to give specific guidance. What follows is an attempt to give answers in the context of what has gone before, and taking into account recent judicial attitudes. It may be that future governments will decide that legislation is necessary to supplement the common law, but so far the attitude of the UK government has been to concentrate on information, counselling and research, rather than the introduction of statutory regulation. United Kingdom policy has also been influenced by discussions on an international level, in particular through membership of the European Union.

The criminal law

Suppose someone is told they are HIV positive. Embittered by this news, they decide to revenge themselves on humanity by having unprotected sexual intercourse with as many partners as possible, hoping that they will thereby infect others with the virus. They are successful in infecting five other people, and within five years one of these has died. Is the person guilty of any crime? (The case of a Birmingham man reported to have infected several sexual partners led to a call from some quarters to enact legislation in this area.)

In 1888 Charles Clarence was charged with unlawfully and maliciously inflicting grievous bodily harm on his wife contrary to s.20 Offences Against the Person Act 1861, or in the alternative, assaulting her occasioning actual bodily harm, contrary to s.47 of the same statute. The accused knew that he was suffering from gonorrhoea. His wife did not know, and if she had known would not have consented to the sexual intercourse which infected her with the disease. On appeal, the accused's conviction was quashed, by a majority of nine judges to four (*R. v. Clarence*). The main justification given by the court for their decision was that both the offences charged required that the act of the defendant constituted a battery in law. A battery is any touching of another without that other's consent. Mrs Clarence had consented to have intercourse with her husband and thus the basic element of the crime was absent.

The main argument of those who dissented was that Mrs Clarence only consented to intercourse because she thought that her husband was free of disease; this was false, so her consent had been obtained by a fraudulent misrepresentation and was therefore no consent. A battery had been committed.

The reason for rejecting this argument was that Mrs Clarence was not deceived as to the nature of the act of intercourse, merely as to its consequences. If, as in *R* v. *Williams*, she had been totally ignorant of sexual matters and had believed that intercourse was a form of medical treatment administered by her singing master to improve her voice, her apparent consent would have been void, but this was not the case. In the view of Mr Justice Stephen, the only cases in which fraud indisputably vitiates consent in these matters are cases of fraud as to the nature of the act done.

However, the legal position is not as clear-cut as this for the following reasons:

(1) Subsequent courts have held that the offence of inflicting grievous bodily harm contrary to s.20 does not necessarily require proof of a battery; you can inflict harm without touching someone, as in the case of the defendant who so terrified his wife that she jumped out of a window to escape him and broke her leg (*R. v. Halliday*; *R. v. Wilson*). These developments may throw doubt on the authority of *R. v. Clarence*.

(2) In recent case law it has been held that no one can give a valid consent to actual bodily harm, e.g. sadistic sexual practices (*R. v. Brown*).

(3) There are other possible criminal offences with which a defendant might be charged. In the case where the person infected develops AIDS and dies, it would be virtually impossible to convict the infecting agent of murder or manslaughter, for apart from the difficulty of proving that the infection was transmitted by the defendant and not from some other source, at common law death must ensue within a year and a day for an unlawful homicide to be committed.

A prosecution under s.18 Offences Against the Person Act 1861 for unlawfully and maliciously causing grievous bodily harm would require proof that the defendant had intercourse deliberately intending to expose another to the risk of disease, and thereby infected his victim.

Yet another possibility is a prosecution under s.23 Offences Against the Person Act 1861 (Fortim & Wauchope 1987; S.H. Bronitt [1994]). The law is different in Scotland (*Khaliq* v. *H.M.A.*). It is an offence unlawfully and maliciously to administer 'any poison or other destructive or noxious thing'. (Liability under this section was not discussed in the case of *Clarence*.) Is HIV a 'noxious thing' within the meaning of the section? Again, it would be difficult to prove beyond reasonable doubt either that the infection of the victim had been caused by the defendant or that the defendant either intended to bring about that result or recklessly had unprotected intercourse knowing that their partner might become infected with the virus (*R.* v. *Cunningham*). Will the publicity given to the HIV threat perhaps influence the judiciary in the direction of imposing criminal liability on those who delib-erately threaten the lives of others? As Mr Justice Hawkins, one of the dissenting judges in *Clarence*, said: 'I can picture to myself a state of things in which a kiss or shake of the hand given by a diseased person, maliciously and with a view to communicate his disorder, might well form the subject of criminal proceedings'. This is already the law in Scotland. In 1994 Dr Gaud, who had practised surgery knowing that he was a carrier of hepatitis B, was convicted of the offence of public nuisance in that he endangered the health of the public. He was imprisoned and struck off the medical register. A similar prosecution might be brought against someone who is HIV positive.

Where the commission of crimes like rape, unlawful sexual intercourse with a girl under 16, or homosexual acts with a man under 18, also carries the risk of infecting the victim with HIV, some judges increased the sentence imposed on convicted criminals, but this has now been discouraged by the Court of Appeal, unless there is evidence that the victim has been infected.

Identification of those infected with HIV

There are basically three groups who need to be able to identify those infected with HIV:

(1)   Public authorities who wish to be able to compile statistics, and possibly controls like the refusal of entry to the UK.
(2)   Individuals who fear that they are infected.
(3)   Individuals who wish to avoid contact with an HIV infected person.

There is no power in English law, even in a judge in a court of law, forcibly to compel any person to give a sample of blood, semen, saliva, urine or other intimate samples. Even where an individual is suspected of a serious crime he may refuse to give a sample, although his refusal may then be admissible against him as evidence of guilt (s.62(10) Police and Criminal Evidence Act 1984; a non-intimate sample, e.g. hair, may be taken without consent. In civil cases, no court has power to order adults to undergo a blood test (*W* v. *W*). A statutory exception is a case where the paternity of a child is in dispute (Family Law Reform Act 1969). But, although there may be no power to insist that any person undergo a blood test, it may be possible for an individual to be faced with an 'either–or' situation; for example,

'Either you submit to a blood test or you don't get the job'. Such an ultimatum may be held unlawful under the anti-discrimination legislation.

There are no laws in the UK which prohibit discrimination against homosexuals of either sex, but there are laws which make discrimination on grounds of sex or race unlawful (Sex Discrimination Acts 1975 and 1986 and Race Relations Act 1976). If it can be shown that in practice most people infected with HIV at the present time are male, the exclusion of those infected with HIV from employment is an act of indirect discrimination against men and therefore unlawful, unless the employer can show that the exclusion is 'justifiable' because the nature of the employment is such that those infected with HIV would constitute a risk to the public or other employees. Since this is rarely the case, the demand for blood tests from prospective employees with the purpose of excluding those infected with HIV is probably unlawful at present.

The Equal Opportunities Commission was able to persuade the airline Dan Air that its policy of excluding male cabin staff was unlawful sex discrimination and must be abandoned; the attempt to justify the exclusion on the ground that those applying for jobs as male cabin staff were more likely to be homosexual men infected with HIV was not legal justification for the policy, since even if it were true they would not constitute any health risk to passengers (Napier 1989). On the other hand, British Airways' policy of testing applicants for jobs as pilots for HIV may be upheld if it can be demonstrated that there is a potential risk of associated brain disease which may create a hazard to the safety of aircraft and passengers.

The Disability Discrimination Act 1995, which came into force in 1996, includes those identified as HIV-positive within the category of the disabled. However, the protection of the Act will only be conferred on those suffering from a substantial adverse effect on day-to-day activities. It will be unlawful to discriminate against disabled persons unless it is 'justified', i.e. the disability renders the employee or job applicant substantially less effective in the job.

Controls on immigration have been held to be outside the sex discrimination legislation (*R.* v. *Entry Clearance Officer*) and by definition are exceptions to the Race Relations Act. If the UK Government wished to insist on blood tests as a condition of entry to the UK of persons who have no right of entry, it would be free to do so. Even in the case of nationals of member states within the European Community, it could be argued that the protection of public health justified the imposition of such controls (Article 48 Treaty of Rome, Directive 641221). The European Union has declared that member states should have a policy of non-discrimination against the HIV-positive: COM (90) 601; AVEC Commission [1994] 3 CMLR 242. The European Court, however, interprets such defences narrowly, and a 1964 EC Directive lists diseases justifying refusal of entry, but does not, of course, mention HIV/ AIDS.

Some insurance companies demand evidence that an applicant for life assurance is HIV negative, at least in the case of some applicants like single men over 35 or two young men who jointly apply for a mortgage. Although that is discriminatory against men, it is not contrary to the Sex Discrimination Act because it can be scientifically proven that individuals infected with HIV have a greatly increased risk of premature death, and it is therefore justified on actuarial grounds (s.45 Sex Discrimination Act 1975). The EOC advocated the repeal of this section in a 1986 consultative document called *Legislating for Change?*. Where insurance policies exclude AIDS-related claims, it is difficult to argue convincingly that the insurance companies need this protection. Some insurance companies even rejected an application for life insurance from someone who had had an HIV test, despite the test having been negative. The government pointed out that this practice was against the public interest, since it deterred people from taking a test (HMSO 1990), and the Association of British Insurers eventually issued a statement of practice to the effect that questions should not be asked about negative tests.

If the individual is an adult, conscious and of sound mind, and is told that they are being asked to give a sample of blood for the purpose of testing it for evidence of HIV, either with their name attached or as an anonymous sample, their consent will give complete authority to the medical and nursing staff who carry out the procedure. It is not necessary in law for such consent to be given in writing, but it is always advisable to have written evidence in case disputes subsequently arise.

The courts have frequently emphasised in recent decisions that consent to medical procedures must be 'informed' – i.e. that the patient must be told of the broad nature of the treatment proposed and of any substantial risks involved (*Sidaway* v. *Board of Governors*). The information which must be given is that which a reasonable doctor or nurse would have given to the patient in question; the courts accept that details may be withheld from an exceptionally nervous patient, but should be given to one with a more stoical attitude (*Bolam* v. *Friern*; *Chatterton* v. *Gerson*).

However, all the informed consent cases concern information about the essential nature of the procedure itself, or about the likely risks or probable outcome of treatment, not about what is to be done with any intimate samples thereby obtained. As with a criminal battery (discussed above), as long as the patient knows of the broad nature of what is to be done and gives a valid consent, no civil liability for battery will arise, even though risks may be concealed from the patient (like a 1% risk of paralysis) which might have led to a refusal of consent had the patient known of them. The patient will be able to sue for damages only if a reasonable member of the medical or nursing profession, following the general practice of the profession, would have given further information. The cause of action will be for negligence, not battery, which means that the patient will have to prove a failure to take reasonable care and that they would have been likely to have refused the treatment had they been properly informed.

If we apply this to a blood test, the consent of an individual to the taking of blood will prevent it from being a battery, even if the patient is unaware that the blood is to be tested for HIV. The patient may be told that it is to be tested for alcohol or drugs or the effects of lead or ionising radiation, or that it is a routine procedure commonly administered. The fact remains that he knows the nature of the process, the taking of a sample of blood, though not the true reason behind it. Unless the courts were willing to invent a new doctrine, there is no action for a civil battery in this type of case. However, if the consent is obtained by fraud – that is the doctor pretended that the test was for one purpose when it was in reality for another – at least one judge has said that the consent will be vitiated.

As to negligence, as there is at present no treatment for HIV disease and as the discovery that an individual is infected with the virus can lead to severe consequences, both financial and emotional, it is probably true that a doctor's duty of care to patients demands that he or she only administers a blood test after warning the patient of the unpleasant consequences if they discover that they are HIV positive. A doctor who knows that the patient is HIV positive may be compelled to disclose that fact to an insurance company at a later date, or if he or she is also the doctor of the patient's spouse, to pass on the information to protect the other patient. Since a test on a patient's blood without the patient's knowledge would exclude the possibility of pre-test counselling, it is possible that it would be negligent not to inform the patient that they were being tested for HIV and to ask for their consent. Even if the doctor did not give the patient the result of the test, the doctor would have knowledge which he or she might later have to disclose to the patient's detriment.

Testing for HIV without the consent of the patient has now been condemned by the General Medical Council (GMC 1995) and the United Kingdom Central Council for Nurses, Midwives and Health Visitors (UKCC 1991) (see also RCS 1990).

The Department of Health is planning to produce guidance on pre-test counselling and this is under discussion at the time of writing by the Expert Advisory Group on AIDS.

The testing of anonymous samples, such that the donor cannot be made aware of the result because the tester does not know his identity, was introduced by the government at the end of 1989. However, the patients are informed of the testing proposed and are asked for their consent. Many ante-natal clinics warn patients that blood taken may be anonymously tested, but assume consent unless specifically notified to the contrary. The Human Fertilisation and Embryology Authority Code of Practice requires that donors of eggs and semen must be tested for HIV, although there is no mandatory requirement to test prospective parents.

Where a patient is unconscious and therefore unable to give or refuse consent, necessary medical procedures may be undertaken without consent. It would be for the medical profession to justify a blood test for HIV as necessary for the patient in the circumstances of the case. The consent of a relative of the unconscious person is not required, nor would it justify the performance of any treatment which was not a real necessity.

Tests may in general only lawfully be performed on children under 16 with the consent of a parent, or if the child under 18 has been made a ward of court, with the consent of the court. If a child under 16 is intelligent and mature enough to understand the nature and implications of the test, they can give consent on their own behalf (*Gillick* v. *W. Norfolk and Wisbech H.A.*).

The mentally ill and adult mentally handicapped can in general only be tested with their consent, as the Mental Health Act 1983 does not cover treatment for physical, as opposed to mental, illness. Recent case law now indicates that there is an exception for procedures imposed for the good of the patient (*F.* v. *W. Berkshire H.A.*) which are reasonably necessary to protect life or health.

Confidentiality

The Hippocratic Oath includes a promise that the doctor will not divulge confidential information about their patient to third parties, but this duty can never be absolute, because sometimes the public interest or the protection of others must take precedence over the rights of the individual. The GMC lists eight circumstances in which confidentiality may be breached, including the sharing of information with other health professionals participating in the care of the patient, disclosure of information by order of a court of law or in pursuance of a statutory requirement, and disclosure in the public interest, for example investigation by the police of a very serious crime or in cases of suspected child abuse.

AIDS is not a notifiable disease under the Public Health (Control of Disease) Act 1984, although certain provisions of that Act have been extended to AIDS by statutory regulation (Public Health (Infectious Diseases) Regs. 1988 (SI 1988/1546). There is at present no obligation on doctors to report cases to the local authority. (The voluntary system of reporting cases without the identification of individuals' details to the Communicable Diseases Surveillance Centre is not a breach of confidence, since the information is anonymous.) A justice of the peace may, on the application of a local authority, make an order for the detention in hospital of an inmate of that hospital suffering from AIDS, or may make an order that an individual with AIDS in the community be detained in hospital. The circumstances must be that proper precautions against the spread of the infection cannot or would not be taken if the patient remained at large. These powers, which relate only to full-blown AIDS, have been used in only one case, in Manchester. The AIDS (Control) Act 1987 obliges health authorities to compile regular statistics of those diagnosed with AIDS and those who have died from the disease. It also requires health authorities to report on facilities and services provided for the treatment, counselling and care of those with HIV disease and AIDS, and on action taken to educate the public about the disease.

There are special regulations relating to sexually transmitted diseases: the NHS (Venereal Diseases) Regulation 1974 SI 1974/29. These provide (Reg. 2) that every health authority shall take all necessary steps to secure that any information capable of identifying an individual, obtained with respect to persons examined or treated for any sexually transmitted disease, shall not be disclosed except for the purpose of communicating the information to a doctor or someone working under his direction in connection with the treatment of persons suffering from the disease or the prevention of its spread. It is assumed that these regulations apply to HIV and AIDS, though arguably neither is in itself a disease, merely a loss of capacity to resist other diseases, and HIV may be transmitted other than through sexual intercourse.

It would seem that a health authority is obliged by the regulations to order STD clinics not to disclose to any person other than the patient's doctor the fact that an individual is HIV positive, even to that person's husband or wife. But the regulations do not control the extent to which the STD clinics may report the situation to the patient's own doctor, nor how far the patient's GP can disclose the information to third parties. If the clinic told a GP that a child of eight was suffering from a disease inflicted on her by her father by means of criminal sexual intercourse (an actual case reported to the author), no law of confidence would prevent the GP revealing the facts to social workers or the police.

If a GP who has both a husband and wife on his or her list is told by the clinic that the husband is HIV positive, should he or she tell the wife? It is probably the law that the doctor's duty to protect the wife's health justifies, indeed obliges him or her to disclose the facts to her, especially as the health of a future child of the couple may also be at risk. Where the GP of the HIV positive patient is not also the doctor of the patient's spouse or sexual partner, there is probably no positive duty in law to make disclosure. But if the GP knows that the patient is sexually active and is ignoring advice to take precautions, it is probably justifiable to break confidence in the general public interest of restricting the spread of the virus (especially if the courts are willing to hold that this kind of conduct by the patient is criminal). The GMC has stated (HIV infection and AIDS: the ethical considerations): 'When a patient is found to be infected ... the doctor must discuss with the patient the question of informing a spouse or other sexual partner. The GMC believes that most such patients will agree to disclose in these circumstances, but where such consent is withheld the doctor may consider it a duty to ensure that any sexual partner is informed in order to safeguard such persons from a possibly fatal infection.'

Medical personnel caring for the patient may be put at risk if precautions are not taken. The same may apply to laboratory workers dealing with blood samples, and domestic staff dealing with soiled clothes or bandages. It is argued that these workers must be told of the condition of the patient so as to be able to protect themselves. Pressure has been brought to bear on managers to make disclosure to all kinds of ancillary staff, like catering and portering staff in hospitals and home helps and meals on wheels helpers in the community, to whom the risk, if any, is small. In consequence, people with AIDS have been subjected to threats and have even had their homes attacked because so many precautions were taken by overzealous health authority employees that the community was alerted to their condition.

It is difficult to find any legal justification for such wide disclosure. Ancillary workers are rarely at risk and could usually be protected by general hygiene precautions which could be applied to all patients, whatever their condition. The ill-informed belief of employees that they are at risk is no justification in law for their employer's breach of confidence, especially when the outcome may be as threatening to the patient and his property as the virus itself.

If a local authority holds a case conference to discuss an AIDS patient, attendance should be confined to those who need to know of the patient's condition because they are giving counselling or medical treatment or because they need to take special precautions. Patients should have the right to decide for themselves whether they wish others to know.

Where an employee wrongly discloses confidential information to a third party, the employer is vicariously liable even if he has given strict instruction that information must be kept a secret. A receptionist who, as in one incident, announced to a crowded surgery, 'Oh my God, it's the man with AIDS', would make both herself and her employer liable to pay damages. Where the fault was all on the employee's side, her employer could both dismiss her and claim reimbursement of any damages paid to the patient (the latter course of action would only be worthwhile where the employee was insured against professional liability – for example, if she was a member of the Royal College of Nursing).

The principles relating to confidentiality and HIV/AIDS were explored in the case of *X* v. *Y* where an employee of a health authority had, in breach of confidence, sold information to a Sunday newspaper about two patients – doctors in general practice who had been diagnosed as HIV positive and were receiving treatment at a clinic under the control of the health authority. The newspaper was threatening to publish the names of the doctors. The health authority asked the court for an injunction restraining publication, in answer to which the newspaper offered to remove the names of the doctors, but proposed to use other parts of the confidential information to discuss the risks to the public of health professionals who are infected and whether they should be barred from practice. It was argued that the public interest justified a breach of the patients' confidence. The judge granted the injunction. He emphasised the overriding importance of confidentiality in limiting the spread of the disease. Patients who feared that details of their condition might be disclosed to others would not seek counselling or treatment. In addition, the risk to patients of contracting HIV from a GP was 'slightly more than negligible'. Maintaining confidentiality made it more likely that the doctor would be under medical supervision and susceptible to advice about reducing the risk of infection even further.

This High Court decision does not preclude the release of confidential information in every case. Where it is known that a health professional who is HIV positive is failing to observe advice about safety precautions, it may be the positive duty of that person's counsellor to inform their superiors in order to protect patients, though selling the story to a Sunday newspaper can never be an advised course of action. Both the GMC and the UKCC advise their members to report to the employer the identify of an HIV positive health care worker who fails to take advice. It is interesting to note that in a few cases the health authority has voluntarily disclosed the HIV status of a doctor to the press, as in the case of a junior surgeon at the Royal Liverpool Hospital in 1992. This could of course be done lawfully only with the consent of the HIV positive surgeon, who is entitled to confidentiality from his employer other than in a very exceptional case where disclosure is necessary in the public interest.

The Royal College of Surgeons recommends that any surgeon who is HIV positive should seek professional advice, which would almost certainly exclude them from further surgical procedures because of the risk of cross infection through the spillage of blood. Comprehensive guidance about dealing with HIV/AIDS infected health care workers was issued by the Department of Health in 1994 (DoH 1994). Guidance was published in 1995 about notifying patients who have been subject to exposure prone procedures performed by an HIV-positive health care worker (DoH 1993).

Cases have arisen of mothers who are HIV positive giving birth to a child and asking for it to be taken for adoption. Such a baby has a 12% to 14% chance of infection (through transmission in the womb), but it is not possible for technical reasons to test the child. The adoption procedure under the Adoption Agencies Regulations 1983 SI 1983/1964 requires the adoption agency (either the local authority or an approved society) to provide a prospective adopter with written information about the child, its personal history and background and its health (Reg. 12). In the course of preadoption investigations, the adoption agency has to enquire into the family history of the mother, including details of any present illness, and any other relevant information (Reg. 7 and Schedule, Part IV). If the mother has been diagnosed as HIV positive it would seem clear that the prospective adopters are entitled to know this, although if the mother refuses to be tested for HIV there is more of a dilemma. Although there is no power to force the mother to undergo a test (the agency must do that which is reasonably practicable to persuade her to do so), the courts would probably hold that the agency was entitled to tell the prospective adopters that the mother was in a high risk group and had refused to be tested, and would probably hold that the agency had a duty to do so, even though it led to the rejection of the child.

The DHSS Circular LAC (84) 3 advises that health information on the natural parents should be sought from a doctor who knows the parents and has access to the relevant records – usually the GP. It states that the prospective adopters must be advised about any health problem. If the placement of a baby direct from hospital is proposed, the medical adviser should ensure that it is carefully explained to the prospective adopters that only preliminary health screening and assessment have so far been possible; the adviser should also ensure that the implications of any particular risk factors are explained. It is essential for the prospective adopters to receive these explanations, so that they can decide whether they wish to go ahead with the placement, and to minimise the possibility of them undertaking more than they feel they can manage.

If the mother's doctor, either her GP or the hospital doctor, knows that she is HIV positive and wants her child adopted, should he or she tell the adoption agency? As the Adoption Agencies Regulations require the agency to obtain medical reports on 'the child and, so far as is reasonably practicable, his natural mother, with the results of any tests carried out during or immediately after pregnancy' (Schedule, Part IV), even a doctor who at the mother's behest refused to disclose medical records would in practice probably prevent the child from going forward for adoption, because the necessary documentation would not be available.

The courts have held that confidence may be broken in the public interest (*Lion Laboratories* v. *Evans*). Unless medical personnel and adoption agencies are able and willing to reveal all the relevant facts, even in breach of the mother's confidence, prospective adopters and foster parents will be deterred from coming forward through fear that they will not be told the whole truth. This cannot be in the public interest or in the long term interest of the child.

Of course the court, which must eventually approve the adoption, has power to order the disclosure of medical records and to order that the child's blood be tested (*S.* v. *S.*), though not that of the mother. Finally, once the adoption is complete, the child becomes the responsibility of its new family who cannot send the child back if it is later diagnosed as HIV positive.

In Re 0 (Minor) (Medical Examination (1993)), Mr Justice Rattee held that magistrates making a care order could require children with both parents HIV positive to be tested for HIV. It has now been ordered that all applications for HIV tests relating to children should come before a High Court judge (Re HIV tests).

The isolation of HIV infected persons

Where a patient has developed AIDS, legal powers exist to confine them compulsorily in hospital if this is necessary to protect others. The Public Health (Infectious Diseases) Regulations 1988 have extended certain provisions of the Public Health (Control of Disease) Act 1984 to AIDS, including the magistrates' power on the application of a local authority to make an order for detention in hospital of a person with AIDS, if that person would not take proper precautions to prevent the spread of disease if allowed to go free.

In 1992 counsellors from South Birmingham Health Authority urged a haemophilic man, who had allegedly infected four women sexual partners with HIV, to adopt more responsible sexual behaviour, but refused to name the man or to apply for his detention in hospital. As the law stands it is likely that the court would have refused to use the Public Health Act to detain such an individual. Only where, for example, the person had open sores carrying a serious risk of infection would the legislation be appropriate. The virtual imprisonment or segregation of asymptomatic HIV positive individuals would be regarded as too great an attack on individual liberty to be authorised without explicit legislation.

If a member of the caring professions discovers that a patient is HIV positive or has AIDS, may he lawfully for that reason refuse to treat him? Where he has already undertaken the care of a patient, as in the case of a GP who has the patient on his list, he will have a duty to take reasonable care of that patient. If the GP fails in his duty by refusing treatment, the patient will be able to sue for damages for negligence if he or she thereby suffers injury. Also, although the NHS regulations governing the doctors' contracts with the Health Authority provide that a doctor may refuse to accept a patient, or may ask for a patient already on his list to be removed, they do not allow him to act unilaterally without following the proper procedures; the Health Authority, which investigates failures by GPs to comply with their terms of service, might take proceedings against him.

If the patient is not registered with a doctor there is no legal obligation to act as a Good Samaritan and come to the aid of a stranger, other than emergency cases arising in the GP's own district.

A hospital doctor or consultant might also be liable for negligence if a patient in the hospital is denied essential treatment because he or she is HIV positive, and thereby suffers injury. The only legal justification for such a refusal is self-defence: that the situation is so dangerous because of a lack of proper precautions that the doctor is being asked to undergo an unreasonable risk. What if a surgeon refuses to perform a non-essential operation like a hip replacement on an HIV positive patient? The patient will suffer extra pain and distress through the surgeon's refusal and would be able to sue for that, but in addition the surgeon's employer, the health authority, could take disciplinary action, and, of course, the GMC might decide that any doctor who refused to treat a patient was guilty of professional misconduct and unfit to be a doctor. (In the case of a nurse, the matter could be reported to the UKCC.) Much would depend in such a case on how the profession as a whole viewed the reasonableness or otherwise of the doctor's conduct. The GMC has warned that it is unethical for a doctor to refuse to treat a patient because of personal risk to the doctor, or moral judgement on the patient's lifestyle.

What about the common situation where an employee is suspected by their employer and fellow employees of being HIV infected? Often workers put pressure on the employer to sack such a person. First, there is no power to force an employee to undergo a blood test or any medical examination, on pain of losing their job if they refuse, unless there is a term in the contract of employment which obliges the employee to submit to such examination. Secondly, if an employee is found to be HIV positive and the employer is informed, it will be unfair dismissal to sack him for that reason unless the employer can show that the presence of the virus or the development of symptoms renders the employee unfit to do the job. It is no defence to a claim for unfair dismissal that the employer was under pressure from other employees, who were either threatening industrial action or actually striking, to dismiss the infected person (s.63 Employment Protection (Consolidation) Act 1978) (DoE 1986).

Where a dismissal is an act of sex or race discrimination, or discriminates against a disabled person the anti-discrimination laws come into play. As has been argued before, inferior treatment given to people with HIV is indirectly discriminatory against men, so that an employer whose policy was to dismiss those who were diagnosed as HIV positive would be acting contrary to the sex discrimination legislation, unless he could prove that for reasons of safety it was necessary to exclude such persons. In addition, the dismissal of an AIDS sufferer who was still competent to do his or her job might be contrary to the Disability Discrimination Act 1995.

Rights and duties of health care workers

Where any person knows or suspects that they may carry a virus which constitutes a danger to others, they are under a duty to take reasonable care to minimise that danger. If they fail to take reasonable care and cause damage, they are liable to compensate anyone who can prove on a balance of reasonable probabilities that they have suffered harm through lack of care. To this extent, both patients and health professionals are governed by the same rules. Patients must take care not to transmit the virus to the health professionals with whom they come into contact, and health professionals must take reasonable care to avoid infecting their patients.

If, for example, a doctor believes that because of his lifestyle he may be infected, he must take all reasonable precautions to protect others against possible infection. The advice of the GMC is that it is unethical for a doctor who knows or suspects that he has AIDS or is HIV positive, to continue working without medical advice. Doctors are instructed to inform health authorities if they suspect a colleague of having the virus but not following advice. The Department of Health has issued guidance on HIV/AIDS infected health care workers (DoH 1994). This recommends that HIV infected health care workers should not perform exposure-prone procedures (procedures where there is a risk that injury to the worker may result in exposure of the patient's open tissues to the blood of the worker). It is likely that the courts would hold that a failure to follow the recommendations of the professional body or the Department of Health was a failure to take reasonable care, giving rise to civil liability in damages. The employer of a negligent professional, usually the health authority, would be vicariously liable to pay any damages, whether or not the health authority had itself been at fault.

The Department of Health guidance recommends that all patients who have undergone exposure-prone procedures, where an infected health care worker was the sole or main operator, should so far as is practicable be notified of this in a 'look-back' study. Guidance has also been issued on the conduct of look-back studies (DoH 1993).

Conversely, the patient who carelessly infects a health professional may be sued. The effectiveness of such a remedy depends, of course, on whether the patient has the finances or insurance to pay compensation. Nonetheless, as has already been discussed, a danger of infection does not justify a refusal to give treatment unless the health professional is being asked to undergo an unreasonable risk without the proper precautionary measures being provided. Though surgeons disagree (Walker 1991), the rules on testing without consent which are set out at the beginning of this chapter apply equally to cases of risks to health professionals as to others.

Health authorities are not vicariously liable for patients. A health professional who contracted the virus in the course of employment would be able to obtain compensation from their employer only on proof that the employer had failed to take reasonable care for the employee's safety, by, for example, failing to provide proper instructions and facilities for the disposal of sharps. HIV, unlike Hepatitis B, is not a prescribed disease under the industrial injuries regulations, although a health care worker who could identify a particular incident through which they had contracted the virus would be able to claim industrial injuries benefits from the Department of Social Security, on the basis of personal injury caused by an accident arising out of and in the course of employment. NHS staff could make a similar claim under the NHS injury benefits scheme.

Though health authorities are not automatically liable for the negligence of patients, they are under a primary duty to take reasonable care for the health and safety of employees while at work. This is a general common law duty, strengthened by statutory regulations – the Control of Substances Hazardous to Health Regulations (COSHH) 1994, made under the Health and Safety at Work Act 1974. Substances hazardous to health include micro-organisms to which a worker is exposed in the course of employment. The employer must assess possible risks and do that which is reasonably practicable to prevent or control exposure. There is a duty to give information and training. Breach of the COSHH Regulations may give rise to a criminal prosecution by the Health and Safety Executive, or a civil action for breach of statutory duty by any person injured by the breach.

A health professional who contracted the virus through employment would have the same job security as if he had contracted it elsewhere; he would be entitled to keep his job unless he constituted an unreasonably high risk to others. In practice, it would be the advice of the relevant professional body which would be examined by the courts to determine such an issue.

The legal obligation of the patient

Once an individual is given the news that they are HIV positive, they are faced with a continuing dilemma to tell or not to tell. If they subsequently wish to take out life assurance they are likely these days to be asked whether they have had a positive blood test. It is pointless to lie, because even if they obtain a policy by suppressing the truth, the contract will not be binding and the insurance company may eventually refuse to pay. Even if the individual is not asked the question, there is a duty in an insurance contract to reveal it. This deters some people in high risk groups from having the blood test; it is financially better to be ignorant.

There is no obligation on an employee to inform their employer that they are HIV positive, nor if they are applying for a new job to reveal the fact to their prospective employer. As a general rule, and subject to the laws against discrimination (see above), an employer choosing employees can ask applicants about their health and refuse to employ them if the answers are unsatisfactory. If an applicant lied in answer to such a question, it has been held that this may justify dismissal when the truth is eventually discovered, but only where the illness or disability actually makes the employee unsuitable to do the job, which is rarely the case with HIV (*O'Brian* v. *Prudential Assurance Co Ltd*).

If a man donates blood to the transfusion service knowing that he is in a high risk group and may be infected, he could in legal theory be sued for negligence if it could be proved that his blood had infected a patient. If he thought that the fact that the blood is tested would exclude infection (where there is a chance that he could be infected but tested negative) that would be a defence unless he had been specifically warned when he gave blood that this was not the case. Identification of the donor would in any event be difficult. In a Scottish case the court refused to order the blood transfusion service to produce records which would have identified an infected donor, in the interest of protecting donor anonymity (*A.B.* v. *Scottish Blood Transfusion Service*).

An individual who has unprotected sexual intercourse or who allows another to use the same drug needle, when they know or have reasonable cause to suspect that they are HIV positive, could be sued for damages for negligence by anyone whom they infect, but in all these cases it would be for the victim to prove that the HIV infection came from that source, which might be difficult if he or she has had several sexual partners.

Compensation for haemophiliacs

People with AIDS who contracted the virus through blood transfusions containing a contaminated supply of Factor VIII purchased by the UK government in the USA, sued the Department of Health alleging negligence. At first the department strenuously resisted these claims but eventually yielded to public pressure and settled the cases out of court. It is likely that the haemophiliacs acted wisely in accepting the out-of-court settlement, since the actions if brought to trial were unlikely to have succeeded. At the time the risks were not fully known and alternative sources of the clotting factor were not available, so that it would have been difficult to prove that the department had acted unreasonably.

Overview

There are many situations in this area of medical and social work practice where the law has yet to be clarified, but counsellors who adhere to the following principles are likely to avoid condemnation in the law courts:

- You have a duty to patients and clients to take reasonable care. If you follow the practice and principles of most of your professional colleagues this will, in law, in the majority of cases constitute reasonable care.
- Your duty to your patients and clients requires that you keep their confidence unless there is a real danger to others, or the public interest demands disclosure.
- It may be a serious disadvantage to an individual to discover that they are HIV positive, because there is no really effective treatment for the condition and the knowledge may prevent them from obtaining insurance and could be passed on by their doctor to their wife. No-one should be tested without their consent, and the possible implications of a positive result should be explained before the consent is obtained. The British Medical Association has received similar legal advice (BMJ 1987). Anonymous testing is probably lawful, whatever the ethical objections may be.

References

A.B. v. *Scottish Blood Transfusion Service. The Independent*, 22 Dec, 1989.
BMJ (1987) *British Medical Journal*, **295**, 911.
Bolem v. *Friern H.M.C.* [1957] 1 WLR 582.
Boyd, K.M. (1992) HIV and AIDS: the ethics of medical confidentiality. *Journal of Medical Ethics*, **18**, 173.
Brazier (1992) *Medicine, Patients and the Law*, 2nd edn. Penguin Books, Harmsworth.

S.H. Bronitt [1994] Crim. L.R. 21.

Chatterton v. *Gerson* [1981] QB 432.

DoE (1986) *AIDS and Employment.* Advisory document. HMSO, London.

DoH (1993) *AIDS/HIV Infected Health Care Workers: Practical Guidance on Notifying Patients.* UK Health Departments.

DoH (1994) *AIDS/HIV Infected Health Care Workers: Guidance on the Management of Infected Health Care Workers.* UK Health Departments.

F. v. *W. Berkshire H.A.* [1990] 2 AC 1.

Fortim & Wauchope (1987) *Law Society's Gazette*, 25 March, p.884.

Gillick v. *W. Norfolk and Wisbech H.A.* [1985] 3 All ER 402.

GMC (1995) *HIV and AIDS*: the ethical considerations. General Medical Council, London.

HMSO (1990) *AIDS and Insurance.* HMSO, London.

Khaliq v. *H.M.A.* 1984 SLT 137.

Lion Laboratories v. *Evans* [1984] 2 All ER 417.

Napier (1989) EOC Formal Investigation Report – Dan-Air, January, 1987. *Industrial Law Journal*, **18**, 84.

O'Brian v. *Prudential Assurance Co Ltd* [1979] 1 RLR 140.

R. v. *Brown* [1993] 2 WLR 556.

R. v. *Clarence* (1988) 22 QBD 23.

R. v. *Cunningham* [1957] 12 QB 396.

R. v. *Entry Clearance Officer*, ex parte *Amin* [1983] 2 All ER 864.

R. v. *Halliday* (1889) 61 LT 701.

R. v. *Malcherek* [1981] 2 All ER 422.

R. v. *Williams* [1923] 1 KB 340.

R. v. *Wilson* [1983] 1 All ER 993.

RCS (1990) *Guidelines AIDS and HIV Infection.* Royal College of Surgeons, London.

Re HIV tests [1994] 2 FLR 116.

Re 0 (Minor) (Medical Examination) [1993] 1 FLR 860.

Sidaway v. *Board of Governors of the Bethlem Royal and the Maudsley Hospital* [1985] 2 WLR 480.

S. v. *S.* [1970] 3 All ER 107.

UKCC (1991) *Statement on AIDS and HIV Infection.* United Kingdom Central Council for Nurses, Midwives and Health Visitors, London.

W. v. *W.* [1963] 2 All ER 841.

Walker A. (1991) Surgeons and HIV. *British Medical Journal*, **302**, 136.

X v. *Y.* [1988] 2 All ER 648.

Chapter 18

Counselling in Developing Countries

John Green

In the years since the first edition of this book was published, there has been a tremendous growth in HIV counselling services in developing countries. The information from published reports on these services has provided a major contribution to our knowledge about the impact of, and constraints on, HIV counselling.

The term 'developing countries' covers a vast range of circumstances. Not only do countries classified as 'developing' differ in terms of income, distribution of wealth and levels of poverty, they also differ in geography, culture and climate. From a health point of view they differ in the levels and types of service available to the population, the percentage of the population with access to health care, and the diseases which are common. Health is not just a matter of the provision of medical services; it is also inextricably linked to adequate nutrition and the provision of a safe water supply.

Because developing countries differ, it is not possible to set out a blueprint for HIV/AIDS counselling services which will fit all countries. Successful programmes in different countries, like TASO in Uganda, the Copperbelt Health Education programme in Zambia or the brothel outreach programme in Belize, have been successful because they have developed to fit local conditions and local needs, building on local strengths. The great failures have been attempts to import wholesale models from the USA or Europe, forgetting that these were themselves built around local conditions in their home countries.

In western countries the model of counselling used is, inevitably, a response to local conditions. It tends to have certain characteristics which can be difficult to apply in most developing countries.

Availability of specialist counsellors

Quite a lot of the counselling in the west tends to be carried out by specialist counsellors, either working full-time with those with HIV/AIDS or working in sexually transmitted disease clinics. Counselling and primary medical care are seldom combined.

Such an arrangement is impossible in many developing countries. There are not sufficient health care staff to make such a model work. A simple calculation shows the problem. A counsellor whose duties go beyond the very simplest pre-test and post-test counselling might, realistically, see 250 cases a year. In a country with three million adults and an annual rate of new infections of 1%, 120 counsellors would be required to see all new cases. With 3% new infections, 360 counsellors would be required working full-time on HIV/AIDS. Of course, not every new infection would turn up, but then the counsellor would be unlikely to see only new infections, and there are partners and seronegatives at risk to deal with. Whatever assumptions one makes in terms of the figures, it is difficult to see most developing countries being able to build a counselling system for HIV/AIDS purely around specialist workers.

In small countries with well-developed health care systems and in large urban areas of other countries, it may be possible to develop a system based around specialist counsellors. In most developing countries it is likely to prove most fruitful if primary care staff are trained in HIV counselling. Any specialist staff may perhaps be used in a training/supervisory/advisory role. In other words, HIV counselling needs to be integrated into other areas of health care.

Geography

Most western countries have well-developed transport systems and most people living in those countries have cars or access to cars. If they do not, they usually have access to affordable public transport. In Europe and most developed parts of south-east Asia most people live in, or within easy reach of, large centres of population. In North America and Australia people may live far from urban centres but they can usually reach them by car, plane or other transport reasonably quickly, and can afford to do so. It therefore makes sense to centralise medical facilities, particularly specialist ones. Patients come to the medical services; medical services do not have to go to them.

The situation in many developing countries is quite different. Roads are poor, large numbers of individuals live in rural areas, public transport is poor, ambulance services are minimal if available at all, and few people have access to cars. Even five miles across rough terrain on foot to reach a hospital can be too far, particularly if one is sick. The nearest medical facility may be much further away than that. Under these circumstances the health services have to go to the patient, rather than the patient to the health services, at least until the patient becomes too sick to manage locally. It therefore follows that training staff who work locally in dispensaries, polyclinics and health centres, or in the community, to provide HIV/AIDS counselling is more likely to prove successful than trying to set up a centralised counselling centre.

In urban areas, of course, the situation may be different again. Central hospitals are likely to be more accessible and it may be easier to centralise resources. Some developing countries are geographically small or do have workable transport systems, but in most cases that is not so.

Risk identification

In most western countries the people most likely to be infected with HIV are likely to be particularly aware of their risk. This is because the highest risk is still associated with people with specific behaviours: injecting drugs or men who have sex with men. This pattern is changing in the USA and Europe as the disease spreads out into the general population, but the spread is slow. The pattern of infection in these countries leads to a situation where most individuals tend to come forward requesting the HIV test because they feel that they have been at risk. Most individuals found to have HIV are identified when they are seropositive and through their presenting themselves for testing.

Most developing countries are areas of type II spread, i.e. most infections are hetero-sexually acquired. In some developing countries infection rates are very high. People may be at great risk without feeling that their behaviour is particularly risky. If the infection rate in a city among young adults is 10%, there is a one-in-ten risk that someone who has had sex with only one other person will have had sex with someone with HIV. Under these circumstances individuals are likely to come forward only when they are ill. Individuals may not feel that they are any more at risk than anyone else, and that probably militates against coming forward to be tested.

Not only is it difficult for individuals in the community to know that they have been at risk, it is more difficult for medical and other health care personnel to assess the risk of infection of any particular patient. However, it is worth bearing in mind that there are degrees of risk. Even in a city where having sex with one partner is a 10% risk of sleeping with someone with HIV, an individual who has ten partners is still at greater risk.

Infrastructure and resources

A large city like London or San Francisco will have a range of voluntary services and statutory services aimed at individuals with HIV infection. Patients have a choice of what services they use. They are able to find a service which matches their needs by 'shopping around'. They can make use of telephone advice lines and counselling services because most people have access to a private telephone line.

Developing countries tend to have lower levels of resources than developed ones, and resources in this case are not simply money, materials and drugs; there is often a lack of trained personnel. But the level of resources is not the only factor. Perhaps the most important difference between developing countries and developed countries is the range of alternatives available. If an HIV counselling service is set up in London and does not work well, there are others to which a patient can go. The money invested in it can, ultimately, be written off and more money produced for another service. The patient who gets poor service from the local hospital can go to another one.

In developing countries there is usually only one of everything. If the Ministry of Health or a non-governmental organisation (NGO) makes a mistake in backing a particular service, it has usually spent all the money available and the service is unlikely to be replaced. It is this lack of scope to experiment and the need to get things right first time which probably most distinguishes service developments in developing countries from those in developed countries.

Culture and language

In most western countries there is a fairly uniform culture across the country. Most countries have a single language or at most two. There is some ethnic, cultural and linguistic diversity in many western countries, but on nothing like the scale seen in many developing countries.

In developing countries national boundaries often fail to reflect cultural, ethnic or religious boundaries. There may be many different languages in a single country, and great diversity in culture and religion from place to place. The counsellor is likely to have to deal with many more problems in terms of understanding the patient, not only in the purely practical matter of understanding a language that they speak, but in terms of understanding the cultural background from which they come.

Developing an appropriate model of counselling for local circumstances

It is clear that simply taking what has been done in many western countries and applying it to developing countries will not provide the best possible service. There are several considerations which seem to predict successful services in developing countries.

Maximisation of the use of existing resources

The scarcity of resources, both economic and human, means that a successful system is likely to have to make the optimal use of existing resources, particularly in terms of trained health professionals but also in terms of making the best use of what systems already exist for delivering health and social care. The counsellor is likely to be someone who is providing more general care to the patient, perhaps a nurse, social worker, doctor or clinical assistant. They may be someone from outside health, perhaps from education or from the churches.

Being pro-active in helping people to change

Many western HIV counselling services are built around counselling and testing programmes. This is probably a poor system in any case, aimed primarily at individuals who have already been infected but tending to neglect individuals at high risk who are uninfected. In most developing countries the numbers of individuals identified through testing programmes (as opposed to identified through symptoms) is likely to be small. It is therefore helpful to try to identify individuals at greater risk and to target at least part of the overall counselling effort at them.

Considering the wider context

In most developing countries it is not hospitals and clinics which provide most of the care for sick patients.

In rural areas it is families who tend to carry the main burden of caring for the sick person. This is likely to include practical care, moral support and financial help. In many developing countries some drugs are only available if the family can pay for them. Under such circumstances it is important to link with families and for the counsellor to work with the families as far as possible. Several services in Africa have taken this approach, for instance the Chikankata hospital; and the Lusaka Home Care Team (Chaava 1990; Chela & Siankanga 1991) in Zambia. Similar approaches have been taken in the Caribbean and Central America.

In urban areas of developing countries the situation tends to be rather different. In many developing countries the cities are growing rapidly as people move from the villages in search of a better life. Very often they leave their families behind when they move. They leave their parents and older generations, but sometimes also wives and children. If they become sick while they are in the cities they have no family to turn to. Under these circumstances support often comes from voluntary organisations, particularly church or other religious groups but also from all sorts of formal and informal groups of people. Clearly, for the counsellor working in an urban environment, there is a need to try to use local community groups to help those with HIV infection and AIDS, both practically and in terms of counselling. Of course the distinction between urban and rural areas is not always straightforward. Some people in urban areas are linked into family structures or their family may come to them when they are ill. Conversely, in villages not everyone has a family.

Sample model

Utilising these basic principles about what seems to work, it is possible to look at a model which might fit one particular context, for example a rural health district in Africa with a hospital, a health centre and dispensary. The model might include the following:

- Maximising use of existing health contacts, including hospital admissions, family planning programmes, maternity services and vaccination programmes, to provide face-to-face health education and health education materials. HIV education and counselling can often be linked to existing programmes; indeed there are many good reasons for trying to link together a range of different programmes. This is one area where rivalries between different services, sometimes backed up by rivalries between donor organisations, can get in the way. There can be difficulties in mixing programmes, however, and some of these are considered later.
- Training staff in the hospital, dispensary and health centre, as well as community staff, to ask the necessary questions to find out who is at high risk, and to provide basic counselling on the prevention of infection. Simply giving staff a list of a few standardised questions can help enormously in this respect.
- Aiming for a limited number of specialist HIV/AIDS counsellors to provide back-up, advice and training to workers and assistance with particularly difficult cases on a referral-on basis. If the hospital offers testing-on-request at a single centre they might also provide the services in that clinic.
- Where resources permit, training community staff who will both provide counselling and support to those with AIDS and their families and also provide a range of simple medical assistance, for instance advice on infection control, anti-diarrhoea medications and pain-killers.
- Training staff to ask simple questions of relatives who may be going to give blood, in order to identify those at high risk and so avoid donations occurring during the 'window period' between infection and seroconversion. This may be the only protection for recipients where equipment shortages or laboratory problems exist and consistent HIV testing of donations is a problem.
- Using existing groups in the community, for instance women's groups, church groups or

other local and national groups to provide health education and support. Many of the most successful counselling services in developing countries are based around such organisations. It is worth considering whether, with appropriate training, members of such organisations might be able to play a role in providing counselling.

● Making a local assessment as to who is likely to be at highest risk currently in the area. This assessment is certain to be imperfect but will allow better concentration of scarce resources than if such an assessment has not been made. The idea that in an area of heterosexual spread almost everyone is at risk, is misleading. In all areas of the world there are gradations of risk.

The model above is only an example. A service for an urban area might look quite different: people would generally be able to reach a centralised facility and greater use might be made of specialised HIV/AIDS counsellors. However, even in an urban area it is doubtful whether all the counselling needs of those with HIV/AIDS could be met through specialist counsellors. In most developing countries there simply would not be the resources available. It would still be necessary to try to come up with a system which maximised the use of existing resources, both in terms of specialist health resources and of voluntary organisations within the community.

Targeting resources

Even in the richest of developed countries resources are not infinite. There is usually a need to take decisions about where to put resources so that they produce the best possible outcomes. In developing countries the problem is even more acute and the margin for error is virtually nil. Targeting scarce counselling resources means thinking hard about where the focus of services should be.

A key part of this task is deciding who is at higher and lower risk of infection. This needs to be done locally on the basis of local circumstances. It is never going to be totally accurate but even a modest improvement in targeting can make a great improvement in the effectiveness of a programme. Assessing relative risk in an area is important because:

● It makes it easier to focus health education efforts and to match the content of these more closely to the specific needs of those at risk.
● It helps health-care staff to pick out from their caseload those individuals with characteristics which suggest that they might be putting themselves at risk. This offers the chance for the health worker to help the patient reduce that risk.
● It helps in diagnosis in terms of deciding which specimens or patients need to be sent to the hospital. Where HIV testing is not readily available and diagnosis of HIV disease is being made on clinical grounds alone, it can help to guide the clinician's thinking.
● It can be used to discourage potentially high-risk donors from giving blood.

In assessing relative risk in an area the first point to decide is the overall prevalence of the disease in the area, because relative risks of different groups of people tend to differ according to the overall prevalence. At very low levels of prevalence individuals with particular characteristics tend to be the ones who are infected. As the incidence of the disease in the general population rises, the characteristics of those infected become less and less distinguishable from the population at large, although even at very high incidences some people are still more at risk than others.

There are several potential sources of information about the incidence of HIV in a population:

- Seroprevalence studies are the most reliable source of information. Because these are seldom carried out on entirely representative samples, however, they can give a misleading overall picture if not treated with some care. Unfortunately HIV levels tend to be very patchy in most countries; for instance, a city may have an HIV incidence in the 15–40 age group of 10% while a rural area 50 km away may have an incidence below 1%. One really needs information from seroprevalence studies in the specific area in which one is working. Generalised figures for a country as a whole or from adjoining areas are seldom very useful. On the other hand it is sometimes possible to make an intelligent guess based on areas with similar characteristics.
- The incidence of AIDS gives a clue to likely prevalence of HIV, although cases of AIDS tend to lag behind HIV infections by some years.
- Data from voluntary testing facilities or from blood donor screening programmes can be used, although unrepresentativeness of those being tested is often a problem.

Data on incidence is doubly useful if it can be matched to some appreciation of the characteristics of those who are infected and how they differ, if at all, from the rest of the population. So seroprevalence studies linked to the collection of demographic and behavioural data are more useful than straightforward seroprevalence data alone. Where there are voluntary testing facilities it is important to collect information on the characteristics of both negatives and positives. All data, however, tends to be subject to a degree of bias and is likely to be, at least in part, unreliable. A certain amount of common sense usually has to be applied to make any sense of the available data. However at worst it is usually possible to identify whether levels of infection in an area are high, medium or low.

In the absence of systematic data on the characteristics of individuals who are infected or uninfected in a population, it is usually possible to make some intelligent guesses based on whether an area has high, medium or low rates of infection.

Areas of low incidence

Those most at risk tend to be:

(1) Those who travel to areas where the incidence of infection is high, for instance truck drivers, businessmen or air crew. Where prevalence varies within a country between rural and urban areas, as is usually the case, those who travel to the cities to work, particularly single men leaving their families or married men separated for long periods, are also likely to be at risk.
(2) Those who have sex with travellers. This will include their wives or lovers, but also prostitutes, 'barmaids' and others.
(3) Migrants from areas of higher incidence. One needs to be cautious about this. There is a temptation for people in a country to wish to see migrants as the source of HIV

infection even where it is clear that the local incidence is high. It sometimes results in nonsensical restrictions on foreign nationals entering countries, or prejudice against immigrants settled in a country or working in a country.

Areas of medium incidence

Those most at risk tend to be:

(1) Those who are the partners of people in group 2 above.
(2) Individuals with higher than usual numbers of sexual partners. For any individual the risk of infection with any sexually transmitted disease depends on the number of individuals with the infection in the population and the number of sexual partners that individual has. The more partners they have the more likely they are to end up having sex with someone with a sexually transmitted disease. Conversely, the higher the rate of infection the less important the number of partners becomes, although it never becomes unimportant.
(3) Individuals whose partners have higher than usual numbers of sexual partners. A woman may have only one sexual partner but if he has many partners then she is at greatly increased risk (Zunzunegui *et al.* 1986).

Areas of high incidence

As the infection spreads through the population, people with fewer sexual partners start to be at risk and particular groups of individuals will be less salient (Goodgame 1990). For instance, if the rate of infection in an area is 1%, a man with five sexual partners per year has a one in twenty chance of having sex with someone infected. If the rate rises to 5%, he has a one in four chance of having sex with someone infected. As the local rate rises, travellers of one sort or another have less and less importance as agents of general spread. However, while rates remain higher in urban than in rural areas (as is usually the case), those travelling to or from the cities remain at most risk of infection. Also, independently of rural–urban differences, in most countries there are quite wide differences in infection rates in different places.

Identifying those with particular risks

Besides the general considerations above, certain groups of people are particularly worth considering when assessing risk or drawing up a list of risk factors to look for in, say, a testing clinic. It can also be helpful to identify particular groups of people for the targeting of health education and preventive counselling programmes. Different countries have different groups of people at risk. However some groups of people tend to appear repeatedly in different countries and it is worth considering these in more detail.

Prostitutes

In any country with significant rates of heterosexual infection, prostitutes are likely to be a risk group unless they act to reduce their risk of infection by consistently using condoms. Prostitutes can also serve as a major element in the spread of HIV (Nzilambi *et al.* 1991).

Condom programmes with prostitutes have often worked very well, a significant proportion of programmes having been successful (Ngugi *et al.* 1988; Fox *et al.* 1993; Asamoah *et al.* 1994). For the prostitute using a condom has few disadvantages, and it has the advantage of protecting against other sexually transmitted diseases and hence against the potential loss of earnings that these can bring. The problem of lack of intimacy, perceived by many heterosexuals, is not a problem for the prostitute – at least with paying customers. Unfortunately not all customers of prostitutes are willing to use a condom. Where competition between prostitutes is fierce and where customers are very resistant, the prostitute may be unable to get customers to use them. It is also not uncommon for customers to offer a premium for sex without a condom.

There is a spectrum of prostitutes in terms of their clients, how much they earn and where they operate. Not all prostitutes in a country are likely to be at equal risk. Which group is most at risk will differ according to local factors. In a country where levels of infection are low it is likely to be prostitutes who cater to travellers who are most at risk early in an epidemic. This includes the prostitutes who service clients in hotels, even though they may have fewer clients than street prostitutes or 'barmaids'. However, street prostitutes who service truck drivers and other travellers are also at high risk if the people they are servicing are coming from high risk areas.

In many countries prostitutes are not local to the area where they are working. They may come from other areas of the country or from other countries. Prostitution is sometimes difficult for women to do in their own area because of social pressure and it is, of course, a job which migrants can do without requiring work permits or visas. Rates of infection among prostitutes can, therefore, reflect those in areas they come from, rather than those in areas where they are working. In countries where injecting drug use occurs, prostitutes are often drug injectors – providing another bridge for the spread of infection.

For every woman who regards herself as a full-time prostitute there are likely to be others who engage in prostitution on an occasional basis, or who have sexual relationships with relatively few men in order to gain money, food or other services. This group of women is particularly difficult to identify or reach. They may be reluctant to identify what they are doing as prostitution and they are less likely to be locatable. In most large cities there are areas where prostitutes congregate – particular streets, hotels or bars. Therefore they are relatively easy to locate for a health education drive. This is likely to be much more difficult with the casual or occasional prostitute.

Travellers

In Africa, truck drivers who travel large distances are particularly at risk because they may pass through areas of high prevalence and have sex there. They are also away from family and friends and therefore away from social restraints and in a position to indulge in sex with new partners in a way that they might not at home. The same is true of long-distance truck drivers in Central America and parts of South America. They may also make use of prostitutes or exchange sexual favours for a lift in their truck, and so may be more likely to have sex with women with multiple partners. The reverse is also true. Women who have sex with travellers are, on average, more likely to be at risk of infection. Truck drivers are not the only travellers; sailors, railway workers and airline staff are also at increased risk. Businessmen and travelling salesmen of various sorts are also at potentially increased risk. While truckers are fairly visible, the contribution of these other groups to the spread of infection is much less obvious but may be much more significant.

As noted above, it is not simply travel between countries which is at risk. Travel within a country can also be an issue, particularly where there are wide disparities in prevalence in different areas.

Those cut off from normal social restraints

All societies act to some extent to regulate the sexual behaviour of their members, whether by explicit rules or by social approval and disapproval. Families also often act as powerful restraining influences on sexual behaviour (although they can, of course, have the opposite effect sometimes). When people are freed from the social constraints of their society and family, they are free to act in ways which would otherwise be unacceptable. In this respect the key group are probably those who move away from their families into cities, either permanently or for extended periods. Not only are they out of sight of those who might influence them, but also in cities opportunity of sexual licence is increased. The anonymity of the city means that no-one in their new setting is likely to worry much what they are doing.

Prisoners

Inmates of prisons tend to be those who are least susceptible to social constraints and many will lead chaotic lives. In areas where drug use is a problem prisoners are more likely to have used drugs, either injecting them, or prostituting in return for drugs or having sex with others in return for supplying drugs. In other words prisoners tend to be at elevated risk of HIV, not because they are in prison but because of their activities before they went to prison. In addition, even in areas where homosexual behaviour is unusual, it may occur in prisons and other all-male institutions where access to women is denied. There are many prisons in the world where, if sufficient money is available, prisoners need not be deprived of female company – often prostitutes.

This is of particular importance because prisons have been used frequently as reliable sources of blood donation, and also because they are natural points at which to intervene with a group at elevated risk.

Those in other all-male institutions

Wherever men are taken away from their families and from normal access to the opposite sex, they are potentially at higher risk. People in the armed forces, men living away from their families in mining camps and people travelling for seasonal work, are all potentially at higher risk. They are away from the restraints of friends and family and are more likely to seek casual or paid sexual contacts.

Young people

Young people are perhaps the most common target of any sexual health education campaign. There are good reasons for this in terms of trying to influence behaviour early before negative patterns can get established. However this issue tends to get mixed up with the question of whether young people are at increased risk.

Whether young people are at particular risk of HIV and other sexually transmitted diseases depends on local sexual mores. In Europe and North America young people, both male and female, tend to experiment with a series of short sexual relationships before finding a more permanent partner. In some parts of the world where virginity is highly prized in women and where young men marry late – perhaps when they have land or money to support a wife – young men may make extensive use of prostitutes. In other cultures pre-marital sex is frowned upon both for men and women (although this does not mean that it does not occur). There are often differences in sexual behaviour between town and country, between different social classes or educational levels, and between different religious and ethnic groups.

It is also worth considering that the majority of young people starting out on their sexual career will be HIV seronegative. In other words, even in a high prevalence area most 15-year-olds will be free from infection. It takes time for HIV to diffuse into a particular age group, usually because of sex by members of that age group with older people. Cultures in which a proportion of young girls tend to have sex with older men ('sugar daddies') or young men with prostitutes, are likely to have young people at much earlier and greater risk of picking up HIV infection. The extent to which young people are particularly at risk, and which groups of young people are particularly at risk, can only be determined by considering the local culture.

Widows, widowers and divorcees

Both men and women separating from their partners tend to show a burst of sexual activity and may have multiple partners. The reasons for this vary with place and circumstance, but several themes can be identified. First, the separated individual may be back in the same role as when they were young, experimenting with different partners to find one to settle down with. The man or woman may be 'making up for lost time' or 'enjoying their freedom'. In cultures where women are very much disadvantaged the woman may have to find a man or more than one man to support her if she has been abandoned. Clearly all these things can lead to a man or woman having several partners in a short time. It should also be borne in mind, of course, that the widow or widower's spouse may have died of AIDS.

Babies of infected mothers

This would include other children in a family where a child had AIDS or known HIV infection.

Recipients of repeated blood transfusions which were unscreened

This might include those with a history of haemophilia, sickle-cell anaemia and surgery.

Sexual partners of those known to have HIV

This would include the sexual partners of those at increased risk, in other words most of the other groups in this section.

Recipients of surgical or other invasive procedures where sterile procedures may not have been followed

This has to be taken on a very much case-by-case basis. Both conventional medicine and traditional medicine, particularly that involving skin cutting or piercing, need to be considered. Ironically, although there are a fair number of cases of suspected transmission through unsterilised needles and syringes in conventional medicine, there is little or no clear evidence of a risk associated with traditional skin-cutting practices. However this may simply reflect a lack of information on the latter. There are similar problems in assessing procedures such as traditional circumcisions.

These are only general considerations. It is important in planning a service to draw up a list of groups at particular risk in the local area. This issue is covered in more detail below.

Assessing who is at low risk

In the same way as it can be helpful to identify those at higher risk, it can be of considerable value to identify individuals at lower risk of HIV infection. There are several advantages to such a process. Deciding where priorities do not lie can be as important as deciding where they do lie. Identifying who is likely to be at lower risk can avoid much unnecessary effort. Estimates of who is at lower risk also have a very specific purpose in targeting potential blood donors.

It is important for most blood donation services to try to find a reasonable pool of uninfected donors. Processing many infected donations increases the risk of infected donations slipping through (for instance during the 'window period') and involves the blood collecting agency in additional work following up infected donors. The blood also has to be discarded, involving a loss of time and money and, worse still, occupying time that might have been used to collect blood from someone uninfected.

As infection rates rise in a country, the pool of potential donors starts to shrink and it becomes very important for blood-collecting services, whether blood transfusion services or local hospitals and clinics, to try to replace this. In some cases this will involve trying to shift away from heavy reliance on relative blood and towards trying to establish a 'panel' or 'pool' or donors. In other cases the aim will be to increase the size of the existing pool or at least keep it stable. Identifying who is at lower risk is an important part of this process. Possibilities include:

- Individuals known or thought to be celibate. This includes the obviously celibate like nuns and priests (although one can occasionally be disappointed here) but also adolescents – depending on the age at which people become sexually active.
- Individuals who are monogamous or in 'closed' polygamous relationships. This group can be difficult to identify but appeals for such individuals to come forward can help.

Unfortunately, while a man or woman can be sure whether they have been monogamous or not, sometimes they cannot rely on the same in their partner.

- Young people very early in their sexual careers in some societies. If young people tend to have sex only, or mainly, with those of their own age group, it takes time for HIV and other sexually transmitted diseases to filter down into newly sexually active age groups. In a culture where individuals tend to have sex with those very different in age from themselves, for instance older men and younger women, this group is not at lower risk.
- In low prevalence areas those with very few sexual partners are at relatively low risk.
- Those who have consistently used condoms during sex.

In particular societies particular groups may be at lower risk because of religious or social customs, but these can only be identified on a case-by-case basis. Nonetheless the process of making such an identification can be very worthwhile.

Organising a counselling service

Identifying those at highest (and lowest) risk in a community is a good first step in trying to organise a counselling service. A successful service will:

- Make maximum use of whatever resources are available, including utilising individuals who are already in contact with those at highest risk. Services sometimes try to build up counselling services *de novo*, without considering how patients will reach them or how other needs of the patients will be met, for instance medical needs.
- Be organised in a way that gives, as far as humanly possible, the initiative to the worker on the ground and minimises unnecessary bureaucracy. Particularly where communications are poor, it is almost impossible to develop a 'top down' system which will work effectively. Services need to be able to be self-sustaining at a local or district level.
- Be pro-active and seek out individuals at risk before they are infected, wherever possible. The ideal is to find individuals at risk before they get infected and help them to reduce their risk of infection.
- Provide services to those who are already infected or ill and their families.

In order to build on assessment of risk it is necessary to go further and ask questions about how those at risk, or those already infected, can be contacted, where they can be contacted and who is best placed to provide counselling input. Counselling input need not be limited to those working in health; it may need to range wider in order to maximise input to individuals. Because it may embrace individuals with little or no knowledge of HIV or sexually transmitted diseases, there is likely to be a need for training and the nature and extent of the training required needs to be identified.

Table 18.1 shows two sections from a listing of these issues put together by workers in one small country. The two sections only represent two of the groups of individuals identified as at risk; truck drivers/business travellers, sex workers, drug users, adolescents, individuals with known AIDS/HIV attending hospital, individuals attending STD clinics and eight other categories of individual at higher risk were also identified. It will be seen that where and how to identify individuals, who was or could be involved in counselling, and what training these individuals needed, were all identified.

Table 18.1   Extracts from a risk assessment listing.

---

(4)   Men who have sex with men

Identification: Where and how
Believed to be a limited number of places of association. Two bars in capital can be identified as particularly frequented by gay and bisexual men. Sexually transmitted disease clinic through questioning all patients about orientation.
Men attending STD clinic with rectal STD infections.

Reason for risk
Known high base rate of infection among men who have sex with men in local population.
Believed particularly likely to have multiple partners.
May be having sex with persons from overseas with high risk or be travelling overseas to areas with high infection rates in this population.
Some individuals known to be engaging in male prostitution.

Persons involved or potentially involved in counselling
STD clinic staff.
Individuals within the subculture who are able to act as peer educators (need to seek to identify and involve such individuals).

Training required
Need to be aware of need to assess risk.
Need to know to identify persons at risk.
Need to be able to help sexual risk modification.
Need to be able to provide basic health education message.

Other potential routes of contact
Via local radio station, one of the programmes known to be popular with this group of individuals.
Distribute leaflets and condoms in known gay/bisexual venues.

(6)   Military personnel

Identification: Where and how
At bases.
Likely to seek medical advice outside the base and unlikely to admit to STDs to staff on the base because of unfavourable attitude to STDs by military; however attend local civilian STD clinics.

Reason for risk
Away from restrictions imposed by family and friends.
Known high usage of sex workers.
Young, usually no settled partner.
Peer pressure towards sex.

Persons involved or potentially involved
STD clinic staff.
Welfare officer on base.
Education officers on base.

Training required
Need to be aware of risk.
Need to be aware of need to assess risk.
Need to know how to identify persons at risk.
Need to be able to help risk modification.
Need to train to provide basic health education message.
Need to know how and when to refer on for more specialist support.
Need policy on how to deal with individuals identified as positive in a more constructive way.

Other potential routes of contact
Via local radio station.
Distribute leaflets on base and arrange for talks and lectures on risks at bases (need to engage active co-operation of senior military staff).
Distribute condoms?

The reasons for increased risk were also identified; without knowing why risk is increased it may be difficult to reduce it. Several groups were initially identified as at increased risk largely on the basis of faulty assumptions, but further thought and the collection of a little basic information showed that they were not, in fact, at high risk.

Other ways of reaching individuals at risk were identified, so that what is often considered as health education was combined with counselling approaches in the overall plan.

Drawing up a list like this can be extremely useful in deciding how to organise counselling services. Indeed, in going through this exercise it often becomes apparent how a counselling service can best be organised. Obviously the interventions to be used are an important part of deciding on a programme, and in deciding these it is important to start from the problems specific to an area. There are many interventions which might be made. Some examples of successful targeted programmes in developing countries include:

- An outreach programme to brothels where health workers distribute condoms and discuss safer sex with the women, as well as offering health checks either immediately or through special sessions at local clinics where the women do not have to wait. Getting the brothel owners on your side is important to the success of such programmes.
- A youth programme aimed at educating adolescents about safer sex and HIV through schools with inter-school competitions and exhibitions and the formation of youth groups around the subject. Getting not just educators but prominent figures in the local community to support (even if only tacitly) such projects is vital to their success. They can easily be spoilt by local opposition on 'moral' grounds.
- A programme to distribute condoms free on a weekly basis to migrant workers in mines.
- A programme aimed at ensuring that every attendee at an STD/dermatology clinic had HIV/AIDS and ways of preventing it discussed with them. It is extraordinary how rarely such an obvious and simple intervention is used, not just in developing countries but also in the west.
- A programme aimed at identifying high-risk attendees at a polyclinic and offering them counselling around risk reduction. This sort of project is often resisted by staff, initially on the grounds that they do not have the time. In the long run preventing infections saves a good deal more time than it uses.

These are some examples of interventions in HIV/AIDS; there are many successful programmes in the world. However, there have been many more failures. Successes, by and large, tend to be geographically limited programmes based on local decisions about local needs and steered by relatively few people. The high failure rate of larger programmes probably reflects the difficulty in managing large programmes over large geographical areas where infrastructure (like telephones, roads and trained manpower) is a problem, and the difficulty of implementing a single solution over a wide area with diverse needs and social structures. There *are* successful programmes at a national or regional level, so it is possible, but it is extremely difficult in practice.

A comprehensive HIV counselling service is one which is likely to operate at several levels. Counselling is often difficult to separate from other issues of service delivery, so counselling and basic health care or blood collection often go together. A comprehensive service is likely to include:

- Health education approaches – while these may not strictly be 'counselling', health education approaches complement counselling services for the individual. Raising general awareness of HIV issues and of the information around HIV in a community makes counselling patients much easier and sets up a sympathetic background against which to try to intervene with the individual.
- Counselling those at high risk, including outreach approaches.
- Testing on request.
- Counselling symptomatic patients.
- Ensuring adequate community support for the infected individual.
- Blood transfusion services.

Health education approaches

Health education approaches set the background against which counselling services can be organised. It is important to get them right.

In many countries there are already mass education campaigns carried out through newspapers, radio and television. However these can usually be backed up through local initiatives, perhaps using local newspapers or radio stations in an area. Posters and local events can be organised and can be very effective in drawing people's attention to the issue of HIV. The great strength of local initiatives over national ones is that they can provide information not only about the disease but also about local services and how to access them.

Often in an area there will be local health education initiatives in existence already. There may be campaigns aimed at other diseases, or immunisation programmes, or even family planning programmes. Successful campaigns in other health areas can be useful, not only in terms of the information they will have gathered about the best way to get health messages across, but also because a certain amount of health education about HIV can be delivered in parallel with other campaigns.

There are sometimes problems with this approach, of course. Mixing HIV education and family planning, for instance, has to be handled carefully. Where family planning pro-grammes are having difficulties there is a danger that promoting the use of condoms for prophylaxis may appear as just another way to introduce an unpopular restriction on family size. It may also get mixed up with the issue of what contraceptive method is best in terms of controlling fertility. Conversely, the association of contraceptives and HIV may make it more difficult to promote family planning. However there is at least a possibility that each cam-paign may benefit from the other.

Family planning is not the only sort of programme which can be used to promote risk-reduction activities. Many other health education campaigns are also suitable for the pro-cedure, including breast-feeding campaigns and immunisation programmes; in fact any occasion on which people are brought face-to-face with health workers alone or in groups can be used. Not only health education programmes but other educational programmes on other topics can also be used. The objective, if possible, is to raise the awareness of the population about HIV/AIDS, get them talking about it, and therefore make them more receptive to individual health messages through counselling.

Besides attempts to influence individuals at risk, there is also a need to try to influence opinion-formers, local politicians, religious leaders, teachers, local officials or village elders, in fact anyone who can influence the public verbally or by example. Not getting such people on the side of HIV health education can lead to efforts failing or even being blocked. Popular entertainers, sports stars, radio personalities and in fact anyone with the ear of the public can also play a key role in getting the message across and keeping it in the public eye. Local groups of one sort or another are common in all societies, whether it is church groups, sports clubs, schools or local clubs. They all provide opportunities to get the message about HIV across and also to spread the message about where to access local services.

Counselling those at high risk of HIV infection

Locating and counselling those at high risk of HIV infection is likely to be a key issue in any country. For the reasons discussed earlier, it is likely to be even more of a problem in a developing country simply because so few people will identify themselves as at high risk. It is worth considering that, while it is time-consuming to identify someone at risk and counsel them, it is likely to be a good deal less time-consuming than treating them for AIDS.

In an area where HIV infection is common, it is important to try to train every health professional in at least the basics of identifying those at increased risk and the sorts of advice which they need to give to reduce that risk. It should be part of routine history-taking to ask questions about risk factors. Asking about sexual behaviour does not always come easily and staff may need help and encouragement to ask the right questions.

In training staff it is important to try to get them to think through how they might identify those at increased risk among their own patients. Sometimes it is possible to improve identification of those at increased risk in quite simple ways which can be of great importance where a health professional has many patients and little time. For instance, in one country where I was involved ante-natal staff were able to identify characteristics which probably indicated increased risk of HIV among their clinic attenders. Women who had children by several different men, who were not able to name the father, or who did not live with the father, were some of the groups which they identified. Of course not all women with these characteristics would be at increased risk, nor would every woman at increased risk be identified in this way; however it allowed them to improve their targeting of health education, advice and history-taking efforts more effectively.

A system does not have to be perfect or foolproof to be worthwhile. This case was also important because it illustrated an important point. The interest was in identifying sexually active women at risk and helping them to modify their risk behaviour to prevent future infection. Even though the work was carried out in ante-natal work, the primary objective was not to identify infected mothers and children; that was a secondary aim.

Making condoms available wherever possible is just as much a part of counselling as talking through the issues with patients. There is no point in advising patients how to reduce their risks when they do not have the wherewithal to do so. This is not to say that condoms are the only way, or necessarily the best way, of reducing risk for all patients, but they are an important part of behaviour change for many.

Distributing condoms can be a problem in many countries. In particular men are sometimes reluctant to collect condoms and, where this is the case, it may be possible to get women to collect them. It is also important that, where condoms are being distributed, staff spend some time explaining how to use them properly. Condoms are reliable if they are properly used, much less so if they are misused. The instructions which come with condoms are often less than helpful, and are totally useless if the user is illiterate or has poor reading skills. Clearly staff need to stress using each condom only once, only putting them on when full erection has been attained, not withdrawing and re-entering during sex, and holding on to the base of the condom during withdrawal after ejaculation. While these measures may appear self-evident they are far from so to someone who has never used a condom. A demonstration using a model, a pen or anything else which is suitable and readily available, often replaces a thousand words.

Of course counselling individuals at risk should not depend on simply waiting for individuals at risk to turn up. Outreach is an important part of many successful programmes, whether to bars and clubs, to brothels or to the families of those affected by HIV. The essence of the issue is working out where individuals at high risk can best be identified and counselled, and if that happens to be outside the hospital outreach is likely to prove a shrewd investment.

HIV testing on request

It is usually beneficial to offer HIV testing on request, if this is possible. There are, essentially, two ways of doing this:

(1) Multiple outlets – offering the test from many different sites
(2) Restricted site – offering testing at only one or a very limited number of sites in a geographical area.

There are pros and cons for each of these models. A multiple outlet fits in well with the idea of as many health care staff as possible being involved in HIV. In this model as many sites as possible, and as many parts of each site as possible, offer HIV testing, so hospitals, health centres, polyclinics, even dispensaries and individual doctors are encouraged to offer tests. This gives good coverage but it is very difficult to maintain quality in terms of counselling, and in terms of clinical aspects of patient handling. There are also major problems in terms of sample transport and handling. In fact, it is usually the latter problem which prevents multiple site models succeeding.

A restricted site aims to provide only a single specialist site or a limited number of sites at which people can get an HIV test. This makes quality control and information about what is going on much more reliable and may be more realistic in terms of laboratory facilities and a reduced need to transport samples. However it restricts access and people may be reluctant to attend a specialist centre; the opportunity to involve a wide range of health-care staff in HIV prevention work may be reduced and there may be real problems with patients being able to travel conveniently to somewhere they can get tested. Where patients are being referred for a test to another hospital or part of the same hospital, they may decide that the effort involved is too great and may never get where they have been referred.

Most services will probably settle on some sort of compromise in terms of venues where the test is available. However it is an important issue to consider as early as possible in organising a service, since failure to resolve it frequently leaves a testing service crippled.

Counselling symptomatic patients

In many developing countries the majority of individuals with HIV infection will be identified not through HIV testing but when they become symptomatic. Indeed, the diagnosis of HIV disease may be made on clinical grounds alone and HIV testing may never be undertaken, particularly where laboratory facilities are not available.

One of the difficulties with AIDS is that it has such a wide range of manifestations that people with HIV infection-related problems can appear at just about any part of the health services of an area. Surgeons, physicians, midwives, health visitors, staff in family planning clinics and a whole range of other staff are likely to be presented suddenly with patients showing signs of HIV infection and AIDS. Patients will present at hospitals, at clinics, at health centres and at dispensaries and community staff; if they are in areas of high prevalence and they have their wits about them, staff involved are likely to turn up further cases.

For this reason it is important that every member of the health care staff in areas of high prevalence should be on the look out for possible HIV disease and that there should be a clear procedure for arranging for possible cases to be reviewed and for a diagnosis to be made. Where HIV testing is not available, an estimate of risk can play an important part in the differential diagnosis.

It is relatively easy to set up a counselling service for those with AIDS-related problems in a district hospital. Providing staff can recognise such patients it is possible for them to pass on the counselling aspects of the work to one or more other staff who take a particular interest in the area.

In rural areas the situation is likely to be very different. It is important that whoever is dealing with the patient should be aware of the basic issues surrounding counselling and should be able to provide at least basic support and counselling. For this to be possible it is important to have staff with greater experience – specialist or semi-specialist staff to provide back-up advice and help to the staff in the field.

At the rural level in larger countries the roles of counsellor and provider of basic medical care are likely to be combined. It may be possible to arrange for the sick individual to be treated at a local dispensary or health centre. However in many cases the health professional is going to be visiting the patient at home and providing both basic medical care, such as treatment for diarrhoea and pain relief, and also basic counselling. In general this will mean that a nurse or other health professional will cover both areas of care.

In rural areas of poor countries, where trained health-care staff are in very short supply and counselling is being provided by other individuals in a community, it is reasonable to ask whether they might not be provided with simple medications and equipment to provide very basic 'first-aid' support to sick patients with known HIV disease, particularly late-stage patients too ill to travel. An individual fulfilling a counselling role without much in the way of medical back-up will have to know how to answer questions that the relatives and patient may have, and how to take decisions about the best way to manage the patient.

In any health care system the point at which the patient is transferred from the care of one worker or team to another is the point at which most of the problems occur. It is vital to provide whoever is taking over the care of a patient with as much information as possible, to ensure that the patient knows who they will be dealing with and to ensure that whoever is taking over care knows who has been looking after the patient so far and feels able to get in contact if anything is unclear.

Community support

Social support is an important element, not just in the mental and physical wellbeing of people with HIV but also in the ability of individuals to make changes in their risk behaviour. Good social support is associated with a much lower incidence of adverse psychological problems in people with HIV (Green & Kocsis 1995). For that reason it is important to ensure that adequate support is in place for the HIV seropositive individual.

In many developing countries the family is often the main focus of social and practical support for the sick person. The family may support them emotionally, nurse them when they are sick at home, take them to and from hospital, pay for their drugs, feed them, house them and support them financially. However not everyone has a family to support them and not all families are supportive, particularly with a disease like AIDS. As mentioned earlier, individuals in urban areas in particular may be far from family and friends. There is often a need for other sources of community support.

Most societies already have groups of various sorts – everything from women's groups to local church groups – and these gatherings can be used not only to get across basic information about HIV infection and ways of avoiding it but also as a starting point for social support. By building up relationships with these groups health professionals can develop a valuable resource for assisting in the care of those with AIDS or HIV infection. People are only likely to provide such support if they understand about AIDS and about the transmission of HIV and the ways that it cannot be transmitted.

Sometimes it may be helpful to try to start up mutual self-help groups with individuals with HIV. There are many potential problems in doing this. Individuals may be reluctant to attend self-help groups or identify themselves to others; this is particularly the case in parts of the world where numbers of infected individuals are low and social disapproval high, but it is not confined to such areas. However, at least in the case of some people at risk it may be possible. The example of prostitute groups was used earlier but there are other groups which can be formed.

Blood transfusion services

Ways of getting blood vary enormously from place to place. In the west generally blood transfusion services tend to rely on mass bleeding sessions with volunteer donors, perhaps supplemented with panels of donors with rare blood types who can be contacted if needed. Many developing countries also have such systems but tend to supplement blood available from such sources with 'relative blood'. Individuals entering hospital are asked to encourage relatives and friends to donate blood. The latter undoubtedly often believe that their blood will go to the patient, being conveniently unaware of the issue of compatibility.

In the west the blood supply is protected by two mechanisms. First, all blood is screened for HIV. Secondly, individuals at high risk are asked to 'defer' (in other words not donate). This reduces the risk of blood being collected in the 'window period' (i.e. between infection and the individual testing seropositive). It also reduces the number of seropositives that the blood transfusion services have to deal with. In fact donor deferral is a much more important element in the western blood transfusion services' overall strategies than identifying positive donations. Donor deferral is much more difficult in countries where it is not so clear who is at greater risk.

For most countries with scarce resources there is a considerable advantage in trying to obtain as much volunteer blood as possible. Volunteer blood can be obtained from populations at lower risk (see above) and so the number of positives can be reduced as much as possible. There is good reason to believe that relatives of hospital patients will tend to be at higher risk than other members of the population, since they may share the lifestyle or the bed of the index patient who may themselves have HIV-related illness.

It may be possible to further screen volunteer donors or relatives by asking them a short series of questions aimed at identifying risk characteristics, although this can be difficult to achieve in practice. A pool of repeat volunteer donors can be targeted with health education materials and information so that they can assess their own risk and so defer.

There is probably nowhere in the world where full pre-test counselling is put in place for blood donors, even though they are, in essence, having an HIV test. There is usually neither the time nor the infrastructure. Under the circumstances it can be particularly difficult to deal with seropositives. Whatever the difficulties, it is important to have a system for recalling positive donors and counselling them. Whether this is done by asking them to come back or by going out to visit them, it still needs to be done. In cases where individuals travel from far away it may be necessary to use counsellors from that geographical area to give the result, meaning that it is important to set up the necessary links with such individuals as early as possible.

Special problems

Whether to actively encourage people to consider being tested

There are settings where it may be desirable to offer the test and to talk to individuals about the potential benefits of being tested. An obvious example is where the HIV test is important to differential diagnosis. It may be helpful to offer the test to all pregnant women but it is only worth doing this if there is some clear potential pay-off to the patient: if some treatment is being offered, or prophylaxis, or a regime of monitoring a parent and child or an adult. This issue is reviewed in more detail in Chapter 9.

It is sometimes argued that encouraging as many people as possible to be tested in itself fulfils a major public health benefit in terms of changing behaviour. The available evidence does not offer much encouragement to this, with most studies either showing no impact on sexual behaviour or relatively modest effects (Dawson *et al.* 1991; Higgins *et al.* 1991; Landis *et al.* 1992; Zenilman *et al.* 1992; Otten *et al.* 1993; Pickering *et al.* 1993; Temmerman *et al.* 1995), although a few studies do show rather better results (Wenger *et al.* 1991; Allen *et al.* 1992). Efforts put into encouraging individuals to be tested might also go into trying to encourage individuals at risk to reduce their risk of infection. You cannot use the same staff time twice, and it is hard not to conclude that if the choice were between, say, a programme aimed at condom distribution in brothels and a programme of mass HIV testing, common sense and available research would back the former. Of course this does not imply that individuals should not be made aware of the fact that the test is available, or that they should be discouraged from having it.

Telling people that they are infected

This chapter assumes that people will, wherever possible, be told that they have HIV or AIDS once this becomes known to the health services. However for those setting up a service this is not necessarily a 'cut-and-dried' issue. One element in the uncertainty is the fear of how the person who has been told that they have HIV will react. There is often a fear that those who are told that they are infected will go out and infect as many people as possible in 'revenge' attacks. There are frequent newspaper reports of such situations arising across the world and they even appear from time to time in scientific papers, in reviews. Tracking down actual cases where this has occurred is extremely difficult. I have tried to follow up a number of cases where this is supposed to have happened and, in each case, have found the rumours groundless. That is not to say that it never happens, but it must be a very rare reaction indeed.

Of course this sort of situation needs to be separated from the situation where an individual is aware that they have HIV infection but is unwilling or unable to change their risk behaviour. This does occur sometimes. There is no reason, overall, to believe that either of these issues should prevent a patient being told that they have HIV or AIDS. Against the theoretical risk of someone deciding to infect others deliberately must be set the advantages in telling the infected person. First, many counsellors would argue that it is the right of the individual to know about their own health. Secondly, there are many practical reasons for telling someone of their HIV status once this is known:

- A person who knows that they are infected is able to take steps to protect their current partner and possible future partners
- They are able to plan for the possibility that they may become ill in the future and make some provision for the support of their family if they should die
- They are able to inform their sexual partner or partners that they too may be infected with the virus
- They are able to take steps to protect their own health, for instance by avoiding other sexually transmitted diseases
- They are able to enter into a sensible dialogue about their treatment prospects and to enter into the decision-taking process.

These considerations provide compelling reasons why, under all but the most extraordinary of circumstances, it is best to tell individuals that they are infected with HIV or that they have AIDS.

Telling sexual partners

This is covered in more detail in Chapter 4. However it is worth summarising some of the issues here in order to look at some of the specific problems in developing countries.

Where a patient is going to inform a sexual partner it is important to rehearse with the patient what they are going to say to make sure that it is factually correct. It is also important to get them to bring in the sexual partner as soon as possible after telling them, so that counselling can take place.

One difficulty with immediate past partners is to know how far back a patient should go in contacting them. A patient will seldom know for sure when they were infected. However there is little point in patients chasing after, and unnecessarily alarming, partners they may have had seven years ago in an area where HIV infection was rare up until four years ago. It is a matter of common sense but in areas where HIV is common it is rarely beneficial to go back beyond immediate past partners.

The extent to which contact tracing should be undertaken on behalf of a patient who does not wish to inform their own partners or whose partners have moved away, is a difficult one. It is even more of an issue in developing countries than in the west. Contact tracing is time-consuming, expensive and labour-intensive. Perceived benefits need to be offset against any reduction in services to individuals already known to be infected. The impact of the diversion of resources to contact tracing from other possible schemes, such as health education, condom distribution, programmes aimed at prostitutes and so on, needs to be evaluated. In other words, the costs as well as the benefits need to be considered. Particularly in areas of high infection it is important to consider that an individual who has had sex with the patient five years ago may have had sex with numbers of other infected individuals since.

None of this is to suggest that a patient should not be helped to inform past partners if they wish to do so, nor that it may be very important to inform some past partners of some patients – for instance those who could not possibly have known that they were at risk, perhaps because they believed they were in a monogamous relationship. However, a consideration of both the costs and the benefits is important in deciding how much effort should be put into contact tracing.

With current sexual partners the situation tends to be more straightforward. Most patients will want to tell their own partners. From time to time they will feel unable to do so even though they want their partner to know. The issue then becomes who will tell the partner. One possibility is for the counsellor to do so. However, it is always worth considering alternatives with the patient. Sometimes an intermediary in the family may be able to do the telling and, because of their social relationship with the partner, may be able to handle the situation better than the counsellor could.

Particularly in extended families there may be an elder member of the family, an auntie or godfather, who fulfils a general advisory role in the family. Sometimes such roles are informal; in some societies they are socially recognised. Otherwise a sister, brother or other relative might be brought in to break the news. Such messengers need to be chosen with care and need to be discreet; it would be a mistake to choose a messenger who then told the whole village about the situation. On the other hand, where resources are scarce and a patient lives a long way from the counsellor's base, it may not be practical for the counsellor to go out.

A man came to a district hospital and was diagnosed as having AIDS. His wife did not believe that he was very sick and would not come to the hospital. He did not want to tell her himself because she was a woman with a sharp tongue and he did not feel he could cope. The counsellor identified an 'auntie' – a distant relative who acted as a sort of general adviser to the women in the family. The 'auntie' then informed the wife, who came to the hospital for advice.

Suppose a patient will not tell his current sexual partner, say his wife, and will not give permission for anyone else to do so. Clearly this is a situation where the counsellor needs to apply all possible persuasion. However, if the patient still refuses, what then? The temptation for the counsellor to tell the wife is strong; however to do so might create difficulties of its own. If people think that if they have a blood test for HIV other people will be told about the result without their consent, they will not come forward in the first place. If they do not come forward there is no way that they can be persuaded to inform their sexual partners. In the end it is this sort of consideration that suggests that, even in a difficult situation, it is best to maintain confidentiality.

Some counsellors feel that they are morally obliged to inform a sexual partner if the patient will not do it himself. This is an understandable view and clearly an acceptable one, providing that they make their position clear to the patients before they take them on. If such a situation is not acceptable to the patient, the case should be passed on to another counsellor.

Although confidentiality is important there can be no obligation for the hospital to lie to a partner about what is wrong with a living patient. If a wife asks what is wrong with her husband and he does not wish the hospital to tell her, all the hospital can do is tell the wife that it is only the patient who can say what is wrong with him. It is then between the two of them to sort it out; there is a limit to what a hospital can do to protect confidence.

Maintaining confidentiality can occasionally present unexpected difficulties.

A woman whose husband was dying of AIDS came to see the hospital. She said that since he had become sick some of his relatives suspected her of poisoning him or engaging in witchcraft.

In some societies it is important that the partner should be able to explain why the patient has died, or even, as in this case, why he is sick. It must be stressed to the patient that confidentiality, where sexual partners are concerned, does not extend beyond the grave. Once someone is dead there is a clear primary duty to look after the living and, whatever the patient wants, the wife must be told. Meanwhile the wife needs to be given at least enough information to allow her to avoid unjust accusations. She can be assured that he is genuinely sick and the relatives, if they can be contacted, can be told the same thing.

Telling other people

Sexual partners are not the only people involved with the person with AIDS. As noted above, in most developing countries it is the family which provides much of the input to a sick individual. The question then arises as to whether the family should be informed as a matter of course, an approach sometimes referred to as 'family confidentiality'. The idea is that a family member's HIV status is confidential to the family rather than simply the individual. It is sometimes argued that this fits in better with family models of illness and health, prevalent in parts of Africa and south-east Asia in particular. There are clear strengths to such a model but also obvious weaknesses. So long as the patient wants their family to know there is no difficulty. But supposing that they do not want their family to know? In all countries I have visited there are examples of individuals being rejected by their families because of their infection with HIV or their having AIDS. For an individual to be rejected by their family may leave them unable to survive.

On balance it seems important to discuss with the patient who else they want to know about their diagnosis. If the arguments in favour of the rest of the family knowing are strong, it should be possible to persuade most patients. If the patient refuses, I feel that it would be necessary to have the most pressing reasons for informing them in spite of the patient's wishes.

It is worth remembering in this context that there is no evidence of casual household transmission. Families may be carrying out what in other contexts would be regarded as basic nursing functions, and they will need to be advised on elementary hygiene measures. However, these do not require that the family should know an individual's diagnosis.

Cultural issues

Every country has its own culture (or often several). One cannot help people to change their behaviour without understanding that culture, which sets some of the expectations and constraints within which the individual operates. This is one of the key reasons why counselling services in developing countries need to be designed from 'the ground up', looking at local issues and local needs, rather than being imported from outside.

Cultural issues affect counselling in many ways. It is not possible to consider all the possible cultural variations here but anyone seeking to establish an effective counselling service should think through which elements of the local culture militate against change, or restriction of risk, and which ones are supportive. In particular it is worth considering any barriers to change in particular sections of the population. It would be presumptuous to try to predict the issues that will arise for every culture, but areas which frequently arise include sexual behaviour, prostitutes, pregnancy, power inequalities between men and women, and drugs. These are dealt with in turn here.

Sexual behaviour

Sexual mores differ widely from place to place. In some places it is acceptable for both men and women to have many sexual partners; in others it is acceptable for men to have many partners but not women; in yet others it is not acceptable for either sex to have many partners. I am not thinking here about the overt rules of the society, about whether the law says a man may be polygamous or monogamous or what it says about divorce, but about what is acceptable to people in a country. Cultures often subtly support certain sorts of behaviour. If a man who is having an affair is ostracised by his male friends he may well give it up; if it enhances his reputation with them he is likely to persist. Expectations about the way a man or woman behaves are important in shaping people's behaviour. If a man considers it natural that he should have several girlfriends, it may be difficult to change this behaviour.

Considering local sexual mores is important. I have seen several places in the world where governments have sought to promote monogamy as the answer to the spread of HIV in spite of local population mores supportive of men having multiple sexual partners. Although there is no harm in promoting virtue, it might have been wiser for them to promote condoms at the same time on the basis that 'if you can't be good at least be safe'.

Prostitutes and near-prostitutes

The use of prostitutes is an interesting issue in HIV. In many countries prostitutes show high rates of HIV infection and low usage of condoms, and it is probable that they are a major element in HIV spread (Simonsen *et al.* 1990; Plourde *et al.* 1992), as indeed they are for the spread of other sexually transmitted infections (D'Costa *et al.* 1985; Rosenberg *et al.* 1987). Particularly (but not exclusively) in societies where men marry relatively late – perhaps because they must make their mark in the world before marrying – the use of prostitutes is often not only commonplace but accepted. This situation is even more likely to arise where a high premium is placed on female virginity at marriage and pre-marital sex is frowned on. In some cultures it is even common for the men in the family – particularly the older men – to take a young man to a brothel for his first sexual experience.

All societies have prostitutes, but the number of prostitutes and the extent to which they are used by the population is determined not only by the demand from men but also by the position of women in that society, and the alternative options available for them to make a living. In some societies a woman without a man to provide for her and without support from her family may have little alternative to prostitution. In many societies women, if they can get paid work at all, are able to earn very little other than through prostitution. Prostitution is not necessarily limited to single women. If a man, through sickness, misfortune or merely the vagaries of the local labour market, is unable to support his family, his wife may have no option but to resort to prostitution.

Not only women are prostitutes; male prostitutes are common in many parts of the world. For every man or woman who would regard themselves as a prostitute there are probably several who exchange sexual favours for goods, services or money. Again, this is particularly common where women find it difficult to provide for themselves financially, and it is not limited to developing countries. The woman may have several male partners at the same time or may move from one to another. In many areas of the world the women tend to be much younger than the men who are supporting them or contributing to their support, and prostitution provides a bridge to take HIV and other sexually transmitted diseases rapidly across the generations.

In the case of both prostitution and near prostitution one of the problems for the woman who finds herself infected with HIV, or at risk, is that she may have difficulty in changing her behaviour without starving, or at least experiencing a dramatic drop in living standards. Where prostitutes come from other countries (very common in many countries), governments tend to try to deal with the problem by deporting them when they become infected, thus moving the problems elsewhere. Sent back to their own home countries most of the women (or men) will have little option but to continue to prostitute.

It may be possible to deal with problems around prostitution by offering women alternative ways of earning a living. These are seldom as lucrative as prostitution, and while it may be effective, and certainly may be worthwhile, for small numbers of women, it is difficult to imagine it being effective as a solution to restricting the role of prostitutes in spreading HIV. This approach is unlikely to work for 'near prostitutes'.

With prostitutes, the main successful steps are likely to revolve around getting them to use condoms. Very often the bar here is the customers; they may not wish to use a condom – very difficult to deal with, particularly where there are considerable numbers of prostitutes in competition – or they may even offer a premium for sex without a condom. Sometimes the main effort needs to be aimed at the customers, not simply the prostitutes.

Pregnancy

Many cultures place a great emphasis on the bearing of children and anything which gets in the way of this is difficult to accept. This sort of situation can be a great problem in getting women (and men) to accept the use of condoms. It can also be a major reason why women who know that they are infected with HIV decide that they will get pregnant, or even simply fail to tell their partner that they are infected (Ryder *et al.* 1991). Most countries have family planning programmes of various sorts and these programmes are often a mine of useful information about the constraints and bars on risk-reduction methods which restrict fertility, and potential ways of overcoming them.

Power inequalities between men and women

In many cultures, perhaps in almost all cultures, a sizeable proportion of women find themselves at a severe disadvantage in relationships relative to men. This is usually because cultural norms restrict the ability of women to assert what they want in relationships. something sometimes even backed up by the force of law. In some cultures women are unable to leave an unhappy relationship because their own families will not have them back and a single woman may be unable to support herself financially. A woman who leaves her husband may be socially ostracised in some cultures. In others women may be easily divorced, whether legally or in practice, more or less at the whim of the man. In still others a woman may fear physical violence if she complains about the sexual behaviour of her partner. These attitudes make it difficult for a woman who finds out, for instance, that her male partner is engaging in other outside relationships, either to get him to stop or to use a condom with other partners or with her.

This sometimes gets mixed up with the roles of men and woman. Men may feel that getting condoms and advice about sex is the role of the woman and yet it may be the man who has the final say as to whether a condom is used. If the HIV counsellor cannot get to the man, they may find that the woman is unable to make necessary changes to reduce risk.

Drugs

Until a few years ago drugs, at least injectable drugs like heroin or highly addictive drugs like cocaine, were rare or unknown in most developing countries. As world prices of most of these drugs have fallen and western markets have become saturated, they have started to find their way into developing countries. Some countries are also on major trading routes for drugs to the west and some of the drugs in passage end up in the countries through which they are passing. Parts of central America, Africa and south-east Asia are particularly affected by this.

The injection of drugs, of course, can be a route for transmission of HIV where injecting equipment is shared. However drugs are linked with HIV in more subtle ways. An expensive drug habit is difficult to support by legal means, particularly for women, but also for many men. Drugs are, therefore, linked to crime and prostitution and to a disorganised, chaotic lifestyle in which reducing sexual risks of HIV infection is a low priority.

Providing a comprehensive and effective HIV counselling service in a country can involve trying to set up services for drug users, both to help individuals to reduce their dependency on drugs and, where injecting is common, to help minimise possible sharing of equipment and consequent infection risks.

Managing an HIV counselling system

In this chapter I have outlined a model of counselling services which is implicitly very much 'bottom up' rather than 'top down' – in other words one that is built around local conditions. In many developing countries the range of local conditions within a single country suggests that a model where counselling services are developed at a regional or local level, within national guidelines, is likely to prove the most effective. The effectiveness of attempts to set up counselling services for HIV via national AIDS committees or similar bodies has sometimes been limited. This is hardly surprising when one considers the difficulties of communications in many countries and the limited information which may be available to national committees about actual conditions on the ground.

In small countries the national AIDS committee (NAC), or its counterpart or sub-committee, may be able to take an executive role, providing it has a membership which involves sufficient of those actually doing the work. In larger countries it is almost always more sensible for the NAC to take a superior planning role and set policy, try to co-ordinate the flow of resources and collect information. The actual role of organising services can be undertaken by local AIDS committees which are also in a better position to link health services aimed at HIV with services aimed at other diseases, and with other providers such as voluntary groups and NGOs.

At the end of the day, perhaps, the most important thing in providing a successful HIV counselling service is getting the right people involved in providing and running it. There is a good deal of luck in this and however good the planning, without that particular piece of luck, providing a really good service is very difficult.

References

Allen, S., Serufilira, A., Bogaerts, J., Van de Perre, P., Nsengumuremyi, F., Lindan, C., Carael, M., Wolf, W., Coates, T. & Hulley, S. (1992) Confidential HIV testing and condom promotion in Africa, impact on HIV and gonorrhoea rates. *Journal of American Medical Association*, 268, 3338–43.

Asamoah-Adu, A., Weir, S., Pappoe, M., Kanlisi, N., Neequaye, A. & Lamptey, P. (1994) Evaluation of a targeted AIDS prevention intervention to increase condom use among prostitutes in Ghana. *AIDS*, 8, 239–46.

Chaava, T. (1990) Approaches to counselling in a Zambian rural community. *AIDS Care*, 2, 81–7.

Chela, C.M. & Siankanga, Z.C. (1991) Home and Community Care: the Zambian experience. *AIDS*, suppl. 1, S157–161.

Dawson, J., Fitzpatrick, R., McLean, J., Hart, G. & Boulton, M. (1991) The HIV test and sexual behaviour in a sample of homosexually active men. *Social Science Medicine*, 32, 683–8.

D'Costa, L.J., Plummer, F.A., Bowmer, I., Fransen, L., Piot, P., Ronald, A.R. & Nsanze, H. (1985) Prostitutes are a major reservoir of sexually transmitted diseases in Nairobi, Kenya. *Sexually Transmitted Diseases*, 12, 64–7.

Fox, L.J., Bailey, P.E., Clarke-Martinez, K.L., Coello, M., Ordonez, F.N. & Barahona, F. (1993). Condom use among high-risk women in Honduras: evaluation of an AIDS prevention program. *AIDS Education and Prevention*, 5, 1–10.

Goodgame, R.W. (1990) AIDS in Uganda, clinical and social features. *New England Journal of Medicine*, 323, 383–9.

Green, J. & Kocsis, A. (1995) Social support in HIV disease. In: *Handbook of Stress Medicine* (ed. C. Cooper). CRC Press, London.

Higgins, D.L., Galovotti, C., O'Reilly, K.R., Schnell, D.J., Moore, M. & Rugg, D.J. (1991) Evidence for the effects of HIV antibody counselling and testing on risk behaviours. *Journal of American Medical Association*, 266, 2419–24.

Landis, S.E., Earp, J.L. & Koch, G.G. (1992) Impact of HIV testing and counselling on subsequent sexual behaviour. *AIDS Education and Prevention*, 4, 61–70.

Ngugi, E.N., Plummer, F.A., Simonsen, J.N. *et al.* (1988) Public health: prevention of transmission of human immunodeficiency virus in Africa: effectiveness of condom promotion and health education among prostitutes. *Lancet*, 2, 887–90.

Nzilambi, N., Laga, M., Thiam, M.A. *et al.* (1991) HIV and other sexually transmitted diseases among female prostitutes in Kinshasa. *AIDS*, 5, 715–21.

Otten, M.W. Jr., Zaida, A.A., Wroten, J.E., Witte, J.J. & Peterman, T.A. (1993) Changes in sexually transmitted disease rates after HIV testing and post-test counselling, Miami, 1988–1989. *American Journal of Public Health*, 83, 529–33.

Pickering, H., Quigley, M., Pepin, J., Todd, J. & Wilkins, A. (1993) The effects of post-test counselling on condom use among prostitutes in The Gambia. *AIDS*, 7, 271–3.

Plourde, P.J., Plummer, F.A., Pepin, J. *et al.* (1992) Human immunodeficiency virus type I infection in women attending a sexually transmitted disease clinic in Kenya. *Journal of Infectious Diseases*, 166, 86–92.

Rosenberg, M.J., Feldblum, P.J., Rojanapithayakorn, W. & Sawasdivorn, W. (1987) The contraceptive sponge's protection against Chlamydia trachomatis and Neisseria gonorrhoea. *Sexually Transmitted Diseases*, 14, 147–52.

Ryder, R.W., Batter, U.L., Nsuami, M., Badi, N. *et al.* (1991) Fertility rates in 238 HIV seropositive women in Zaire followed for three years post-partum. *AIDS*, 5, 1521–2.

Simonsen, J.N., Plummer, F.A. & Ngugi, E.N. (1990) HIV infection among lower socio-economic strata prostitutes in Nairobi. *AIDS*, 4, 139–44.

Temmerman, M., Ndinya-Achola, J., Ambani, J. & Piot, P. (1995) The right not to know HIV-test results. *Lancet*, 345, 969–71.

Wenger, N.S., Linn, L.S., Epstein, M. & Shapiro, M.F. (1991) Reduction of high-risk sexual behaviour among heterosexuals undergoing HIV antibody testing: a randomised clinical trial. *American Journal of Public Health*, 81, 1580–5.

Zenilman, J.M., Erickson, B., Fox, R., Reichart, C.A. & Hook, E.W. (1992) Effect of HIV post-test counselling on STD incidence. *Journal of American Medical Association*, 267, 843–5.

Zunzunegui, M.V., King, M.C., Coria, C.F. & Charlet, J. (1986) Male influences on cervical cancer risk. *American Journal of Epidemiology*, 123, 302–7.

Chapter 19

Relaxation

Agnes Kocsis

Learning the skills of relaxation is valuable for many people who are under stress. People with HIV infection and AIDS are no different in this respect. Many patients to whom we have taught relaxation techniques have found them very helpful and positive.

If relaxation were easy we would all do it. Ironically, the more stressed one is, the harder it is to relax. It is therefore pointless to tell a stressed person to go away and relax. While it is possible simply to give them a relaxation tape and tell them to play it, a large proportion of people will fail to gain benefit from it without further preparation. If someone is often, or has become, chronically tense, that is no accident – they have learned to be that way. Often tension is perceived as a necessary survival tactic, as summed up in the plea, 'Don't tell me to relax – it's my tension that's holding me together'. Teaching someone to relax, therefore, requires several stages.

The value of relaxation

It is helpful to review with patients why relaxation is valuable:

- By reducing anxiety and counteracting stress, it improves subjective wellbeing
- It has direct beneficial effects on bodily functioning by relieving the physical effects of anxiety and stress, for instance it can reduce blood pressure
- Stress in itself can result in lowering of immune system responses and therefore counteracting it is likely to be beneficial.

Preparing the ground

The objections

While accepting that relaxation is a good idea in principle, individuals often give reasons as to why they cannot practise it. They may say that they do not have time, that those around them would not approve if they were 'not active', or that relaxation is 'self-indulgent'. Or they may feel that their anxiety 'keeps them together'.

Some people get more reward from their stress or busyness than they imagine. Being stressed and always 'busy' may fit in with their ideal image of themselves, whereas taking time to relax may not. Therefore the counsellor who is preparing a stressed person for relaxation has to start at the basics if the client is to comply with the programme. Aspects which prevent the person taking up relaxation need to be discussed and confronted. Some issues that can be explored include:

- Priorities – the choices between health or stress, work or personal wellbeing
- Giving oneself permission to look after oneself and one's health
- Others would probably prefer a person who takes time to relax but is well, rather than someone who is perpetually stretched
- Being realistic – real efficiency and productivity usually come with a calm mind and are not necessarily produced by a busy body.

The aim is that the patient will give themselves permission to relax and that they can identify times and places during the day when it will be possible to do so.

Defining stress

It is important for the counsellor and the patient to agree what is stressful for the patient; what is stressful for some people is not stressful for others. They also need to explore how the patient recognises that they are stressed; different people recognise when they are under stress in different ways. A list of these can be drawn up jointly for a particular patient. It may be increased irritability, or making more mistakes, or showing symptoms of anxiety, or simply feeling unable to cope, or some other set of symptoms.

The next step is to identify times of day and situations when the symptoms of stress are worst for the patient. This can be done by going back over the past few days, recalling and writing down the situation together with the tension experienced, and rating the tension on a scale of 1 to 5, where 1 is no tension and 5 is very high tension (Chapter 12).

Building on existing forms of relaxation

Most people will already have ways of relaxing in their lives and these can be built upon first before suggesting new ways of relaxing. The counsellor must beware of deciding for the patient what is going to be relaxing, just because it comes under that heading for the counsellor. Violent exercise, hang-gliding, washing floors or watching flowers grow can all be relaxing occupations for different people. Progress will be much easier if you work with these first, before suggesting other kinds of relaxation to try.

It is important to identify with patients the ways in which they relax. There are various general categories to explore:

- Active physical activities, e.g. squash, jogging, swimming, dancing, going for a walk, doing the housework, tidying up
- Sensuous physical activities, e.g. having a bath, going for a sauna, having a massage, sex, playing a musical instrument, preparing a special meal, eating and drinking, yoga

- Stimulating mental activities, watching television, listening to the radio, going to the theatre or cinema, listening to music, reading, conversing, doing the crossword
- Mental activities which reduce stimulation, e.g. locking oneself away in the bathroom or in the home, taking the phone off the hook, day–dreaming, dosing.

These are all constructive ways of relaxing. However, individuals may have ways of relaxing which, in the long term, can cause more problems than they solve; for instance, excessive use of alcohol or drugs. These need to be elicited and talked through.

A list of ways in which the patient can relax will help you and the patient decide whether they tend to relax more through muscular activity or through mental processes. This is of value later.

The next step is to discuss how they are currently using these relaxing activities in their life and to find ways in which they can enhance them or incorporate them more frequently and consciously. When people are relatively cheerful and coping, they will partake in relaxation often without labelling it as such. They will also spontaneously use activities to cheer themselves up and to unwind at the end of the day. Unfortunately, when people get anxious and depressed, instead of stepping up the amount of relaxing activities they often do not bother about relaxation or put it low on their list of priorities, and spend all their time worrying or feeling low. It needs a conscious decision then not only to remember that the enjoyable parts of life still exist, but that incorporating them into everyday life is a sensible way of coping – not meaningless self-indulgence.

Preparing a relaxation tape

The use of a relaxation tape can help someone to relax. Finding out about the patient's preferred forms of relaxation will have given an indication of whether the patient has a preference for physical or mental relaxation, or whether perhaps both are enjoyed. This preference will affect the preparation of the tape.

There are many commercially available relaxation tapes. These vary in quality, but the main problem is that they tend to be too general and not to take individual variation into account. There are two advantages in the counsellor and the patient working on developing a tailor made relaxation tape together:

- The patient will end up with a tape to suit them personally
- During its preparation the patient will have had to consider, experiment and choose what they find relaxing, in the process becoming more aware of relaxation as an important activity.

It will probably be most reassuring for the patient if, when the content has been agreed, the tape is recorded by the counsellor. Occasionally the patient may prefer to ask a friend to do it, or even to record their own voice.

In the instructions below, pauses will be required. The counsellor will have to use judgement on the length of pause. There are several possible components for a relaxation tape, and which should be included and the balance between them will vary with individual patient preference.

Breathing exercises

Control of breathing is a crucial skill for anyone who experiences anxiety with physical symptoms. There are several ways to learn control breathing, two of which are given below. Try each of these out with the patient in the session and send them away to practise. When the patient has chosen what suits them best, record instructions for that exercise on the tape.

Hands on stomach

This method is useful in social situations because the patient can quite comfortably keep their hands folded on their stomach without anybody noticing they are practising relaxation. The following are example instructions.

Place your hands flat and touching, with fingers laced, on the lower part of your stomach, just above your pelvis. Spend a few moments noticing how your stomach is moving as you breathe. Now exaggerate the movement slightly, so that you can really feel your stomach move upwards as you breathe in and downwards as you breathe out. Now imagine something slow and peaceful and comfortable. You are strolling down a country lane on a sunny day and you are listening out for the distant sound of the sea. You can just hear the regular comforting sound of the waves breaking on the shore. There is no wind and the waves make a slow, infinitely regular sound. Breathe in time with the waves.

This image can be adapted according to the patient's preference. If the patient cannot easily visualise, they could think of a slow piece of music or could count. The disadvantage of counting is that when people are anxious it is difficult for them to count slowly. An alternative is to say a phrase when breathing in, and another when breathing out, for example: 'Now, be calm' (breathe in); 'Relaxation is a balm' (breathe out).

Breathing out and up

Example instructions:
This is best done lying flat. Lie down in a warm, convenient spot and make your body comfortable. Place your hands with fingers splayed on your ribcage, just under your nipples or breasts. Now half breathe in by pushing your chest up to the ceiling, and then finish the breath by pulling your ribcage towards your head. Hold the breath for a moment, and let go. Do this just three times. (Pause.) Then breathe normally and feel the pleasant lightness in your head. Let yourself float.

Muscular relaxation

There are two ways of relaxing muscles, which can be done while lying still. Both involve going over the body systematically and relaxing each muscle or group of muscles in turn. It is usual to start at one end of the body and work towards the other, but this is not essential. Some people like to start with, say, their back, because that is such a nerve-packed area.

The first method is especially valuable for those who have never really thought about relaxing and do not have much awareness of how tense or relaxed their body might be. It involves, paradoxically, tensing each muscle even more – and then letting go. This method means that everyone can achieve the sensation of letting go some of the tension, even if just a little. It is helpful to synchronise each muscle relaxation exercise with breathing in and out. Example instructions are given below for the upper torso. Each muscle group is repeated twice. The instructions should be extended by simply replacing the parts of the body referred to with the muscles of the lower back, the upper thighs, the knees, the calves, the ankles and the toes. The instructions should be read at a slow, comfortable pace, attempting to impose a rhythm on the exercises:

Start with your hands. Focus on your hands. Feel the tension in your hands. Now start to breathe in and curl your fingers up into a fist. Tense them three-quarters tense; tense, but not too tense. Hold – and let go. And again. Start to breathe in. Curl your fingers into a fist. Tense them, but not too tense. Prepare to breathe out and let go the tension. Feel the tension move out of your hands. Now your arms. Prepare to breathe in. Now tense your arms and breathe in. Tense up, but not too tense. Hold – prepare to breathe out – and let go. Say goodbye to the tension. And your arms again. Prepare to breathe in. Tense – feel the tension. And prepare to breathe out. Let go the tension. Now your shoulders. Prepare to breathe in. Now move your shoulders back as far as they will go. Push them back under you. Hold – prepare to breathe out – and let go. Now the shoulders again. Prepare to breathe in. Now push the shoulders back, push them against one another. Hold – prepare to let go – and breathe out.

The second method of muscle relaxation is for those who have a sense of muscle tension and already know how to manipulate it. This can be done lying in any comfortable position, on the front or back. The body must feel well supported. A high pillow is not helpful for most people. Unless very uncomfortable it is probably best to lie quite flat. Example instructions follow:

I want you now to make a journey through your body. You are journeying to the different parts of your body to relax them. As your journey goes on, more and more of your body will feel comfortable. Start at your head. Make your head go heavy. Let it sink into the floor. You do not have to support any part of your head. The floor is there to support it for you. Give your head to the floor to support. Now your arms. Stop holding your arms. Let them go. Let the floor support your arms for the moment. Feel now that you have no responsibility for your arms. Now your upper body. Let your upper body go completely. Let it sink into the floor. Your body is sinking deeper and deeper, is being held by the floor.

The instructions can be extended for the legs and the feet.

Sensuous imagery

For those individuals identified early on as enjoying mental stimulation and day-dreaming, imagery and visualisation can be a potent form of relaxation. The essence is to discover images which the patient finds soothing and pleasurable. The images should be texturally rich and detailed, with colour, shape, sound touch and even smell if this can be achieved. People vary enormously in their ability to visualise scenes or sensations, and not everyone will find this pleasurable or possible. It is of course vital to explore which images will be pleasant. Some people for example hate lying on a beach and listening to the seagulls, while others do not enjoy the countryside. Example instructions are given here:

It is a warm day in early summer and you are waiting for a friend in the countryside. You are anticipating having a happy day together. You are lying on some new grass, close to a willow tree. There is a stream alongside you and you can sense the coolness of the water as it runs past to a small waterfall. As you lie there with your eyes closed and the sun warming your eyelids, you can hear the soft whisper of the waterfall. The water makes you feel thirsty. You take an orange from your bag and run your fingers over its cool skin. It is a beautiful, vibrant colour. You peel it slowly with your fingers, feeling the moistness of its thick flesh and smelling the oil as it spurts on to your fingers. You part the orange segments and feel their silky surface. You can anticipate the sweetness of the juice you are about to taste, the coolness and sweetness.

Memories of happiness

Along similar lines, you can discuss a moment in the client's life when they remember being particularly happy. This can either be described in detail on the tape, or if the patient prefers to remember it privately, they can be prompted to do this for a few minutes.

Incorporating music or sounds

Moods are generally very responsive to music and even particular sounds. Patients can be encouraged to identify music which they associate with happiness or relaxation and to incorporate this on the tape. Flutes, pan-pipes and harps are often used to create a soothing ambience, but again this is idiosyncratic. It can be quite interesting to try to identify your most soothing piece of music.

Poems, uplifting words

Those who like poetry may wish to record particularly meaningful pieces. Those with HIV are sometimes interested in 'talking to the virus' in their body. Any statements that they wish to use could also be incorporated. Alternatively, the following statements could be used:

● I am becoming a more relaxed person
● I am enjoying taking control of my body, and my life

Preparing to use the tape – setting the scene

When the tape has been prepared, discuss with the client when they are likely to use it, and where. It should be used daily if possible. Sometimes patients pose difficulties: 'My flatmate is there, I can't disturb her'; 'I'm too busy to listen to the tape every day'; etc. These excuses have to be confronted. It is a question of priorities. Friends are usually fascinated by relaxation tapes and if anything want to join in.

Dealing with panic attacks

If the client experiences panic attacks with overbreathing, and is planning to try to return to the situations feared most (Chapter 12), it is helpful to discuss the strategies they are going to use. The breathing, and to some extent the muscle relaxation, are likely to be most helpful. The example instructions here are for someone who tends to panic in the supermarket.

On your way there, I want you to prepare your body. You are preparing your breathing and your muscles. You are going to keep relaxing the muscles of your neck, your shoulders and your chest – your upper chest and your lower chest. You are going to walk out, feeling the strength in your body. You are going to walk confidently and with suppleness. Keep checking your breathing and your muscles. Think of the exercises. Now you are taking control. Do not take any notice of your heart beating or any of your body's fear responses. You are going into the supermarket and you are going to beat your anxiety. It is not a dangerous place. If you feel your anxiety rising, practise your breathing. Aim for a natural, smooth rhythm. Remember the rhythm of the waves, beating on the shore.

Although it is usual to listen to the tape in a private place and lying comfortably, some people have used their tapes in a personal stereo while on the street or in the underground. This can be very helpful for people who are worried about experiencing panic attacks or who are practising getting back into their feared situations. Additional comforting thoughts can be pre-recorded. Examples are:

- 'I'm not alone in this. My counsellor is going to be really pleased that I've done this. *I'm* going to be really pleased that I've done it.'
- 'Even if I panic, it's only my body playing up. I've got to reassure my body. There's no real danger. There are no lions in this supermarket.'
- 'My heart's beating very fast, but it's not doing me any harm. Physically I am quite all right. This just shows my body knows how to react to danger if it has to. But here it doesn't have to.'

Monitoring the programme

The whole relaxation programme comprises two, or possibly three parts:

- The incorporation of relaxation into everyday life
- Preparation and use of the relaxation tape
- Preparing to deal with a panic attack.

In order for the patient and counsellor to monitor how the programme is going, it may be helpful to keep a daily diary. This can be in the form of a check-list incorporating the relaxing activities discussed, to be filled in every day:

Monday

	Time	How relaxed
Tape	11PM	5
Jogging	8PM	3
Listened to music	10PM	4
Spent time with friends	6–8PM	2

Alternatively, if someone's anxiety varies a great deal during the day and they wish to practise incorporating relaxation as much as possible, a fear 'thermometer' chart can be used for each day, marking shifts in state of relaxation (Fig. 19.1).

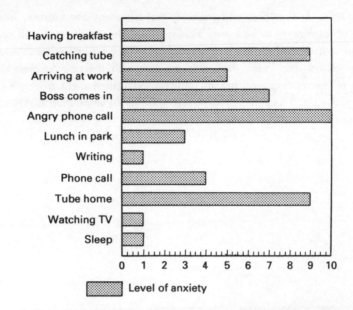

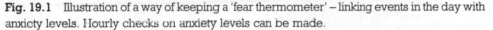

Fig. 19.1   Illustration of a way of keeping a 'fear thermometer' – linking events in the day with anxiety levels. Hourly checks on anxiety levels can be made.

Modifying and perfecting the programme

As the patient becomes increasingly skilled at relaxing and using the relaxation tape, some of the exercises will become second nature and the patient will be able to do them without the tape. This applies particularly to the muscles exercises. The patient may then prefer to use the tape only for imagery or music. They may wish to prepare another tape.

The diary keeping should not be continued for so long that it becomes a chore. Sometimes it is better to keep a diary every third week.

General points to remember

During the whole relaxation work with the patient, it is important to emphasise monitoring of tension. The more tense someone is to start with, the harder it is to relax. It is therefore important for them to get into the habit of monitoring their level of tension, so as to be able to intervene early enough. This may mean checking and relaxing as often as every minute in some situations, every few hours in others. Relaxation must become an integral part of life.

People who have been anxious for many years, prior to HIV infection rather than just in response to becoming seropositive or being diagnosed as having AIDS, may find relaxation itself quite anxiety-provoking at first. It should be pointed out to them that this is not surprising, since they have been using anxiety to cope, as a sort of attempt at survival. The trouble is that the attempt was counterproductive. Now they will be learning a more effective survival method. But for a while they will feel anxious about letting the old one go. This is normal and they should just practise regularly. The anxiety will fade quickly.

It is crucial to emphasise that relaxation takes time. All the exercises have to be learnt and practised regularly. At first they will probably feel laborious and clumsy, like the initial awkwardness of learning to drive a car. This is inevitable and patients will only feel disappointed and discouraged if they are allowed to expect an immediate, heady sense of relaxation. It will certainly come. But daily practice with the tape, as well as the active incorporation of the relaxing pastimes and activities identified at the beginning of the sessions, will be necessary. The aim is to allow relaxation to permeate their lifestyle, not simply to be added on top of an existing lifestyle.

Chapter 20

Staff Stress, Occupational Morbidity and Burnout: Current Understanding and Models of Care

David Miller

Introduction

There has been much discussion about the importance of burnout in management of HIV, particularly because of the potentially damaging effects on staff members of working in HIV, and the consequences this may have for staff morale, sickness, absenteeism and turnover in vital care facilities (Miller 1991). In the UK there was an instance of the closure of high-profile and unique care service for people with AIDS (PWAs), partly due to poor recognition of the need to accommodate the unique burdens that work in HIV/AIDS may generate for those working in this field (Moreland & Legg 1991). However, discussions of burnout in the HIV literature have tended to rely on anecdote and speculation rather than solid data and clear use of terms, with the result that when burnout has been discussed, more heat than light has been generated and suggestions for constructive ways forward have remained rooted more in hope than proven experience or empiricism.

This chapter aims to clarify terms, to identify the main themes in staff stress and care from the experiences of researchers and clinicians in HIV/AIDS, to identify why prevention of staff stress may be particularly necessary in HIV/AIDS, and to characterise some models for intervention. It should be stated from the start, however, that in this particular area there are few studies that have tested the real value of staff stress management or emotional support.

Background: the problems of definition

Considerable literature was generated in the decade before the AIDS era on the subject of burnout and its manifestations. The most influential work was that of Maslach and Jackson, particularly because they developed a theoretical and empirical base that has been the starting point for much subsequent research activity. Maslach and Jackson (1982) identify burnout as a multidimensional process with three central constructs:

- Emotional exhaustion – having no capacity left to offer psychological support to others
- Depersonalisation – a negative and callous attitude to colleagues and patients
- Reduced sense of personal accomplishment – playing down or disregarding positive job performance and past achievements.

The significance of this for contemporary HIV/AIDS work is not entirely clear. While many studies use the Maslach burnout inventory (MBI) (Maslach & Jackson 1982) as a basis for identifying potential or actual burnout in health, educational and industrial workers, deriving a score relative to norms with such an instrument may not be the same as identifying real or potential burnout. I suspect that the constructs employed in the MBI and similar much less standardised and validated instruments, together reflect a relatively rare syndrome of increasing occupational dysfunction and decline. It may well be the case that health workers, including those involved with HIV/AIDS, carry into their occupations varying levels of sub-clinical morbidity that affect their efficiency or psychosocial state to varying degrees at different times. There is a suspicion arising from a recent study by Wallace and Brinkeroff (1991), for example, that in a 'human service worker' only one of the MBI scales (emotional exhaustion) is a reliable and valid measure, and that burnout therefore requires reconceptualisation theoretically and operationally.

Aside from research initiatives that have endeavoured to create a reliable theoretical framework for investigation and management of staff burnout, clinical reports have also described an often spectacular phenomenology associated with burnout in its most extreme sense (e.g. McElroy 1982). While such descriptions are compelling, it is again unusual to observe the full spectrum of described features all together. Rather, it seems that most health workers subjected to stressful (particularly clinical) working circumstances will identify some symptoms that recur and come to characterise their perceptions of health work. These are, in most circumstances, manageable to the extent that their most conspicuous features can be contained, although not necessarily cured. Commonly reported symptoms of staff stress, and those commonly reported in association with staff burnout, are listed in Table 20.1.

It may well be the case, therefore, that those symptoms and constructs that may contribute to an eventual occupational dysfunction are not quite as dramatic or as frequently observed as earlier burnout reports have suggested; and that instead, occupational staff care and management should be focusing on basically sub-clinical psychosocial and psychological morbidities that have hitherto been carried by individual health workers as burdens that 'go with the territory' of commitment, care for the community, and peer engagement for public health. In other words, the concept of burnout may helpfully be discarded as being too unclear, too dramatic, too emotive, and not reflecting the clinical realities of health care staff stress.

This does not mean that the previously-described sub-clinical morbidities should remain unacknowledged by health managers. On the contrary, where recent reports have indicated, for instance, that staff sickness and absenteeism may be costing the UK hundreds of millions of pounds per year in lost production, the appropriateness of mounting or improving staff care is undeniable.

If such consequences for production are acknowledged, why are the possible stresses giving rise to them so often sub-clinical; why is there such a reluctance to individually and institutionally acknowledge that our work can and does generate psychosocial and psychological difficulties for many of those doing it? Surely this could only make matters worse? The case for clear and unprejudiced acknowledgement and characterisation of health care staff stress becomes increasingly irresistible.

Table 20.1 Reported symptoms of staff stress and burnout.

Physical
- Physical exhaustion
- Lingering minor illnesses
- Headaches and back pain
- Sleeplessness
- Gastro-intestinal disturbances
- Malaise

Behavioural
- Readiness to be irritated
- Proneness to anger
- Increased alcohol and drug use
- Marital and relationship problems
- Inflexibility in problem-solving
- Impulsivity and acting out
- Self-righteousness
- Withdrawal from non-colleagues

Cognitive/affective
- Emotional numbness
- Emotional hypersensitivity
- Over-identification with patients
- Grief and sadness
- Pessimism and hopelessness
- Boredom and cynicism
- Indecision and inattention
- Depression

What causes staff stress and occupational morbidity?

Received understanding from non–AIDS settings is that work stressors can appear on many levels, and may be substantially interrelated; for example, Cooper (1983) identifies six major categories of work stressor:

(1) Job-specific factors, such as dangers, work satisfaction and work load
(2) Role within the organisation and problems with this, including role ambiguity, conflict, and role territoriality
(3) Career structures and processes, including prospects for promotion and job security
(4) Work-based relationships, including levels of emotional and social support from colleagues, bosses and subordinates
(5) Organisational structures and flexibility, including real participation in decision-making
(6) Pressures on family life resulting from work.

Findings from health care literature reinforce these categories and suggest that stresses associated with them are ubiquitous (Kahill 1988; Miller 1991). In studies of mental health professionals, including family therapists and clinical psychologists, stress (and the presumed potential for burnout) has increasingly been found to be a function of denial of the health worker's own emotional needs while continuing to give all care possible to others (e.g.

Maynard 1985; McCarthy 1989; Walsh 1990). Walsh found that clinical psychologists face considerable obstacles to admitting and responding to occupational stress, including:

(1)   The 'debilitating nature of professional values' associated with the job, involving the threat of lost credibility, lost equality with non-support-receiving colleagues, and lost job security
(2)   The fear of becoming a client; having needs for emotional support is construed as being unfit to work in the profession.

If such results can be generalised, it is easy to see how personal needs in response to stress at work can be minimised and may lead, if unresolved, to serious personal difficulties. Walsh importantly identified the need to distinguish between receiving professional (case management) support and receiving emotional support.

Findings from cohorts of oncology staff suggest that specific elements of oncology care, including administration of toxic and illness-inducing chemotherapy, managing the psychosocial needs of dying patients and their families, and unit administration, are major causes of stress (e.g. Bailey *et al.* 1980; Gray-Toft & Anderson 1980, 1981). The Bailey study also paradoxically revealed that patient care and interpersonal relationships were among the elements giving greatest work satisfaction. Clearly, individual perception of work stressors and their meanings is the critical mediator of experienced stress, according to these findings. A further issue raised in these studies is the importance of giving health staff adequate preparation and training for management of such stress issues. Experience has been shown to buffer potentially stressful work circumstances in a number of recent studies (e.g. Bennett *et al.* 1991).

Other studies have found that stress and (MBI-defined) burnout may be a consequence of unrealistic demands on clinical expertise, time, availability and limited resources, often in a context of workers having similarly unrealistic expectations about what they can achieve (Lyall 1989). Gladding (1991) describes mental health counsellor self-abuse as not learning from the past or not setting proper boundaries for themselves with their clients and colleagues. Burnout can result, along with unethical behaviour and inappropriate countertransference behaviours being manifest.

Increasingly health care is multidisciplinary and this can lead to significant clashes of professional culture resulting in work stress, especially where line management and professional roles and responsibilities become blurred. Further, there is some controversy over the importance of institutional affiliation for development of staff stress; Farber (1990) suggests that institutionally based and inexperienced psychotherapists are most at risk, while non-school counsellors (those away from institutions) had a greater concern for burnout in a survey by Housley *et al.* (1990). From a survey in the UK, it is clear that pressures associated with institutional management and resources are a significant factor in the development and recognition of work stressors among HIV/AIDS workers (Miller 1993). It also seems increasingly the case that specific institutional dynamics are reflected in different mean scores in the MBI and other instruments (e.g. Bennett *et al.* 1991), suggesting that management of institutional stressors should be localised.

What extra burdens do HIV workers face?

Although it is not proven that the burdens faced by HIV/AIDS health care workers are unique (Kleiber *et al.* 1992), the attention given to the potential for staff stress in this area probably is. It is nevertheless clear that stresses in HIV/AIDS work are compounded by the high profile and often contradictory media emphases the epidemic has attracted. Studies have highlighted the pressures in HIV/AIDS care associated with:

- Anxieties over safe working practices and fears of contagion (Gordin *et al.* 1987)
- The intensity of staff–patient relationships over long term health care and episodic, often eventually fatal, decline (Morin & Batchelor 1984; Miller 1987; Ross & Seeger 1988; Bennett *et al.* 1991)
- Self-identification with people with HIV/AIDS (Horstman & McKusick 1986)
- Perceived lack of support among volunteer care populations whose roles and expectations for care are often less clear than in statutory service personnel (Guinan *et al.* 1991; Maslanka 1992)
- Care-role expansion, particularly in domestic care-givers, i.e. loved-ones and family (Pearlin *et al.* 1988).

Further, as noted in Miller 1992b, the potential for occupational stress in HIV care workers can be expected to increase in the near future, in developed and developing countries, for the following reasons:

- Numbers of people with recognised HIV and AIDS are rising rapidly, mortality in many areas is more frequent and overwork is increasing
- Resources in many areas are proportionally decreasing
- In many parts of the world whole communities are increasingly becoming implicated and so there is less possibility in such places for health care workers to find distance from the disease
- Patient-presenting characteristics are altering; the 'patient' increasingly is the whole family, or groups and communities of orphans, etc.
- Many management uncertainties remain unresolved or are growing – treatment options, care capacity, resource-building capacity etc.
- Many overt psychological pressures are being increasingly recognised as evident and important in care and management, and in communities without the specialised resources to manage such manifestations (although community mechanisms for psychosocial management and care may be well-established in related contexts)
- Many HIV/AIDS carers are complaining of stress and recognising the need for care for themselves.

Increasing numbers of reports describe the psychological toll of working in a context of multiple loss of patients and bereavement within peer groups:

- Being unable to 'escape' from work
- Feeling a lack of trust in colleagues and finding problems in moving from the supportive role to being supported
- Working within a relatively young staff population
- Experiencing an increasing lack of resources

- A lack of ability to participate in decision-making about management of individuals or the wider social aspects of epidemic administration.

Health workers on lower scales of the career ladder may find themselves trapped in positions with high expectations placed upon them, feeling the weight of responsibility without sufficient authority to perform in the way they would wish. And always, the pressure to fight against time, political inertia or lassitude, social stigma, media fashion, and sometimes bewildering role expansion, follows the daily routine of many HIV/AIDS workers, exerting further expectations on and by HIV/AIDS health workers.

This is not to say that such work is unremittingly negative for those doing it; if that were so, no-one would do it. Studies by Horstman and McKusick (1986), and Ross and Seeger (1988) revealed in particular how increased intellectual stimulation and work satisfaction may be an important sustainer for HIV workers in the face of the potentially negative experiences already described.

It is also important to recognise that the potential for burnout or occupational stress and morbidity may be an institutional experience, as well as an individual one. A review of the stages of response made by the drug abuse treatment system to HIV/AIDS in New York (des Jarlais 1990) identifies institutional stages of denial, panic and coping as the realities of the HIV epidemic are avoided, recognised and accommodated. However, a potential fourth stage is described as burnout where perhaps the combined and unremitting imperatives of HIV/AIDS responses, care and management overwhelm services and the personnel within them. The experience of the closure of a major peer-led community service for people with AIDS in London, called Frontliners, highlighted the particular vulnerabilities of volunteer and peer-led bodies that struggle to accommodate the burgeoning demands placed on them by a grateful public. In many instances it will be community based, focal programmes that tackle the acute needs of people at risk, perhaps in a manner that is more accessible and even more relevant to the needs of those for and by whom they have been developed. However, when the shape of the epidemic changes, and responses need to change with them, problems may arise that can eventually cripple the organisation. This was part of the reason for the closure of Frontliners. The three key factors identified were:

- The lack of relevant management experience in those leading the organisation
- The very rapid expansion of the organisation in response to the demands of members and funders
- The transition from self-help (for people with AIDS by people with AIDS) to service provision undertaken without sufficient research or planning (Moreland & Legg 1991).

Systems or institutions can look after their own staff by ensuring that they are appropriately equipped with skills and with clear roles with which to express them (Kleiber *et al.* 1992), as well as with support on an emotional and professional level. Those that do so will, it is assumed, be able to provide a better quality of care for people affected by HIV/AIDS over the longer term. However, even that may not be sufficient, particularly where seroprevalence is still relatively low:

- Where there are fewer identified people with HIV, stigma may correspondingly be higher
- Prevention activity may be taking place in a context of indifference

- There may be a greater tendency to externalise responsibility for HIV prevention and care, making HIV activities undervalued
- Where responses to HIV identification are infrequent, there may be no clear occupational network or management structure, so professional expectations, roles and boundaries may be unclear
- Lack of experience may be reflected in a lack of confidence, in a context of insufficient work
- Where facilities are eager to learn and develop HIV/AIDS expertise, there may be competition for resources, skills and patients
- Existing professional skills and established procedures are frequently being challenged
- Every new case may be seen as a crisis.

What obstacles exist to implementation of effective health staff care?

In addition to the burdens listed above, current research reveals that major obstacles exist to implementation and usage of appropriate staff support programmes; for example:

- Staff may often not know precisely what they want when they say they want staff support or when they are offering it
- Professional supervision and monitoring are frequently confused with emotional support
- Many assumptions are being made about the degree of trust that colleagues may have for each other; frequently, it seems, staff refuse to disclose their emotional vulnerability to others because they do not know how that information will be perceived or subsequently be used
- There remains a prevailing view that disclosure of vulnerability is dangerous because it will be seen as indicative of non-professionalism or unsuitability to do the job
- Staff may feel unable to move from the supportive role to being supported in the workplace, even for brief periods
- There may be insufficient time or staff cover to allow regular or reliable support sessions
- Health professionals in HIV/AIDS are working within a culture of secrecy while facing the acute and complex needs of their patients
- There may be assumptions made about the appropriate development and maintenance of interventions designed to improve staff morale, but which may actually be counter-productive, e.g. support groups may have very limited effective duration, yet may be carried on to the point of adding to staff tensions rather than reducing them.

Suggestions and models for staff stress management and prevention

The need for effective models of staff stress management and prevention is more pressing than ever. Such models are generally absent or have yet to be clearly characterised. As a result, suggestions for interventions rarely have outcome data upon which to assess their efficacy or value (and/or their potential for making things worse!). Table 20.2 gives guidance rather than providing hard recommendations for intervention.

Table 20.2   Models for staff stress management and prevention.

	Professional supervision	Emotional support/ therapeutic counselling	Stress reduction/ management	Context management
Facilitator	External or internal	External or internal	External or internal	Not applicable
Nature	Individual or group ('Team')	Individual or group ('Team')	Individual or group ('Team')	See below
Regularity	Regular or irregular (on demand)	Regular or irregular (on demand)	Regular or irregular (on demand)	Continuous
Duration	On-going	On-going or limited duration (e.g. crisis management)	On-going or limited duration (e.g. crisis management)	Continuous
Frequency	Weekly, fortnightly or monthly	Weekly, fortnightly or monthly, or on request	Weekly, fortnightly or monthly, or on request	Not applicable
Composition	Same or mixed professions	Same or mixed professions for groups	Same or mixed professions for groups	Applies to all staff
Content	Case review, professional monitoring, skills assessment	Ventilation, emotional support, team-building and restoration	Relaxation strategies, including meditation, visualisation/ imagery, massage, shiatsu and exercise, seminars and classes in, for example, time management, team-building, etc.	See text

Staff stress management may be divided into four types:

(1)   Professional supervision
(2)   Emotional support/therapeutic counselling
(3)   Stress reduction/management programmes
(4)   Context management

These are discussed in turn below.

Professional supervision

This is the intervention provided to monitor and enhance the clinical and professional activities of health care workers. It may be provided to teams, such as ward staffs or community care units, or to individual health professionals. It may be provided by supervisors from within or outside the setting in which people are being supervised, and where groups or teams are being supervised they may be of either the same or mixed professions. Such intervention may also be regular or irregular.

As the intention of professional supervision is usually to maintain standards of professional care, it will most commonly involve reviewing case or patient management, monitoring professional understanding and practices, and evaluating professional procedures and skills. In voluntary contexts where codes of professionalism cannot necessarily be enforced, professional supervision may more appropriately be thought of as 'supervision of appropriate standards of intervention', perhaps by a professionally qualified and experienced health professional.

Emotional support/therapeutic counselling

As Table 20.2 illustrates, the format of emotional supervision/therapeutic counselling for health workers contains few major differences from those for professional supervision. There are important differences, however, in the aims and therefore content of each. In providing emotional support or therapeutic counselling to health staff, the intention is to relieve or support the health worker facing the stresses of their job. This implies an acceptance that:

(1) Their work contains stresses that may need to be addressed or ventilated
(2) Expression of emotional vulnerability associated with work is seen as a legitimate circumstance, rather than a sign of weakness or unprofessionalism.

The intention, therefore, includes ensuring that stresses do not become issues of crisis or, if they do, that crises can be localised and managed effectively for all concerned. Interventions under this general heading thus can contribute effectively to team-building or restoration, even when health workers are seen individually.

Examples of the type of interventions that may come within this model include that reported by Kesler (1990), in which Lazarus' BASIC ID schema for formulating psychological distress and interventions form a useful basis for understanding and resolving burnout. Maynard (1985) suggests that during crisis intervention staff seldom stop and identify their own feelings, but will mask them to maintain effectiveness with clients, although this will make it more difficult to stay attuned to their own feelings. Maynard describes the use of support groups to enable regular and free ventilation of suppressed/masked feelings to avoid build-up and burnout. In a similar vein, Friedman (1985) reports working with family therapists, giving attention to expectations, role definition, sharing of feelings and therapeutic ambition (and patients' versus therapists' responsibilities in this), to ease strain on the therapist.

Stress reduction/management

Once again the format of such interventions is relatively similar to those for professional supervision and emotional support/therapeutic counselling, yet the aims determine substantial differences in content. This mode of health worker care aims to directly reduce or prevent the experience of work-related stress, and usually employs active relaxation and stress-reduction techniques, and/or development of skills to prevent stress arising. These may take place within or outside work time, and to groups or individuals.

Recent approaches to stress reduction, management and prevention have been described by Strassmeier (1986), using a systems theory perspective to develop an ecosystem approach toward social networks, social development crisis intervention and help-seeking behaviour. Bair and Greenspan (1986) describe 'Training in Effectiveness through Assertiveness in a Medical Setting' (TEAMS) – a programme of workshops for multidisciplinary communication building and restoring. The aims are to increase collaborative practice, leadership skills, and knowledge of team-building and stress management. Pierey and Welchier (1987) have reported on a didactic-experiential workshop programme to examine and sort out issues from family therapists' own families and relationships, to enable them to avoid burnout which may otherwise result.

Context management

This mode of stress management or prevention involves environmental or contextual initiatives that assist in raising staff appreciation, and reducing staff stress. They may involve procedural initiatives such as limiting allowable working hours for health staff, or environmental initiatives such as the provision of quiet rest areas for staff, or refurbishment of facilities to make working environs more pleasant. Such interventions may also include:

- Organising working practices to encourage and facilitate a team spirit and teamwork
- Discouraging working alone
- Institutional provision of pre-work training which includes expectations of employees and acceptance of limits to such expectations (e.g. by setting realistic criteria for productivity and success in HIV-related work)
- Providing means for expressing and articulating successes in HIV care
- Institutional training in stress recognition and management for individuals, including advice on how to pace work once signs of stress are experienced
- Institutional acknowledgement of work stress and encouragement (without prejudice) to have stresses managed appropriately within the work framework – especially by providing structures and mechanisms for confidential staff support
- Ensuring task variation where possible
- Institutional encouragement for personal planning of work and non-work time, ensuring there remains a recognition of the difference between work and home, and the value of that difference
- Recognition of the need to grieve losses
- Institutional opportunities for refresher training and skills development
- Allowing holidays and actively encouraging that they be taken
- Avoiding an excessive focus on burnout and normalising the experience and expression of stress.

In this context it is interesting to speculate on the possible value of institutional structure and hierarchy in helping to reduce stress on health workers. Wilcoxon (1989) found that agencies with administrators with high initiative and consideration and a good structure had reduced reported therapist burnout in rural community health centres. Good structure was seen to be associated with reduced deterioration of therapist–client relations, presumably because everyone knew clearly where they stood. This notion of high institutional and/or professional structure resulting in lowered role ambiguity and therefore lowered occupational and role-related stress, is certainly deserving of closer study in future, perhaps by comparing health workers in the armed forces with those in the outside world. A similar assessment of the value of a clear institutional ideology would also shed important light on the potential for avoidance of occupational morbidity associated with health care, in religious contexts for example. Such lessons would be of particular value in settings such as many developing countries, where significant proportions of health care are provided by mission hospitals.

Implications for planning stress prevention

Perhaps the main point to be made about the divisions of stress prevention is that they are often confused, precisely because the different aims of each are not clearly considered in stress prevention planning. This is particularly so in observing the differences between professional supervision and emotional support. For example, where professional supervision is being given by a higher-ranking colleague (who themselves may be responsible for much of the stresses experienced by the junior colleague – especially where clinical and management responsibilities overlap), it may often be unrealistic to expect that emotional vulnerability will be admitted. Emotional stresses will not be expressed and may thus be seriously compounded (including stresses and pressures on the institution). There may also be considerable overlap between emotional support and stress management regimes, and while understandable and reasonable, it is important for such crossovers to be acknowledged by facilitators and staff where necessary.

Similarly, it is reasonable to assume that stress management will only be effectively taken up if it is seen to have the active support of management. In this way, health professionals may lose the fear that using such facilities exposes them to the charge of being professionally suspect or weak, or vulnerable. Such institutional and managerial endorsement may also help to reduce staff fears that their use of staff support facilities to express any occupationally-derived emotional vulnerability will result in their 'professional exposure' because of a lack of confidentiality of an institutional condition that all details be made known to managers. Support facilities will only usually succeed when confidentiality can be guaranteed.

It is also clear that these models for staff stress management and prevention are not mutually exclusive and can be employed in any combination. Although there is so little empirical data on efficacy of any approach, it seems likely that where more strategies are available to the individual health worker, one or some are more likely to be taken up, and the likelihood of effective beneficial outcome will be greater.

Finally, each of these general models conveys responsibilities both for the institution and the individuals involved. For the institution, a main responsibility is to make such models available, singly or in combination. For the individual a main responsibility is to make use of the models or, where they are not available, to argue coherently and appropriately for their establishment.

What more do we need to know?

Findings and impressions regarding staff stress, occupational morbidity and burnout – in HIV/AIDS and all other health staff – cannot yet be stated with full confidence. There are many methodological problems with research, including the lack of a rigorous operational definition of burnout. It is clear that health workers do experience levels of stress in their work, some of which relate to their specialist roles and some directly to the clinical versus administrative demands they face, for example Bailey *et al.* (1980); Gray-Toft & Anderson (1980, 1981); Stewart *et al.* (1982). But whether such studies can be said to be measuring burnout is often doubtful.

Many studies have employed different measures and may not all be measuring the same thing. Sample sizes in burnout research are often too small to achieve powerful measures of significance, and data-gathering instruments are frequently unclearly specified, making replication difficult. More recent studies in HIV/AIDS run the risk of imposing definitions of burnout which are then confirmed by the researchers using instruments that look only for the phenomena that the definition demands, and do not examine the wider roles of life outside the workplace, personality and other variables that may be critically important (Miller 1992a). Further, the temporary nature of burnout and occupational stress has been seriously neglected as a study issue (Cherniss 1992). How long does burnout last, and why?

As already stated, the value of prophylaxis needs urgent clarification, and the roles of contextual factors, including expressed ideology and structure, need re-examination. The merits of age and experience are increasingly being stated and deserve closer review, as do the specific stressors faced by volunteers and those working within peer-led community organisations – for too long the unsung slave labour behind the edifice of HIV community care. More needs to be learned from those who have experienced burnout so their experiences are not repeated. And models of stress management and prevention urgently need empirical examination so that their effectiveness can be characterised and repeated in those areas where it is most needed.

Finally, in this context it seems especially valuable to look outward to the experiences and findings of colleagues in non-health disciplines, to see if there are any measures that may be adopted from industry and other public service spheres. The importance of doing so and of taking up all the challenges stated here cannot be overstated when HIV still has no cure, no effective treatment, no demonstrated reliable obstacle to its remorseless social corrosion, and where experience is still our most valuable ally. Health workers without a sense of history and experience are health workers without a sense of achievement or hope. If we lose our colleagues because of avoidable stresses, we deplete one of our most vital potentials for epidemic control. Knowledge is responsibility, and for the sake of all our patients we have a responsibility to avoid such unnecessary waste.

References

Bailey, J.T., Steffen, S.M. & Grout, S.W. (1980) The stress audit: identifying the stressors with ICU nursing. *Journal of Nursing Education*, **19**, 15–25.

Bair, J.P. & Greenspan, B.K. (1986) TEAMS: Teamwork training for interns, residents and nurses. *Hospital and Community Psychiatry*, **37**(6) 633–5.

Bennett, L., Mitchie, P. & Kippax, S. (1991) Quantitative analysis of burnout and its associated factors in AIDS nursing. *AIDS Care*, **3**(2) 181–92.

Cherniss, C. (1992) Long-term consequences of burnout: an exploratory study. *Journal of Organisational Behaviour*, **13**(1) 1–11.

Cooper, C.L. (1983) Identifying stressors at work: recent research developments. *Journal of Psychosomatic Research*, **2**, 369–76.

Farber, B.A. (1990) Burnout in psychotherapists: incidence, types and trends. *Psychotherapy in Private Practice*, **8**(2) 35–44.

Friedman, R. (1985) Making family therapy easier for the therapist: burnout prevention. *Family Process*, **24**(4) 549–53.

Gladding, S.T. (1991) Counsellor self-abuse. *Journal of Mental Health Counselling*, **13**(3) 414–19.

Gordin, F.M., Willoughby, A.D., Levine, L.A., Gurel, L. & Neill, K.M. (1987) Knowledge of AIDS among hospital workers: behavioural correlates and consequences. *AIDS*, **1**, 183–8.

Gray-Toft, P. & Anderson, J.G. (1980) The nursing stress scale: development of an instrument. *Journal of Behavioural Assessment*, **3**, 11–23.

Gray-Toft, P. & Anderson, J.G. (1981) Stress among hospital nursing staff, its causes and effects. *Social Science and Medicine*, **15A**, 639–47.

Guinan, J.J., McCallum, L.W., Painter, L., Dykes, J. *et al.* (1991) Stressors and rewards for being an AIDS emotional-support volunteer: a scale for use by care-givers for people with AIDS. *AIDS Care*, **3**(2), 137–50.

Hortsman, W. & McKusick, L. (1986) The impact of AIDS on the physician. In: *What to do About AIDS* (ed. L. McKusick), pp.63–74. University of California Press, Berkley.

Housley, W.F., McDaniel, L.C. & Underwood, J.R. (1990) Mandated assessment of counsellors in Mississippi. *School Counsellor*, **37**(4), 294–302.

Des Jarlais, D.C. (1990) Stages in the response of the drug abuse treatment system to the AIDS epidemic in New York City. *Journal of Drug Issues*, **20**(2) 335–47.

Kahill, S. (1988) Symptoms of professional burnout: a review of the empirical evidence. *Canadian Psychology*, **29**(3) 284–97.

Kesler, K.D. (1990) Burnout: a multimodal approach to assessment and resolution. Special issue: Multimodal theory, research and practice. *Elementary School Guidance and Counselling*, **24**(4), 303–11.

Kleiber, D., Gusy, Enzmann, Beerlage (1992) Paper presented at international conference on AIDS, Amsterdam July 1992.

Lyall, A. (1989) The prevention and treatment of professional burnout. *Loss, Grief and Care*, **3**(1–2) 27–32.

Maslach, C.H. & Jackson, S.E. (1982) Burnout in health professions: a social psychological analysis. In: *Social Psychology of Illness* (eds. G.S. Saunders & J. Suis). Lawrence Erlbaum, London.

Maslanka, H. (1992) Poster presented at International Conference on AIDS, Amsterdam July 1992.

Maynard, E.D. (1985) The intervener: managing personal crises. *Emotional First-Aid: A Journal of Crisis Intervention*, **2**(3) 39–46.

McCarthy, M. (1989) Burnout: what price care-giving? *Loss, Grief and Care*, **3**(1–2) 67–71.

McElroy, A.M. (1982) Burnout – a review of the literature with application to cancer nursing. *Cancer Nursing*, **5**, 211–17.

Miller, D. (1987) *Living with AIDS and HIV*. MacMillan Press, Basingstoke.

Miller, D. (1991) Occupational morbidity and burnout: lessons and warnings for HIV/AIDS carers. *International Review of Psychiatry*, **3**, 439–49.

Miller, D. (1992a) Staff stress in HIV health care workers. *AIDS Care*, **4**(4), 429–32.

Miller, D. (1992b) Stress, burnout and coping of HIV/AIDS health care workers – a review and a challenge. Poster presented at IX Conference of AIDS in Africa, Yaounde, Cameroon, November 1992.

Miller, D. (1993) Berlin conference paper.

Moreland, L. & Legg, S. (1991) *Managing and Funding AIDS Organisations*. Department of Health/Compass Partnership.

Morin, S.F. & Batchelor, W.F. (1984) Responding to the psychological crisis of AIDS. *Public Health Reports*, **99**, 4–9.

Pearlin, L.I., Semple, S. & Turner, H. (1988) Stress of AIDS caregiving: a preliminary overview of the issues. *Death Studies*, **12**(5–6), 501–17.

Pierey, F.P. & Welchier, J.L. (1987) Family work interfaces of psychotherapists. *Journal of Psychotherapy and the Family*, **3**(2) 17–32.

Ross, M.W. & Seeger, V. (1988) Determinants of reported burnout in health professionals associated with the care of patients with AIDS. *AIDS*, **2**, 395–7.

Stewart, B.E., Meyerowitz, B.E., Jackson, L.E., Yarkin, K.L. & Harvey, J.H. (1982) Psychological stress associated with outpatient oncology nursing. *Cancer Nursing*, **5**, 383–7.

Strassmeier, W. (1986) Early intervention and ecology. *Fruhforderung-Interdisziplinar*, **5**(4), 151–62.

Wallace, J.E. & Brinkeroff, M. (1991) The measurement of burnout revisited. *Journal of Social Science Research*, **14**(1–2), 85–111.

Walsh, S. (1990) *Personal and Professional Threat: A Model of Self-Care for Clinicians*. MSc thesis, Exeter University.

Wilcoxon, S.A. (1989) Leadership behaviour and therapist burnout: a study of rural agency settings. *Journal of Rural Community Psychology*, **10**(2), 3–14.

Chapter 21

Making Choices about Diagnosis, Treatment and Care: Counselling Approaches

Riva Miller

Introduction

For those infected with HIV, choice over a wide range of issues may be perceived to be diminished or taken away, as HIV is a life threatening, lifelong, incurable condition. Doctors likewise may consider that they have little choice but to encourage their patients to accept all available investigations and treatments, which in turn can put pressure on patients to accept what is offered.

The period from infection with HIV to illness can be 10 years or more, and for some it may be even longer (Phillips *et al.* 1991). Although it is not yet proven that all those infected will develop AIDS, over 50% have done so (Moss & Bachetti 1989). Decisions about being tested, and about the advantages and disadvantages of treatments during all phases of infection and illness, take place in an atmosphere of evolving knowledge and changing information. The management of HIV infection in the 1990s has moved from responding to medical crises to monitoring and early intervention.

Decisions on what choices to make about testing and treatment are influenced by the availability, specificity and reliability of diagnostic tests, prognostic markers, clinical signs, and treatment advances. Patients' beliefs in conventional or alternative medical care, the spiritual domain, and societal and family pressures are also important factors. Parents of young children and adolescents with HIV, and sexual partners and families of those infected, also have choices to make about transmission risks, treatment and care. This chapter discusses how the use of counselling skills as part of care and treatment can enable patients to recognise their choices and can increase their perception of available options, thereby enabling them to make more informed decisions (Miller & Bor 1988).

Counselling about choice

Patients who have HIV infection are increasingly well informed about treatment options and clinical drug trials. Counselling can help them think through their options at all stages of HIV infection. This helps to:

- Give back some feeling of control for as long as possible, in a condition that can diminish physical and mental ability
- Reduce the fear of declining options and pressure to make decisions, by accentuating that they do have choices, even if limited
- Show respect for their beliefs, particularly about conventional and alternative medicine
- Provide opportunities to review decisions from time to time, particularly important for those who decide against conventional medication, or who opt for a combination of alternative and conventional treatments – their views may change from one stage of illness to another
- Give patients another view of any situation and increase their perception of choice by challenging ideas and beliefs; in this way patients may feel less 'trapped'
- Enhance trust and co-operative understanding between patient and doctor by sharing the responsibility for decision-making with patients and appropriate close contacts; clarifying the doctor's rationale for offering available treatment increases understanding and reduces pressure on doctors for decision-making when difficult situations arise, such as medical crises.

Counselling approaches

The counselling techniques described in this chapter are based on systemic family therapy and adapted from the Milan School of Family Therapy (Bor, Miller, Goldman, 1992). Focus is placed on identifying concerns, giving information, creating balance, maintaining hope and using questions therapeutically to enable informed decision-making on the part of patients, their close contacts and treating physicians. Approaches for addressing the certainties and uncertainties of HIV disease, such as the use of hypothetical future-orientated questions, can enhance patients' perception of choices (Penn, 1985).

The stages of HIV infection and illness

Counselling patients about actual and perceived choices should be an integral part of treatment and care, from decisions about HIV testing to wishes about care during the terminal phase of illness. Although the stages of HIV disease are here considered under separate headings, they are part of a continuum of choice and decision-making.

Prior to infection

Routine conversations about HIV infection, as part of health education and medical history-taking in a wide variety of settings, can help to reduce fear and stigma and provide information important for increasing choice. For example:

'We talk to all women attending the clinic about HIV and other sexually transmitted diseases. What do you know about how HIV is passed from one person to another?'
'I talk to all my young patients about using condoms. If you had the choice of persuading your partner to use a condom or risking some infection how would you deal with it?'

Those who are tested for screening purposes, such as blood donors, also have choices as they are informed about HIV testing in leaflets and can decline to donate if they wish.

Prior to HIV antibody testing

Those who voluntarily seek the HIV antibody test, or patients who are tested to establish a differential diagnosis, should have the opportunity to weigh up the personal advantages and difficulties to ensure 'informed consent' is given for HIV testing (WHO 1990). Informed choices about testing cannot be made unless the patient has knowledge about HIV infection and has understood and considered the meaning and implications of the test result, whether positive or negative. Information about HIV monitoring, available treatments and care must be clarified, as choice about HIV testing is only a first step. Knowing their HIV status enables some people to choose safer sexual and drug using practices, and to consider how to deal with relationships. Making a decision about testing, for example, can be facilitated:

COUNSELLOR: 'You say that you are not ready to cope with the certainty that you might be infected with HIV. How would you know that you were ready?'

PATIENT: 'I don't want to be trapped by knowing for sure. I can't make up my mind yet.'

COUNSELLOR: 'What would help you to make up your mind?'

PATIENT: 'Knowing that if I was positive I would still be able to do the things that I do now.'

COUNSELLOR: 'What things do you think you could not do?'

Travel and insurance are among the practical considerations that can limit choices. People can be helped to view these limitations differently.

COUNSELLOR: 'If you were unable to travel or to get the insurance cover that you had hoped for, how would you view that?'

PATIENT: 'I would use what money I have to secure my accommodation.'

Early discussion about the person's greatest fears, such as dealing with relationships or choices about pregnancy, death, dying and debilitation, can help to prepare him or her for the results of testing. Although anxiety may initially be raised, more considered choices are made if some thought is given to the results prior to testing.

Diagnosis of HIV infection

Despite preparation people may experience shock and despair following the diagnosis of HIV infection. It is not uncommon to believe that all choices have immediately been taken away. If patients 'switch off' in shock they will not take in information, limiting receptiveness to available choices. Asking questions rather than 'flooding' patients with information, can 'reactivate' them and enable expression of their main concerns.

COUNSELLOR: 'What is the main thing on your mind now?'

PATIENT: 'I just feel shocked and it all seems so hopeless and futile.'

COUNSELLOR: 'What seems most futile?'

PATIENT: 'That I am going to die.'
COUNSELLOR: 'What would help you most right now?'
PATIENT: 'To know that I'm not going to die soon.'
COUNSELLOR: 'If you were not to die soon what would you like to know about HIV?'
PATIENT: 'I'm not sure.'
COUNSELLOR: 'What do you know about what treatments and care we can offer you?'
PATIENT: 'Nothing, at least I can't think now.'
COUNSELLOR: 'That's all right. When you are ready we can begin to discuss what you want to know, and what we believe might be important for you to know.'

It is important at the start not to make assumptions about what patients know or want to know. If patients are given the choice whether they would prefer to be given information immediately or to consider issues and receive information slowly, step by step, some measure of control is regained.

There is a strong pull to reassure newly diagnosed patients that they do not have AIDS. Such reassurance cannot be given until further clinical and laboratory information has been obtained. At the same time it is important to maintain hope, for example by opening up discussion about future choices.

PATIENT: 'So it means I have AIDS.'
COUNSELLOR: 'I cannot say whether you have AIDS, but from what you have told me you are feeling well. What do you remember about the meaning of the antibody test?'
PATIENT: 'Not much, except that I know I've had it.'
COUNSELLOR: 'I'm not sure what you mean by "had it". There are treatments for infections. Do you know anything about them?'

The main challenge at the time of diagnosis may be to pre-empt extreme despair, such as suicide threats. Imaginative use of time and responding to what the patient presents, help to expand the range of possibilities and can prevent the counsellor from mirroring the patient's despair. Patients can be helped to think about other options, and the consequences to others of choices such as suicide.

Choices about who to tell about HIV, such as sexual partners, family, friends, employers and other professionals, including the GP and dentist, can be major concerns. Having the perception of choice, and not feeling trapped, can facilitate this decision-making. Some questions to lead the discussion are:

- 'Who do you think you ought to tell?'
- 'Is there anyone you want to tell?'
- 'Is there anyone that you would like to tell, but cannot for any reason?'
- 'Who will it be easiest/hardest to tell?'
- 'What would make it easier/more difficult?'
- 'What might be the implications for you of not telling your GP?'

Asymptomatic phase of HIV disease

The asymptomatic phase of HIV disease can last for many years. Patients may find decision-making difficult because of swings between hope and hopelessness, certainty and uncertainty, and thoughts of living and dying. It is important to be in touch with where patients are at any time and to help them prepare for changes, enabling them to recognise that they have choices, however limited. Consideration of the following aspects are important during the asymptomatic phase of HIV infection:

- If patients perceive that they have choices – including using alternative and/or conventional medical treatment – adherence to follow-up, monitoring, treatments and care is likely to be better. In any event, many will turn to alternative therapies without telling the treatment team. If their choices are openly discussed they are more likely to return when the need or wish for conventional care arises.
- Reactions to regular monitoring affects what choices patients make. For some it increases fears of having HIV infection, and for others the regular contact with the medical and social care team is reassuring.
- Keeping the balance between maintaining hope and preparing patients and their close contacts for changes in their health, becomes important during this phase of HIV infection. Discussion of the pros and cons of early treatments can help patients to choose whether to take a risk of remaining well, or to accept prophylactic treatments with both known and unknown risks of side effects.

> PATIENT: 'I don't see the point of taking AZT as it isn't proved to really be any good.'
>
> DOCTOR: 'We don't yet have the full information about the efficacy of this anti-retroviral treatment for people who have no clinical symptoms. From the results of trials so far no clear advantage has been established. However, if we continue to monitor your health carefully we can give you other preventative treatments for infections such as pneumonia and candida. Whilst taking these drugs to try and maintain reasonable health, new antiretroviral treatments might be found.'

- Change and transition from being asymptomatic to symptomatic may be perceived as diminishing choices. A balance has to be achieved between addressing fears early, which can in the short term raise anxiety, or only discussing the future when crises occur and choices are diminished.
- Some patients can be immobilised by fears for the future, such as the uncertainty of when and what illnesses will occur, and of becoming dependent. Others, knowing that they are infected, are able to live more positively and to make choices more easily.

> COUNSELLOR: 'You say that it is difficult coping with the uncertainty of not knowing when you might become ill. What are your greatest fears about becoming ill?'
>
> PATIENT: 'That I will lose my job and become dependent in every way.'
>
> COUNSELLOR: 'Have you thought about how you would cope if you had to stop working?'

PATIENT: 'Not really. But sometimes I wish I could stop now and do all the things I want in case I have no time.'

COUNSELLOR: 'If you decided to stop now what practical steps would you have to take?'

Some examples of questions addressing other fears are:

● 'If you decided not to risk transmitting HIV to a child, and did not become pregnant, how do you see yourself coping with this choice?'
● 'If you became unwell and needed someone to help you, who would you like it to be?'
● 'Have you thought about who you would want to look after your child if you were unable to do so?'
● 'If you were to become ill, would you prefer to be at home or in hospital?'
● 'What are your views about mechanical ventilation if this ever became necessary?'

Hearing the questions is as important as the answers, which patients may find in their own time. Their fears and views can change and must be checked from time to time, otherwise their choices are limited.

Consideration of secrets and confidentiality about what and when information is shared with others can pre-empt some difficulties that might arise when patients become ill.

COUNSELLOR: 'Who else knows that you have HIV?'

PATIENT: 'No one except my partner. My parents do not even know that I am gay.'

COUNSELLOR: 'Would you like them to know?'

PATIENT: 'Yes, but I couldn't tell them now. They would be angry with me and very upset.'

COUNSELLOR: 'Do you think it would be easier to tell them now whilst you are well or when you might be ill?'

Specific aspects of monitoring and treatment which can influence patient choice include laboratory tests and clinical investigations. An understanding should be reached between doctor and patient about each patient's rationale for accepting or rejecting laboratory tests and investigations for monitoring. Some of the following questions may help to achieve this:

● 'What do you want to know about the range of tests and investigations that are done to monitor your health?'
● 'Do you want to be told about the results regularly, occasionally, when you ask, or only when treatment could be offered?'
● 'Is there anything that you do not want to know?'

The CD4+ count is the main prognostic marker of immune functioning and can be used in combination with other tests to guide decisions about when to start prophylactic treatments (Phillips *et al.* 1991). Patients should be given the option of knowing or not knowing the result of the CD4+ count. Some only want to be told when something can be offered. Others do not want to know the results at all. Such a choice can be detrimental to the patient's wellbeing, leaving the doctor with the responsibility for decision-making. If left unchallenged the situation can lead to less than optimal care for that patient.

DOCTOR: 'As you do not want to know the results of your CD4+ count when you come to see me, what should I do if the results are such that I would want to offer you some treatment?'

PATIENT: 'I'm not sure.'

DOCTOR: 'Do you know when and why we might offer treatments to try and prevent infections?'

PATIENT: 'I suppose you had better tell me, although listening to all these explanations only makes me more anxious.'

DOCTOR: 'Which explanation might make you most anxious?'

PATIENT: 'Hearing about all the possible illnesses.'

DOCTOR: 'I would feel less concerned myself if you understood the reason for offering you treatments for one particular infection, pneumonia. Early treatments can prevent this particular illness. However, you can tell me when you decide that you are ready to talk about it.'

Drug trials are used to assess the efficacy of new drugs. Many patients with HIV infection are well informed about new drugs and put pressure on doctors to give them an early chance of trying them (Lee *et al.* 1991). Participating in a trial can give access to a drug that is not otherwise available, and can offer a measure of hope to those patients wishing to take whatever measures they can to prevent the onset of illness. To make informed choices patients must be informed about:

- Their eligibility for a particular drug trial
- The time involved in monitoring and length of trial
- Side effects of drugs
- Conditions of exiting and ending the trial.

Opportunities for discussion should be part of pre-enrolment, enrolment, monitoring, and ending the trial. The regular monitoring which accompanies drug trials may permit earlier diagnosis and treatment of symptoms. For some this is outweighed by too much focus on, and the inability to forget, HIV because of tablet-taking. Early discussion about withdrawal from the trial for medical reasons, or because patients want to stop, paves the way for choices at a time when patients may feel trapped. If the patient chooses not to enter the trial, other options should be considered.

Choices about primary and secondary treatments can be difficult, particularly when patients are feeling well. Some fear that drugs may exacerbate deterioration in health. Others fear the side effects and the possibility of becoming resistant to the drug so that when treatment is needed the drug will be ineffective. Information should include:

- Whether the side effects are reversible if the drug is stopped
- The possibilities of reduced dosage.

Symptomatic stage

As patients become symptomatic, maintaining hope and retaining control over their lives becomes increasingly difficult. They may be more prepared if there has been prior discussion of their fears and their wishes about when and if they will accept medication, how they wish to be informed, and who else they will involve about a range of issues. Some of the following aspects should be reviewed:

- The available investigations and medication
- What symptoms might be important and when to report them
- How they wish to be managed medically
- What they would wish for in terms of treatment and care should they not respond to medication
- Who is around to help
- Who else knows about their condition
- Who they think they now ought to tell
- Naming a next-of-kin
- Who would they wish to make decisions for them if they were unable to do so themselves
- How the team should respond to enquiries from close contacts and family.

Many health care workers fear that such discussions will immediately heighten the patient's anxiety, but protecting patients from these issues may mean not giving them the opportunity to voice their fears, and leaving important life and death decisions until patients are too weak and debilitated to make choices easily.

During the symptomatic stage, invasive investigations may be needed. Patients should be fully informed and feel that they can make choices. If they refuse investigation or treatment it is important that the doctor clarifies how such a decision may limit what can be offered. In some instances patients may be faced with fewer choices than expected; in others counselling can help them to view problems differently and thus provide choices where none seemed possible. Patients, their close contacts and family can be better prepared for the terminal stages of illness.

Terminal care phase

Once the terminal phase of illness has been reached the patient's range of choices has been further reduced, but under many circumstances they are still able to participate in decision-making. Ensuring that this happens is one way of maintaining hope and increasing their ability to cope, even in the face of great losses. Some unresolved issues are likely to surface to be exacerbated when the patient becomes very ill. These include secrets and confidentiality, which can be a source of stress and tension for the patient and the health care team if there are people who do not know of the patient's status.

NURSE: 'Your mother telephoned to know how you are. She asked me what was wrong with you. Does she know about the HIV?'

PATIENT: 'No, I haven't told her and I don't want her to know'.

NURSE: 'Would you rather tell her now or that she found out later when perhaps you won't be able to talk to her?'

PATIENT: 'I'm not sure. She may hear from one of my friends and I'd hate that.'

NURSE: 'Until you have decided what to do, what should we tell her if she asks again?'

PATIENT: 'Pneumonia. I think I should tell her soon. She doesn't know that my partner is more than a good friend and that is another problem. He wants to tell her and is upset with me for keeping it secret.'

Pre-existing conflicts between family of origin and family of affiliation can reappear. The patient should be enabled, as far as possible, to continue to make choices. Despite views that resolving conflicts and settling affairs is important for a more peaceful death, this is not necessarily so. Patients may not be able to, or wish to, settle all their affairs prior to death. It is important, however, that they are given the opportunity to do so if they wish. No assumptions should be made; some patients may choose to let others decide for them. Some business may go unfinished, for example not making a will or ensuring future care of dependent children.

Not everyone wants to 'come to terms with death and dying'. Patients should be given the opportunity to talk about death and dying if they wish, by placing emphasis on identifying and addressing, if appropriate, their fears and beliefs. Some questions that can be used are:

- 'Is there anything of concern to you right now?'
- 'How do you want us to look after you now that you are not so well?'
- 'You say that you are worried about pain. Did you know that there are ways to keep you more comfortable?'

Patients should be enabled, if possible, to make choices until they die. Although patients become increasingly physically dependent, whilst they are mentally alert they can be consulted as to their wishes about active investigations and palliative care. Some patients may have indicated that when they reach a stage of dependency they do not want to be 'kept alive'. It is important to review such decisions as their views may be different in the terminal stage. Practical aspects, such as physical dependency, may come to the fore and may be embarrassing and difficult to accept. Patients may perceive that they have no choices. Small statements can ease the situation:

NURSE: 'You seem to be very uncomfortable depending on us for all your needs. I want you to know that this is part of our role as nurses. However, if there is anyone else you would rather be helping you, do tell me.'

Even during the terminal stage, hope has to be maintained. At the same time it is important now to falsely reassure patients or close contacts. When active treatment has ceased patients can still be asked:

- Who they want to be with them
- Whether they wish to be alone
- How they want to be treated
- What would help them most
- What measures they want taken for pain control.

Overview

Choice is only possible when views of a situation are expanded. This is especially so when there is a life threatening, incurable condition. The challenge to patients, their close contacts and the health care team is to find ways of increasing choices and avoiding making people feel trapped. Too much discussion about choices can also impede decision-making. No assumptions should be made about what patients should or should not decide on a range of issues. Finding the balance between maintaining hope and preparing for the future is vital throughout all stages of HIV disease.

References

Bor, R., Miller, R. & Goldman, E. (1992) *Theory and Practise of HIV Counselling: A Systemic Approach.* Cassell, London.

Lee, C., Miller, R. & Goldman, E. (1991) Treatment dilemmas for HIV infected haemophiliacs. *AIDS Care*, 1, 2.

Miller, R. & Bor, R. (1988) *AIDS: A Guide to Clinical Counselling.* Science Press, London.

Moss, A. & Bachetti, P. (1989) Natural history of HIV infection. *AIDS*, 3, 55–61.

Penn, P. (1985) Feed forward: future questions, future maps. *Family Process*, 24, 299–310.

Phillips, A., Lee, C., Elford, J., Jannosy, G., Timms, A., Bofill, M. & Kernoff, P. (1991) Serial CD4 lymphocyte counts and development of AIDS. *Lancet*, 337, 389–92.

Phillips, A.N., Sabin, C.A., Elford, J., Bofill, M., Janossy, G. & Lee, C.A. (1994) Use of CD4 lymphocyte count to predict long term survival free of AIDS after HIV infection. *British Medical Journal*, 309, 309–13.

WHO (1990) *Guidelines for Counselling People about HIV.* World Health Organisation, Geneva.

Chapter 22

HIV, Mental Health and Community Care: a Psychiatric View

Una McDermott and Peter Tyrer

Introduction

The direct effects of HIV on the physical health of those infected have been well documented. However, in recent years there has been a great deal of interest in the effects of HIV on the psychological wellbeing of the individual and in the direct effects of HIV on the brain. Different workers in the area have written about the issue from different perspectives, including psychosocial (Ostrow *et al.* 1986; Miller 1987; King 1989), neuropsychiatric (Catalan 1988; WHO 1988; Maj 1990a), psychodynamic (Vamos 1992) and intrapsychic (Krikler 1988; Hildebrand 1992). The psychiatric consequences of infection have been also described (Faulstitch 1987; Ostrow 1987; Catalan *et al.* 1989; Catalan 1990; Maj 1990b).

As the number of cases of HIV infection rises worldwide, so the need for appropriate psychiatric services aimed at those who are infected will increase. The way that services are organised will depend in part on local circumstances; for instance, in the UK, psychiatric care is moving increasingly into the community and this is a pattern in many other countries across the world too. In this chapter some issues are discussed – such as resource needs – that will inevitably arise in the years to come in the context of this disease.

Mental health is a difficult term to define. In its positive sense it implies a state of wellbeing that is more than the absence of illness. Caplan (1961) incorporated into his definition an idea of mental health which allows for an individual or a community to live as full, productive and happy a life as is realistically possible within a given cultural framework. Implicit to this idea is the notion of a healthy individual's capacity to confront the problems which are inherent to the human condition. These include coping with imperfection, inequalities, losses, aging, and death. In keeping with this definition, disordered mental health indicates reduced capacity to deal with life's vicissitudes, resulting in impaired productivity, unhappiness and, in its most severe forms, a condition in which reality testing is lost and replaced by disordered false tenets (the psychoses).

The term community care has become what the philosopher Wittgenstein would have called a 'portmanteau' phrase, i.e. one which is made to carry a number of poorly defined and overlapping meanings. Community care could refer to care of the community or care in the community. Here it refers to the assessment, treatment and follow-up of patients in the community by therapeutic teams. In psychiatric settings such teams commonly comprise several disciplines and cater for defined groups of patients.

Those with HIV infection are not yet numerous enough and do not have sufficiently high levels of psychiatric disturbance to merit specific community psychiatric teams for their care; thus in many cases there will be a need for existing services to adapt their pattern of care to a new patient group. However, we believe that the point is being reached, and in some areas may already have been reached, where serious consideration needs to be given to specialist community psychiatric teams for HIV patients.

Aspects of the epidemiology of psychiatric disorder in AIDS

At the time of writing, in the western world the groups predominantly infected with HIV are gay and bisexual men, IV drug users and haemophiliacs, in other words mainly men. Much smaller numbers of women and babies have also been infected. There is only a limited, impressionistic picture of the epidemiology of this disease because studies have been largely limited to particular high-risk groups in large cities. In most parts of the world HIV is mainly heterosexually transmitted, with almost as many women as men (Maj *et al.* 1991).

The World Health Organisation Global Programme on AIDS and the Division of Mental Health conventions (WHO 1988, 1990) concluded that the epidemiology of functional psychiatric disturbance in people with HIV has not yet been reliably determined. Studies to date, despite their considerable number (Fenton 1987; Ostrow 1987; Catalan 1988; King 1990) are often little more than anecdotal case reports and represent largely non-systematic studies of small numbers of patients from non-representative samples. Little or no account of selection factors is made, diagnostic criteria of syndromes are poorly defined, and there is little information on outcome; they are therefore inadequate as epidemiological data. Mental health disturbances of haemophiliacs and women and children infected with HIV have generally been neglected. There is also little research on the psychiatric aspects of AIDS in sub-Saharan Africa.

The role of the psychiatrist in HIV

Psychiatrists, as physicians, have a background in the medical sciences, a grounding in physical medicine and should have received a specialised training in the full range of psychological disturbances and their treatments. It can be argued, not without contention, that they are the practitioners ideally placed to espouse a biopsychosocial model (Engel 1977) of patient care.

For the psychiatrist, AIDS presents many challenges in that it requires the assessment, diagnosis and treatment of psychiatric disturbances in the context of underlying or concurrent physical pathology. Iatrogenic psychological disturbances must also be borne in mind as HIV patients are often receiving several physical treatments, many of which are novel with side effect profiles that are only partially known. Many of the drugs used affect mental state adversely (Wurtz *et al.* 1989) and such unwanted effects may be misinterpreted as signs of HIV/AIDS infection. HIV/AIDS demands that the psychiatrist has a particular understanding of the psychological processes associated with terminal illness (Hinton 1967), in order to help patients face possible severe illness and death.

All of us live in some relation to a social network. In respect of AIDS patients recognition must be given as to how this devastating and stigmatising condition influences patients' social relationships. The psychiatrist (preferably working in the context of a multi-disciplinary team) must support and help the families and carers of patients in an appropriately sensitive and understanding manner. At times families and carers may need psychiatric treatment in their own right.

It has long been recognised that health workers, particularly those working in intensive treatment environments or with terminal illness (Vachon *et al.* 1987), suffer high levels of stress because of the nature of their work. Health staff working with AIDS patients require help both in terms of education about the psychological needs of their terminally ill patients, and in terms of supporting them in their own emotional responses to seeing many young patients die despite their efforts to save them (Klimes *et al.* 1989). At times, staff working with this potentially frightening (Ross & Seager 1988) and poorly understood (Gordin *et al.* 1987) disease may need psychiatric intervention, either on an individual or group basis (Volberding 1989) (Chapter 20).

Psychiatric disorder in AIDS

Broadly speaking, the range and type of psychiatric disorder in this group of patients are not unlike those found in patients with terminal cancer (Derogatis *et al.* 1985) or other life threatening illnesses (Holland & Tross 1985) which have some cerebral manifestations. The majority of presentations arise from stressors related to knowledge of personal infection (Dilley *et al.* 1985; Miller & Riccio 1990).

The prevalence of psychiatric disorder in those referred to psychiatrists is said to vary greatly from 31–65% (Perry & Tross 1984; Atkinson *et al.* 1988; King 1989). This probably reflects different patterns of referral to different services, which are likely to depend on a number of factors in the patient, the referrer and the particular AIDS service. This is not surprising as different units use different models of psychiatric liaison care. The need for inpatient psychiatric admission is generally said to be low (Catalan 1988; Miller & Riccio 1990), though overall figures nationally or internationally are not readily available. In the service where we work an average of ten to twelve HIV/AIDS patients per year have been referred to the psychiatric services for inpatient treatment. The remainder of the patients are treated as psychiatric outpatients or receive psychiatric consultation while inpatients on the medical wards.

Psychiatric syndromes in HIV infected patients

The most frequently recognised psychiatric disorders are discussed and classified using the International Classification of Diseases (ICD 10, WHO 1992). This classification is phenomenological in describing certain symptom clusters which by consensus are agreed to constitute specific syndromes, and is operational in that a diagnosis requires a certain number of 'diagnostic guidelines' to be scored positively. Psychiatric manifestations of HIV may:

(1) Occur as a result of the direct effect of the HIV virus on the brain
(2) Be secondary to the effects of opportunistic cerebral infections in the immunosuppressed host
(3) Be related to the indirect toxic cerebral effects of severe systemic infections or other metabolic or drug induced disturbances
(4) Be reactive to the overwhelming psychosocial stresses of HIV illness and its consequences
(5) Have any mixture of causations from 1 to 4
(6) Occur coincidentally because of the high prevalence of both mental illness and AIDS in the population.

One major section of mental disorder in ICD 10 is organic mental disorder (FO). This also includes symptomatic mental disorder in which the form of presentation is indistinguishable from nonorganic disorder (e.g. anxiety, depression, hallucinosis) but the cause is organic. The true aetiology of the presenting psychiatric condition may only become clear with time. Polymorphism of psychiatric presentation has been recorded, with changes in psychopathology within an admission as well as between admissions (Baer 1989; Seth *et al.* 1991). Rapid response to medication has also been noted (Baer 1989). Both these characteristics may be suggestive of an underlying organic pathology. Considerable difficulties in diagnosis (Miller & Riccio 1990) may therefore arise. Given all these factors, the cause of psychiatric disturbance cannot always be identified with certainty.

In such a situation of uncertainty a psychiatrist may use a 'working diagnosis', i.e. a diagnosis which is open to revision and which is updated as the amount of available information about a particular patient's problems grows. Obviously it is important to be careful about making long-term plans on the basis of a working diagnosis. Having made this proviso it is useful to consider the possible psychiatric problems which people with HIV may develop, and the ways in which they can be helped.

Stress related disorders

Acute stress reactions (F 43.0)

These are transient reactions to acute stress and occur in HIV patients particularly in response to initial diagnosis. They also occur at times of change of diagnosis from HIV to AIDS. Reactions are varied and include despair, anxiety, protest, denial, depression, confusion, disorientation, a narrowing of attention, constriction of field of consciousness, impotence, withdrawal, fear, anger, and suicidal ideation and suicide attempts. To qualify for the diagnosis of an acute stress reaction in ICD 10, the symptoms have to become manifest within one hour of the stressful stimulus. The disorder is normally a short lived condition (two to three days). The prevalence and incidence are not reliably quantified in this patient group but are reported in up to 90% of subjects with recent diagnoses (WHO 1988).

To adjust to a diagnosis of a life threatening illness is a gargantuan task for the individual involved. Personal psychological reactions to physical illness vary widely in their nature and severity, with no clear division between normal and abnormal (Lloyd 1991). Reaction is morbid if it interferes with adjustment to illness or if the reaction itself is a source of distress.

The AIDS patient confronts the same existential issues as patients with any other terminal illness, including thoughts of facing the death itself, the meaning of (their) life, and the realisation of time running out, goals not achieved and unfinished business remaining (Wiseman & Worden 1976). There are, however, particular difficulties for AIDS patients. These may relate to sexuality or drug-taking habits which can be socially stigmatised and frowned upon. Consequently the sympathy and support from others, including those close to the patient such as other family members, is sometimes less than in other terminal illnesses. Sometimes distressed patients can take up some of the negative views of those around them. Feelings of responsibility may bring about fantasies of divine retribution (Dilley *et al.* 1985), a latter day damnation of Faust for succumbing to the evils of temptation. Social stigma may aggravate feelings of guilt and despair (Vamos 1992). Fears of contagion and social marginalisation may increase feelings of isolation.

Particularly difficult also for these patients is the uncertainty about when, or even if, they will develop full blown AIDS. The estimated mean time is now thought to be 10 years (Beck 1991), but this says little about the individual case. Once a patient has developed AIDS there is the marked uncertainty of rate of progress of the condition.

There is evidence that the acute response of the patient to HIV or to a diagnosis of AIDS will be determined, at least in part, by prior coping style (Namir *et al.* 1987; Sensky 1990). The phenomenology, severity and duration of the reactions seen is reportedly similar to those seen in the context of other major life events or disease diagnoses (Derogatis *et al.* 1985; Dilley *et al.* 1985).

While most acute stress reactions are brief and self-limited, this does not mean that they should not be managed to reduce, as far as possible, their intensity and duration. Appropriate management measures include psychosocial support and counselling (Green & McCreaner 1989) discussed elsewhere in this book. Preventive measures include pre and post HIV test counselling (Miller & Green 1986).

Adjustment disorders (F 43.2)

These are states of subjective distress and emotional disturbances which interfere with social functioning and performance. They occur secondary to identifiable psychosocial stressor(s) – usually HIV/AIDS in this context. Onset is usually within one month of onset of stressor(s) and persists no longer than six months (ICD 10).

The psychopathological features are similar to those found in an acute stress reaction, but these are more intensive, persistent and chronic and are in excess of a normal expectable reaction. These disorders are characterised by impairment in interpersonal, occupational and social functioning. The incidence and prevalence are unknown but these disorders are said to be more common in symptomatic non-AIDS patients. A possible explanation for this may be that the stress of uncertainty as to likelihood and rate of disease progression is greater than that of knowing the worst.

Management interventions are usually non-pharmacological and consist of mixtures of counselling, cognitive, behavioural and other psychotherapeutic interventions. Short term drug treatment can be used where necessary, usually by intermittent use of small doses of anxiolytic drugs such as the benzodiazepines or tricyclic antidepressants in low dosages.

Care must be exercised with some drug treatments as there have been anecdotal reports of increased sensitivity to unwanted effects in many patients, possibly because of undetected underlying organic impairment. The risk of respiratory depression with benzodiazepines, especially in the presence of *Pneumocystis carinii* pneumonia infection, must be borne in mind, as well as the risks of dependence. At times brief admission to hospital may be indicated. A prior psychiatric history has been strongly associated with the occurrence of adjustment disorder (Catalan 1988); this is, however, a view not without contention.

Mood (affective) disorders (F30– F39)

Depressive disorders

Depressive disorders are fundamentally characterised by a lowering of mood, with or without accompanying anxiety, and are usually accompanied by a change in the overall level of functioning (ICD 10). Other symptoms, such as loss of interest in pleasurable activities (anhedonia), social withdrawal, loss of hope, self criticism, somatic symptoms and suicidal ideas, are usually secondary to or easily understood in terms of these changes in mood and activity. Depression has a tendency to recur, and in differing levels of severity. Onset of individual episodes is often related to stressful events or situations.

In the HIV patient group, depression is reported commonly but it is rarely quantified. Depression as a symptom can occur as part of an acute stress reaction or adjustment disorder and may indeed be the predominant feature of either. Major depression has been particularly associated with later stages of disease (Seth *et al.* 1991). As with other patient groups, depression has been described secondary (F06.3) to dementia, opportunistic brain infections and cerebral tumours (Holland & Tross 1985). Iatrogenically induced depression also occurs, for example the well recognised depression secondary to steroid treatment or anti-neoplastic drugs (Vogel-Scibilia *et al.* 1988).

In common with all hospital-based liaison psychiatry, an assessment for the symptoms of depression is the request most frequently made of psychiatrists by clinicians looking after physically ill patients. In addition, depressive syndromes are the most frequently recorded diagnoses made by psychiatrists when assessing referred HIV patients (Dilley *et al.* 1985). This is in part explained by the possibility that many patients suffering from stress reactions may be directly referred to psychologists instead of psychiatrists (Seth *et al.* 1991). This reflects the practices and resources of any particular service, and prevails in the situation in which we work. Depression is, in any case, a common disorder in hospital patients (Rosen *et al.* 1987) (Chapter 12).

It is often thought that depression is 'understandable' in a condition characterised by uncertainty of disease progression, multiple devastating losses including patients' own decline, and frequently the deaths of friends and lovers through the same disease (Miller 1988). However, this does not mean that it should not be rapidly and effectively treated. Psychosocial influences are frequently cited as predictors in the onset of depression in this patient group. Factors implicated include:

- Lack of social support or health care
- Accommodation

- Financial or employment difficulties
- Guilt and feelings of lack of acceptance of sexuality or lifestyle.

Depression is a recurrent disorder and as with other groups of patients, AIDS patients are no exception (Dilley *et al.* 1985).

Vegetative or somatic symptoms (e.g. weight loss, reduced libido, anorexia) are not the reliable diagnostic indicators found in other depressive disorders, since in AIDS patients physical symptoms (e.g. bowel disturbance, weight loss, anorexia, sleeplessness) may understandably result from the underlying physical conditions (e.g. oesophageal candida).

A particular difficulty in differential diagnosis with individuals with AIDS can lie in separating the symptoms of depression from those of organic brain problems. Symptoms of early dementia, particularly slowed thinking, decreased alertness, affective flattening, social withdrawal, disturbance in concentration, forgetfulness and psychomotor retardation and loss of libido, can mimic those seen in depression (Holland & Tross 1985; Faulstich 1987). To further complicate matters, it is worth bearing in mind that both functional and organic aetiologies of mood disorder can co-exist and differentiation can often be very difficult (Vogel-Scibilia 1988).

The most important point in the management of mood disorders in this group is that no matter what the presumed underlying cause or causes for depression may be, the psychiatrist works empirically and uses a similar range of interventions and treatments as in other depressive disorders. Accepting that a condition can be understood in terms of life context is no argument for failing to treat depression adequately. AIDS related depressive disorder is usually responsive to standard anti-depressant treatment (Ostrow 1987; Baer 1989).

Care needs to be exercised in the choice of anti-depressant because of an increased sensitivity of these patients to the anti-cholinergic side-effects of tricyclic antidepressants (Set *et al.* 1991). Tricyclic antidepressants have been claimed to be associated with the onset of delirium through their central anti-cholinergic effects. In theory, therefore, one should attempt to use antidepressants known to have low anti-cholinergic potential, commencing them at a low dosage and making gradual incremental increases in dosage while monitoring clinical response. In practice the antidepressants used are tricyclic antidepressants with a low incidence of side effects (e.g. lofepramine), or with sedative properties (e.g. dothiepin), or the selective serotonin reuptake inhibitors (SSRIs), fluoxetine, fluvoxamine, sertraline and paroxetine. Overcaution may lead to under-treatment (Miller & Riccio 1990) and unnecessary prolongation of suffering. ECT and lithium have also been used to treat mood disorder in this patient group, reportedly with good effect. As with depressive syndromes generally, in conjunction with pharmacotherapy, psychotherapeutic approaches may also be indicated.

Manic disorders

Various degrees of disturbance of mood, characterised by elation and an increase in quantity and speed of physical and mental activity, have been reported in this patient group, though much less commonly than depression. Mania in this patient group is thought to be associated with a poor prognosis (Seth *et al.* 1991) and in our experience is often associated with organic brain syndrome (i.e. is an organic affective disorder (F06.3) in ICD 10 terms).

Management consists of treating or minimising the effects of underlying cerebral problem(s) where possible, together with adjunctive use of antipsychotic medications for their tranquillising effects. Care must be taken to avoid unwanted extrapyramidal effects secondary to dopamine blockade. In this patient group there have been several reports of increased Parkinsonian side-effects (Edelstein & Knight 1987; Maccario & Scharre 1987; Vogel-Scibilia *et al.* 1988; Baer 1989), acute dystonic reactions (Seth *et al.* 1991), and one case of suspected neuroleptic malignant syndrome (Gabel *et al.* 1986).

Suicide

Suicide risk must always be assessed in patients with mood disorders as it is known that some 45% (Robins *et al.* 1959) to 66% (Barraclough *et al.* 1974) of completed suicides occur in the context of sufficient evidence for a diagnosis of depression. Increased rates of suicide have been found in many medically ill patient groups, for example renal dialysis patients (Haenel *et al.* 1980) and patients with Huntingtons disease (Schoenfeld *et al.* 1984).

Although good epidemiological data is not yet available concerning suicide in HIV disease, it would not be surprising if it was of at least the same frequency, or possibly greater, than in the above groups, since it is also a chronic disorder requiring complex treatment interventions. Marzuk *et al.* (1988), from a sample found in New York City in 1985, estimated the relative risk of suicide in men with AIDS to be 36.6 times that for men without AIDS in the age group 20–59, and 66 times that of the general population. Predictive factors for completed suicide are not unlike those for other groups of patients. They include:

(1)   The presence of multiple social stressors
(2)   Perceived social isolation and lack of support
(3)   Tendency to see oneself in the victim role
(4)   Reliance on denial as sole mental defence mechanism
(5)   The co-existence of substance abuse
(6)   Feelings of hopelessness
(7)   Low levels of problem solving skills (Rundell *et al.* 1992)
(8)   In some African cultures shame has also been implicated.

While suicide in the terminally ill is sometimes thought of as a 'natural' reaction, in practice it is usually thought to be associated with treatable psychiatric disorder, commonly depression. A prior history of psychiatric morbidity or deliberate self-harm in gay men or drug addicts is said to be a better predictor of suicide than the presence of HIV infection. It has been suggested that the suicide risk is increased at times of change – e.g. change to being sero-positive or developing an AIDS defining diagnosis – and at times of disease progression. Losses have also been implicated: loss of physical integrity and capabilities, loss of partner(s) or friends through death, and loss of family or social supports (often reported). The risk is also said to be higher in those with personality disorder.

It has even been suggested by some authors that patients who put themselves at risk of contracting HIV are exhibiting suicide-equivalent types of behaviour (Flavin *et al.* 1986), although such an interpretation needs to be viewed with enormous caution given the range of circumstances under which individuals put themselves at risk.

Because the risk of suicide is high, great care should be taken to anticipate feelings of hopelessness and despair. For example, the sensitive handling of a positive HIV test and avoidance of social isolation and consequent feelings of hopelessness, by introducing support systems, can prevent depression from becoming overwhelming and ending in suicide.

Schizophrenia and delusional disorders

Schizophrenic disorders are characterised by fundamental and characteristic distortions of thinking and perception, and effects that are blunted or inappropriate. Patients may present with:

- Delusional beliefs, i.e. false unshakeable beliefs which may be persecutory or grandiose
- Hallucinations, i.e. false perceptions which may be auditory or visual
- Abnormal behaviours.

When psychotic episodes occur in AIDS, uncertainty as to the contribution of 'organic or functional' factors is ever present. It is often debated whether such conditions are prodromal appearances of neuropsychiatric disturbances, are reactive, or are purely coincidental. If there is no past history of schizophrenic disorder in an HIV positive patient, it is a reasonable working hypothesis to regard a schizophrenic episode as organic in origin until proved otherwise.

The true incidence and prevalence of psychotic symptoms or syndromes in patients with HIV infection, as compared to the general population, is unknown (Maj 1990a). They are rarely reported in the early stages of infection (Miller & Riccio 1990) but are not infrequent in the later stages of the disease. There are, however, anecdotal reports of AIDS patients presenting with psychosis (Maccario & Scharre 1987; Vogel-Scibilia *et al.* 1988). It is generally accepted that psychosis unassociated with dementia or delirium is uncommon in this patient group. Cerebral diseases may initially present as indistinguishable from functional disorder (Lishman 1987). In AIDS also, organic psychoses may present initially as indistinguishable from functional psychoses, only revealing their true organic origin later (Buhrich *et al.* 1988; Halsread *et al.* 1988).

There are five possible explanations for psychotic symptoms arising in the context of HIV infection:

(1) Psychosis is independent of HIV infection
(2) Psychosis is secondary to neuropathic properties of HIV virus (Halsread *et al.* 1988)
(3) HIV has acted as a non-specific stressor in an already predisposed individual (Buhrich *et al.* 1988; Vogel-Scibilia *et al.* 1988)
(4) HIV has acted as a psychological stressor which triggers a psychosis (Rundell *et al.* 1986)
(5) Symptoms are secondary to drug treatments for AIDS related disorders (Cambell 1987) or the concomitant use of non-prescribed drugs (e.g. LSD).

Psychotic symptoms also occur as mood congruent delusions in severe affective disorders, and secondary to HIV dementia and organic brain syndromes. Symptomatic response to treatment is generally favourable (Vogel-Scibilia 1988). As stated previously, these patients are overly sensitive to the unwanted effects of neuroleptics.

Organic, including symptomatic, mental disorders

Dementia in human immunodeficiency (HIV) disease (F02.4)

The term dementia is used in a looser way in AIDS patients than in the rest of psychiatry, and includes conditions variously called chronic brain syndrome, subacute encephalitis, AIDS dementia complex (Price *et al.* 1988) and HIV encephalopathy.

Dementia is a syndrome characterised by impairment of multiple higher cortical functions including memory, thinking, orientation, comprehension, calculation, learning capacity, language and judgement. This occurs without clouding of consciousness (ICD 10). Classically AIDS dementia occurs secondary to direct infiltration of sub-cortical brain structures (Pumerola Sune *et al.* 1987) by the neurotropic HIV virus (Navia *et al.* 1986) which is known to occur early in infection (Marshall *et al.* 1988). Dementia is thought usually to require marked immunosuppression for its development (Maj 1990a).

The point prevalence of dementia in HIV positive patients varies in different studies between 7% and 16% (WHO 1988). Initial fears (in the 1980s) that psychiatric services would be overwhelmed by the demand for long stay beds for countless numbers of young demented AIDS patients have not been realised. Dementia is said to be more common in full blown AIDS, but there is great difficulty in generalising from research studies as sample sizes have been non-representative or small. The pathogenesis is uncertain. Onset is usually insidious and the course is variable. There are currently no predictors of disease progress rate (Maj 1990a). Some degree of impairment may be present in most patients as brain pathology has been found in 88% of examined post mortem brains of AIDS patients (Lantos *et al.* 1989).

Clinically this sub-cortical dementia is characterised by cognitive dysfunction, and by behavioural, motor and affective signs. Cognitive signs include the classical feature of memory impairment (maximal for recent learning), poor concentration, mental slowing, impaired abstract thinking and decreased performance on complex mental tasks. Behavioural signs include apathy, decreased spontaneity and emotional responsivity, social withdrawal, early fatiguing and malaise. Motor signs include loss of balance and co-ordination, clumsiness and leg weakness. Atypically these patients may present with affective or psychotic symptoms or seizures. Unlike Alzheimers dementia there is an absence of the classic symptoms of dysphasia (i.e. difficulty in understanding the spoken word, expressing words or naming objects), dyspraxia (i.e. difficulty in spatial orientation) and agnosia (i.e. difficulty in recognition).

As in other patients with sub-cortical dementias (e.g. Parkinsons disease) and in contrast to patients suffering from a cortical dementia (e.g. Alzheimers disease), these patients may be able to acknowledge their subjective feelings of incapacity. They have difficulty remembering appointments or names, feel the need to make lists to aid their memory, get lost in conversations, particularly when talking with more than one person, and may show indifference to usual personal, social and sexual interests. Later the disease can progress to severe global dementia, mutism and death.

Dementia is recognised as also occurring in the AIDS patient group secondary to opportunistic cerebral infections and cerebral tumours (Rosenblum *et al.* 1988). In terms of clinical presentation, progression and psychiatric management, these dementias are similar. The possibility of a potentially treatable contributory disorder must be investigated and managed appropriately. Such investigations include thorough physical examination, including CT or MRI scans to rule out treatable conditions such as toxoplasmosis or lymphoma.

There is no effective drug treatment for dementia caused by HIV itself. Management is supportive toward patient, family and carers. One of the distinctive characteristics of dementias in the AIDS patient group, as opposed to patients with Alzheimer dementia, is that AIDS dementia is relatively short-lived. It is often rapidly progressive with survival times from diagnosis to death measured in weeks to months. In many aspects it requires a model of terminal care rather than chronic management. The range of services required clearly will vary according to the functional state of the patient and the degree of social support and resources already available. The range of care packages which need to be considered can include home care support, which may involve help with housework, shopping or meal preparations; meals on wheels; respite care; day centre care; and residential care in hospice, hospital or nursing home. Not unlike other groups of patients with dementia, most patients with AIDS dementia are cared for in their own homes (Adler 1987). Death is usually secondary to inanition, aspiration pneumonia or systemic opportunistic infection.

Mild cognitive disorder (F06.7)

This disorder may precede, accompany or follow a wide variety of infections and physical disorders, both cerebral and systemic, including HIV. The main features are complaints of memory impairment and forgetfulness, learning difficulties, and a reduced ability to concentrate on a task for more than brief periods. New learning is found to be subjectively difficult, even when objectively the test result is within the normal range.

There has been much debate and controversy concerning the occurrence and management of mild cognitive impairment in HIV infected patients. The results of studies of neuropsychometric testing of patients are unclear for many reasons. Studies do not take account of confounding factors such as the lack of control groups, the presence of psychiatric disorder or symptoms, the non-comparability of groups studied in terms of background intelligence etc, the effects of prescribed or non-prescribed medications or alcohol, and the validity and reliability of the tests used (Joffe *et al.* 1986; Wilkins *et al.* 1990). Empirical observations are hard to correlate in any meaningful way with demonstrable neuropathology on brain scans.

There is some suggestion that the anti-viral drug zidovudine partially reverses brain scan cerebral changes with improved cognitive function (Schmitt *et al.* 1988), though this remains as yet unclear. The WHO (1988) has concluded that there is no evidence of increase in clinically significant neuropsychiatric abnormalities in asymptomatic seropositive people.

It is not at all clear, at the time of writing, that mild cognitive impairment inevitably leads to more severe impairment or dementia later, and there is a need for further work in this area.

Delirium (F05.0)

Delirium is 'an acute organic reaction whose clinical picture is dominated by impairment of consciousness along with intrusive abnormalities delivered from the fields of perception and affect' (Lishman 1987). Delirium is an aetiologically nonspecific syndrome characterised by concurrent disturbances of consciousness and attention, cognition, psychomotor behaviour, emotion, and the sleep–wake cycle. It may be superimposed on, or progress into dementia (ICD 10). There is no definite knowledge or estimate of prevalence or incidence but it is said to occur more frequently in the later stages of HIV infection. As many as 35% of hospitalised AIDS patients have been reported to show signs of acute brain syndrome at one time or another (Perry & Tross 1984).

The cardinal feature of delirium is a fluctuating clouding of consciousness which is worse at night and is associated with time disorientation (in more severe cases disorientation also for place and person). Other symptoms include:

- Excess tendency to startle reaction
- Decreased capacity to shift, focus and sustain attention
- Impaired comprehension
- Disorganised thinking
- Transient delusions (commonly paranoid or related to feelings of imminent mis-adventure)
- Impairment of immediate and recent memory
- Increased or decreased psychomotor activity with unpredictable shifts between both extremes
- There may also be aggressive behaviour.

Disturbances of perception include fleeting illusions, false identifications (unfamiliar recognised as familiar) and hallucinations, especially visual ones. Emotional disturbances include anxiety, fear, irritability, apathy, wondering perplexity, insomnia or reversal of sleep–wake cycle and disturbed dreams and nightmares.

Delirium usually develops over hours or days and carries a poor prognosis in all patient groups. Delirious states can occur secondary to organic disturbance originating in any system of the body (Davison 1981) and, in a complex multisystem disease like AIDS, these are common. Risk factors for the development of delirium include:

(1) Underlying brain damage (F05.1)
(2) Coexistent alcohol or drug abuse
(3) The complex prescribed drug regimes frequently used for both treatment and pro-phylaxis in this patient group.

In our view, insufficient attention has to date been given to iatrogenic factors in delirium in AIDS (McDonald *et al.* 1987), and a careful review of the possibility of such causation needs to be undertaken in each case. In terms of specific disease-related causations, acute brain syndromes associated with a good prognosis for the delirium itself, have been described secondary to the aseptic meningitis which may develop at the time of seroconversion (Carne *et al.* 1985). This needs to be borne in mind in an individual at risk with sudden onset of acute symptoms.

Management consists of:

- Treating the underlying cause
- Maintaining fluid and electrolyte balance and nutrition
- Sedation
- Correction of the sleep–wake cycle
- Provision of a quiet, appropriately lighted environment
- Nursing support aimed at helping the patient with orientation.

Neuroleptics may be used cautiously (see earlier) to sedate patients when necessary. Delirious patients in this group who have underlying dementia have been noted to have considerable intolerance of haloperidol (Baer 1989).

Psychiatric disorder in non-HIV infected patients

Mental health professionals may become involved in the management of patients uninfected with HIV who exhibit excessive concern about infection. In some cases this occurs despite the absence of risk factors in their lives and in the presence of clearly demonstrated negative HIV tests. These patients require thorough psychiatric assessment as their symptomatology could be indicative of a number of important psychiatric disorders such as depressive illness, AIDS phobia, obsessive–compulsive disorder, somatoform disorder, and schizophreniform disorder. It is dangerous to apply the popular term 'worried well' to any such patient who has not been thoroughly assessed, as it is essential that any underlying psychiatric disorder be appropriately treated.

This does not in any way preclude the use of more specific cognitive–behavioural therapies (Green & McCreaner 1989; Hedge 1989) aimed at teaching patients to recognise their symptoms as those of anxiety rather than AIDS (Chapter 12). These strategies can be used alone or in conjunction with psychiatric treatments where necessary.

Psychiatrists are also involved in the treatment of psychotic patients in whom AIDS has become incorporated as a psychopathological theme in their delusions (Mahorney & Cavenar 1988; Todd 1989). This is hardly surprising when such has been the fate of many other significant world preoccupations through time, such as religion, technology, space travel and, most recently, satellite TV dishes!

AIDS in the context of developing community psychiatry

AIDS poses a serious public health problem – probably the most serious of the second half of this century – and will be of major importance for at least the next half century. The World Health Organisation's global programme on AIDS predicts that by the year 2000 there will be 18 million people HIV positive and six million people suffering from AIDS (Chin *et al.* 1990). This represents a doubling of estimates of numbers of HIV positive people and a more than fourfold increase in the numbers estimated to have AIDS worldwide up to 1990.

These figures are very large and represent an exponential increase in rate of spread of the AIDS pandemic. However, even these figures already seem overoptimistic and it would surprise no-one if the true figure in 2000 was substantially higher. The implications for future services are that they will need to expand accordingly. Future services depend to a large extent on today's planning. We need to be planning now for the services of the 21st century.

Realistic planning is impossible without epidemiological data based on good research. This is particularly relevant in the case of a new disease, like AIDS, the natural history of which is as yet incompletely understood. Over the last ten years it has been shown that the mean survival time from AIDS diagnosis has increased. With this increase has come a concomitant increase in patient morbidity and a marked shift from inpatient episodes to outpatient care (Beck *et al.* 1991).

Most HIV and AIDS patients receive most of their care while remaining in the community (Adler 1987; Beck 1991). In many ways this is desirable, particularly from the point of view of quality of life for the patient. Mental disorder is known to account for the greatest cost of any single group of conditions to the Department of Health (1991) in terms of days off work (14%), use of NHS inpatient beds (23%) and GP pharmaceutical bills (25%). Despite limited epidemiological data on psychiatric disorder occurring in AIDS patients, there is agreement that it is a significant problem. One would expect the need for psychiatric services to increase as the numbers of people becoming infected increases, but the rate of increase cannot be predicted easily.

It has already been stated that the need for in-patient psychiatric admission in these patients is generally low. In a condition where patients require treatment from both the medical and psychiatric disciplines, difficulties can and do arise as to where the patient is most appropriately admitted. Staff in psychiatric settings express anxiety about seriously physically ill patients being on their wards where facilities for intensive physical care are not available and where by definition there is a high level of disturbance in the patients in their care. Staff on busy, intensive medical wards often underestimate their skills in managing psychiatric disturbance and express concern that other frail patients may be put at risk from such behaviour.

For these reasons it often happens that AIDS in-patients who develop a psychiatric component to their illness receive their psychiatric treatment while remaining on the medical ward. This is often made possible by the special provision or secondment (on the medical ward) of psychiatric trained nurses. Medical psychiatric wards do not exist in the UK, in contrast to certain centres in the US (Stoudemire *et al.* 1987). There will be cases where it will be necessary or preferable to admit psychiatrically ill AIDS patients to a psychiatric ward, as for example with a dangerously disturbed patient.

It is difficult to predict the way in which psychiatric services will develop for the care of AIDS patients. At present the stigma of the disease, together with its relative infrequency in most parts of the country, has led to the development of highly specialised units in which primary and secondary care have been combined. In the immediate future this pattern of care is likely to continue.

In the longer term this will almost certainly change. As HIV/AIDS becomes more widespread, and according to predictions, gradually affects the heterosexual population to a much greater extent, services will need to be devolved to give more appropriate care. The fears that many patients would need to be treated (long term) in psychiatric hospitals have not been realised, and as better treatments are developed, progressively more treatment can be given away from hospital settings. Nevertheless, the particular problems posed by the infection are such that some specialisation is likely to be necessary in treatment.

The nature of the psychiatric intervention required, including knowledge of psychodynamic mechanisms, neuropsychological functioning, psychosocial function and neuropsychiatry, makes an ideal case for the establishment of multidisciplinary teams in the community psychiatric care of HIV/AIDS. Such teams need the skills of counselling, cognitive and behaviour therapy, psychotropic drug treatment and careful neurological and psychological assessment. These cannot be provided from one discipline, and teams in the future will need psychologists, psychiatrists, social workers and occupational therapists within their structures if they are to provide comprehensive care. At present these skills are provided in many units but they are too detached from one another, and integrated treatment is difficult. One could envisage specific HIV psychiatric teams for busy health districts with high HIV patient loads, although in areas of lower prevalence regional teams might be more appropriate.

Such teams would have an advantage over attempts to add skills to existing community psychiatric teams. Some aspects of the psychiatry of HIV infection are new and professionals in the subject are all feeling their way forward with relatively little past knowledge to go on. This helps to create an appropriate degree of humility and a greater willingness to share resources and skills. It could also represent a useful collaboration between patients and their carers, as those with HIV/AIDS are highly active in organising and planning services for themselves.

References

Adler, M.W. (1987) Care for patients with HIV infection and AIDS. *British Medical Journal*, **295**, 27–30.

Atkinson, J., Grant, I., Kennedy, C., Richman, D.D., Spector, S.A. & McCutchan, A. (1988) Prevalence of psychiatric disorders among men infected with human immunodeficiency virus. A controlled study. *Archives of General Psychiatry*, **45**, 859–64.

Baer, J.W. (1989) Study of 60 patients with AIDS or AIDS-related complex requiring psychiatric hospitalisation. *American Journal of Psychiatry*, **146**(10) 1285–8.

Barraclough, B., Bunch, J., Nelson, B. & Sainsbury, P. (1974) A hundred cases of suicide: clinical aspects. *British Journal of Psychiatry*, **125**, 355–73.

Beck, E.J. (1991) HIV infection and intervention: the first decade. *AIDS Care*, **3**(3) 295–302.

Beck, E.J., McKevifl, C., Whitaker, L., Wadsworth, J. & Miller, D.L. (1991) *Hospital Service Provision for People with AIDS and HIV Infection*. A report for the Department of Health. Academic Department of Public Health, St. Mary's Hospital Medical School, London.

Buhrich, N., Cooper, D.A. & Freed, E. (1988) HIV Infection Associated with Symptoms Indistinguishable from Functional Psychosis. *British Journal of Psychiatry*, **15**, 649–53.

Cambell, A. (1987) Aggressive psychosis in AIDS patient on high dose steroids. *Lancet*, **i**, 750–51.

Caplan, G. (1961) A community approach to preventive psychiatry, a conceptual framework. In: *An Approach to Community Mental Health*. Tavistock Publications, London.

Caring for People, Community Care in The Next Decade and Beyond (1989) Government White Paper. HMSO, London.

Carne, C.A., Smith, A., Elkington, S.G. *et al.* (1985) Acute encephalopathy coincident with seroconversion for anti HTLV-III. *Lancet*, **ii**, 1206–8.

Catalan, J. (1988) Psychosocial and neuropsychiatric aspects of HIV infection: review of their extent and implications for psychiatry. *Journal of Psychosomatic Research*, **32**, 237–48.

Catalan, J. (1990) Psychiatric manifestations of HIV disease. *Bailliere's Clinical Gastroenterology*. **4**(2) 547–62.

Catalan, J., Riccio, M. & Thompson, C. (1989) HIV disease and psychiatric practice. *Psychiatric Bulletin*, **13**, 316–32.

Chin, J., Sato, P.A. & Mann, J.M. (1990) Projection of HIV infections and AIDS cases to the year 2000. *Bulletin of the World Health Organisation*, **68**, 1–11.

Davison, K. (1981) Toxic Psychosis. *British Journal of Hospital Medicine*, **26**, 530–37.

Department of Health (1991) *Health of the Nation*. HMSO, London.

Derogatis, L.R., Morrow, G.R., Fetting, J., Denman, D., Piasetsky, S., Schmale, A.M. & Carniclee, C.L.M. The prevalence of psychiatric disorders among cancer patients. *Journal of the American Medical Association*, **249**, 751–7.

Dilley, J.W., Herbert, N., Ochitill, M.D., Peri, M. & Volberding, P.A. (1985) Findings in psychiatric consultations with patients with acquired immune deficiency syndrome. *American Journal of Psychiatry*, **142**, 82–6.

Edelstein, H. & Knight, R.T. (1987) Severe Parkinsonism in two AIDS patients taking Prochlorperazine. *Lancet*, **ii**, 341–2.

Engel, G.L. (1977) The need for a new medical model: a challenge for medicine. *Science*, **196**, 129–36.

Faulstich, M.E. (1987) Psychiatric aspects of AIDS. *American Journal of Psychiatry*, **144**(5) 551–6.

Fenton, T.W. (1987) AIDS related psychiatric disorder. *British Journal of Psychiatry*, **51**, 579–88.

Flavin, D.K., Franklin, J.E. & Frances, R.J. (1986) The acquired immunodeficiency syndrome (AIDS) and suicidal behaviour in alcohol dependent men. *American Journal of Psychiatry*, **143**, 1440–42.

Gabel, R.H., Barnard, N., Norko, M. & O'Connell, R.A. (1986) AIDS presenting as mania. *Comprehensive Psychiatry*, **27**, 251–4.

Gordin, M., Willoughby, A.D., Levine, L.A., Gure, L. & Neill, K.M. (1987) Knowledge of AIDS among hospital workers and behavioural correlates and consequences. *AIDS*, **1**, 183–8.

Green, J. & McCreaner, A. (eds) (1989) Counselling in HIV infection and AIDS. Blackwell Science, Oxford.

Haenel, T., Brunner, F. & Battegay, R. (1980). Renal disease and suicide in Switzerland and Europe. *Comprehensive Psychiatry*, **21**(2), 140–45.

Halsread, S., Riccio, M., Harlow, P., Oretti, R. & Thompson, C. (1988) Psychosis associated with HIV infection. *British Journal of Psychiatry*, **153**, 618–23.

Hedge, B. (1989) Worried Well and psychological issues. *AIDS Care*, **1**(2), 193–4.

Hildebrand, P. (1992) A patient dying with AIDS. The International Review of Psycho–Analysis, **19**(4) 457–69.

Hinton, J. (1967) *Dying*. Penguin Books, Harmondsworth.

Holland, J.C. & Tross, S. (1985) The psychosocial and neuropsychiatric sequelae of acquired immunodeficiency syndrome and related disorders. *Annals of Internal Medicine*, **103**, 760–64.

Jeffries, D. (1986) Virology. In: *The Management of AIDS patients*, (eds D. Miller, J. Weber & J. Green). Macmillan Press, London.

Joffe, R.T., Rubinow, D.R., Souillace, K. *et al.* (1986) Neuropsychiatric aspects of AIDS. *Psychopharmacology Bulletin*, **22**, 684–8.

King, M. (1989) Psychosocial status of 192 out-patients with HIV infection and AIDS. *British Journal of Psychiatry*, **154**, 237–42.

King, M. (1990) Psychological aspects of HIV infection and AIDS. *British Journal of Psychiatry*, **156**, 151–6.

Klimes, I., Catalan, J., Bond, A. *et al.* (1989) Knowledge and attitudes of health care staff about HIV infection. *AIDS Care*, **1**, 313–17.

Krikler, B. (1988) Homosexuality in the Eighties. *Journal of British Association of Psychotherapy*, **19**, July, 23–54.

Lantos, P.L., McLaughlin, J.E., Scholtz, C.L., Berry, C.L. & Tighe, J.R. (1989) Neuropathology of the brain in HIV infection. *Lancet*, **i**, 309–11.

Lishman, W.A. (1987) *Organic Psychiatry*. Blackwell, Oxford.

Lloyd, G.G. (1991) Psychological consequences of physical illness. In: *Textbook of General Psychiatry* (ed. S. Crown), pp. 27–57. Churchill Livingstone, Edinburgh.

Maccarlo, M. & Scharre, D.W. (1987) HIV and acute onset of psychosis. *Lancet*, **ii**, 342.

Mahorney, S.L. & Cavenar, J.O. Jr. (1988) A new and timely delusion: the complaint of having AIDS. *American Journal of Psychiatry*, **145**, 1130–32.

Maj, M. (1990a) Organic mental disorders in HIV-1 infection. *AIDS*, **4**, 831–40.

Maj, M. (1990b) Psychiatric aspects of HIV-1 infection and AIDS. *Psychological Medicine*, **20**, 547–63.

Maj, M., Janssen, R., Satz, P., Zaudig, M., Starace, F., Boor, D., Sughondhabirom, B., Bing, E.R., Luabeya, M.K., Ndetei, D., Riedel, R., Schulte, G. & Sartorious, N. (1991) The World Health Organisation cross-cultural study on neuropsychiatric aspects of infection with the human immunodeficiency virus (HIV-1), preparation and pilot phase. *British Journal of Psychiatry*, **159**, 351–6.

Marshall, D.W., Brey, R.L., Cabill, W.T., Zajac, R.A. & Boswell, R.N. (1988) Spectrum of CSF findings in various stages of human immunodeficiency virus infection. *Archives of Neurology*, **45**, 954–8.

Marzuk, P.M., Tierney, H., Tardiff, K., Gross, E.M., Morgan, E.B., Hsu, M-N. & Mann, J. (1988) Increased risk of suicide in persons with AIDS. *Journal of American Medical Association*, **259**, 1333–7.

McDonald, E.M., Mann, A.H. & Thomas, H.C. (1987) Interferons as mediators of psychiatric morbidity. *Lancet*, **ii**, 1175–7.

Miller, D. (1987) *Living with AIDS and HIV*. Macmillan Press, London.

Miller, D. (1988) HIV and social psychiatry. *British Medical Bulletin*, **148**(44) 130.

Miller, D. & Green, J. (1986) Counselling for HIV infection and AIDS. *Clinics in Immunology and Allergy*, **6**(3), 661–83.

Miller, D. & Riccio, M. (1990) Editorial review. Non-organic psychiatric and psychosocial syndromes associated with HIV-1 infection and disease. *AIDS*, **4**, 381–8.

Namir, S., Wolcott, D.L., Fawzy, F.L. & Almbaugh, M.J. (1987) Coping with AIDS: psychological and health implications. *Journal of Applied Social Psychology*, **17**, 309–28.

Navia, B.A., Jordan, B.D. & Price, R.W. (1986) The AIDS dementia complex: 1. Clinical features. *Annals of Neurology*, **19**, 517–24.

Ostrow, D.G. (1987) Psychiatric consequences of AIDS: an overview. *International Journal of Neuroscience*, **32**, 647–59.

Ostrow, D., Joseph, J., Monjan, A. *et al.* (1986) Psychosocial aspects of AIDS risk. *Psychopharmacological Bulletin*, **22**, 678–83.

Perry, S.W. & Tross, S. (1984) Psychiatric problems of AIDS patients at the New York Hospital: preliminary report. *Public Health Reports*, **99**, 201–5.

Pinching, A.J. (1988) Clinical aspects of AIDS and HIV infection in the developed world. *British Medical Bulletin*, **44**(1), 89–100.

Price, R.W., Sidtis, J.J., Navia, B.A., Pumarola-Sune, T. & Ornitz, D.B. (1988) The AIDS dementia complex in AIDS and the nervous system, (eds. M.L. Bosenblum, R.M. Levy & D.E. Bredesen), pp. 203–19. Raven Press, New York.

Pumarola-Sune, T., Navia, B.A., Cordon-Cardo, C., Cho, E-S. & Price, R.W. (1987) HIV antigen in the brains of patients with the AIDS dementia complex. *Annals of Neurology*, **21**, 490–96.

Robins, E., Murphy, G., Wilkinson, R. Gassner, S. & Kayes, J. (1959) Case histories of 134 completed suicides. *American Journal of Public Health*, **49**, 888–98.

Rosen, D.H., Gregory, R.J., Pollock, D. & Schiffman, A. (1987) Depression in patients referred for psychiatric consultation. A need for a new diagnosis. *General Hospital Psychiatry*, **9**, 391–7.

Rosenblum, M., Levy, R. & Bredesen, D. (eds) (1988) *AIDS and the Nervous System*. Raven Press, New York.

Ross, M. & Seager, V. (1988) Determinants of reported burnout in health professionals associated with care of AIDS patients. *AIDS*, **2**, 395–7.

Rosser, R. (1990) From health indicators to quality adjusted life years: technical and ethical issues. In: *Measuring the Outcomes of Medical Care* (eds A. Hopkins & D. Costain). Royal College of Physicians Publications, London.

Rundell, J.R., Wise, M.G. & Ursano, R.J. (1986) Three cases of AIDS related psychiatric disorders. *American Journal of Psychiatry*, **143**, 777–8.

Rundell, J.R., Kyle, K.M., Brown, G.R. & Thomason, J.L. (1992) Risk factors for suicide attempts in a human immunodeficiency virus screening programme. *Psychosomatics*, **33**(1), 24–7.

Schmitt, F.A., Bigley, J.W., McKinnis, R., Logue, P.E. *et al.* (1988) Neuropsychological outcome of Zidovudine (AZT) treatment of patients with AIDS and AIDS related complex. *New England Journal of Medicine*, **319**, 1573–8.

Schoenfeld, M., Myers, R.H., Cuppies, Berkman, B., Sax, D.S. & Clark, E. (1984) Increased rate of suicide among patients with Huntingtons disease. *Journal of Neurology, Neurosurgery and Psychiatry*, **47**, 1283–7.

Sensky, T. (1990) Patients' reactions to illness. *British Medical Journal*, **300**, 622–3.

Seth, R., Granville-Grossman, K., Goldmeier, D. & Lynch, S. (1991) Psychiatric illnesses in patients with HIV infection and AIDS referred to the liaison psychiatrists. *British Journal of Psychiatry*, **159**, 347–50.

Stoudemire, A., Hales, R.E. & Thomas, C.R. (1987) Medical–psychiatric units: an economic alternative for consultation-liaison psychiatry. *Hospital and Community Psychiatry*, **38**(8) 815–18.

Todd, J. (1989) AIDS as a current psychopathological theme, a report on five heterosexual patients. *British Journal of Psychiatry*, **154**, 253–5.

Vachon, M., Lyall, W. & Freeman, S. (1987) Measurement and management of stress in health professionals working with advanced cancer. *Death Education*, **1**, 365–75.

Vamos, M.J. (1992) MANIA and AIDS: a psychodynamic emphasis. *Australian and New Zealand Journal of Psychiatry*, **26**, 111–18.

Vogel-Scibilia, S.E., Mulsant, B.H. & Keshavan, M.S. (1988) HIV infection presenting as psychosis: a critique. *Acta Psychiatrica Scandanavia*, **78**, 652–6.

Volberding, P. (1989) Supporting the health care team in caring for patients with AIDS. *Journal of the American Medical Association*, **261**, 747–8.

Weber, J. & Pinching, A. (1986) Clinical Management of AIDS and HTLV-III infection. In: *The Management of AIDS Patients* (eds D. Miller, J. Weber & J. Green). Macmillan Press, London.

Wilkins, J.W., Robertson, K.R., Van der Horst, C., Robertson, W.T., Fryer, J.G. & Hall, C.D. (1990) The importance of confounding factors in the evaluation of neuropsychological changes in patients infected with Human Immunodeficiency Virus. *Journal of Acquired Immunodeficiency Syndrome*, **3**(10) 938–42.

Wiseman, A.O. & Worden, J.W. (1976) The existential plight in cancer, significance of the first 100 days. *International Journal of Psychiatric Medicine*, **7**, 1–15.

WHO (1988) *Report of the Consultation on the Neuropsychiatric Aspects of HIV Infection*, 14–17 March 1988. World Health Organisation, Geneva.

WHO (1990) *Neuropsychiatric Aspects of HIV-1 Infection: A Review of the Evidence*. Draft report of the consultation held in Geneva, 11–13 January 1990. World Health Organisation, Geneva.

WHO (1992) *10th Revision of the International Classification of Diseases*. World Health Organisation, Geneva.

Wurtz, R.M., Abrams, D., Becker, S., Jacobson, M.A., Mass, M.M. & Marks, S.H. (1989) Anaphylactoid drug reactions to ciprofloxacin and rifampicin in HIV-infected patients. *Lancet*, **i**, 955–6.

Index